'Knowledge is power and, in the disem[...] gling to conceive, this book is an absol[...] you're brand new to the world of fertili[...] while, this book is a beacon of clear, de[...] ... it is an amazing resource and I would highly rec[...]mend it to anyone who is even considering having a go at conceiving!'
DR XAND VAN TULLEKEN, TV presenter, Honorary Associate Professor, University College London

'This unique, patient-centred book provides high-quality clinical and scientific information, but with an emphasis on a holistic approach that seeks to empower readers. Comprehensive and authoritative, it is written in an easy, accessible style that makes it a pleasure to read and understand. Everyone concerned about their fertility should read it – and so should the clinicians looking after them!'
DR RAJ MATHUR, Chair, British Fertility Society

'An utterly brilliant book. Fully comprehensive and reader-friendly. I wish it had been around when I was on my own fertility journey.'
JESSICA HEPBURN, founder of Fertility Fest

'Inability to conceive is tremendously stressful for many couples. Whilst there is no shortage of information, it is difficult to separate what is credible and evidence-based from wishful theories and anecdotes. This is where *The Fertility Book* makes a unique contribution, by synthesising and presenting credible evidence to inform one's fertility journey. If you are struggling to have a baby, make time for this book. It will help you.'
PROF ARRI COOMARASAMY, Director, Tommy's National Centre for Miscarriage Research, University of Birmingham

'This book has all that most need to optimise their fertility. It clearly explains the science in ways that should help couples feel empowered when it comes to making what could be some of the most important decisions of their lives.'
DR EDWARD MORRIS, President, Royal College of Obstetricians and Gynaecologists

'I absolutely love this book. I have learnt so much. It is an ideal read for non-medical professionals who wish to gain an understanding of the medical side of fertility treatments.'
ANGELA PERICLEOUS-SMITH, Chair, British Infertility Counselling Association

'A comprehensive and easily understandable text for couples who wish to take a proactive approach, optimising their chances of starting a healthy family. Highly recommended for women and men.'
PROF BASKY THILAGANATHAN, Clinical Director, Tommy's National Centre for Maternity Improvement

'*The Fertility Book* is a comprehensive and reliable source of information for those with fertility problems and an essential read in a time when medical fictions spread faster than medical facts.'
SARAH NORCROSS, Director, Progress Educational Trust

'Balen and Dugdale have managed to distil a huge amount of complex information about fertility into an easily accessible read which includes a lot to help men, who are often overlooked. I highly recommended this book'
PROF ALLAN PACEY, MBE, Professor of Andrology, Head of Oncology and Metabolism, Sheffield University

'Having such high-quality and up-to-date information on reproductive health all available in one place is really important for women's health and well-being.'
SHAISTA GOHIR, OBE, Chair, Royal College of Obstetricians and Gynaecologists Women's Network

'*The Fertility Book* is a thorough and comprehensive guide to the issues that can cause fertility problems. It helps readers navigate a pathway through the tests and treatments they may face.'
KATE BRIAN, Fertility Network UK

'Taking care of your own health is really powerful, but that needs evidence-based, reputable sources of information, and the help of medicine and science when necessary. *The Fertility Book* is all of that. It's a comprehensive, easy-to-understand guide to preparing for the road to conception, whether natural or assisted.'
CATHERINE NESTOR, former Vice-Chair, Royal College of Obstetricians and Gynaecologists Women's Network

'This book is an invaluable resource for those on their fertility journey. An essential read!'
CAROLINE ANDREWS AND RACHEL HAWKES, Secretary and Chair, Verity, the PCOS patient representative organisation

Professor Adam Balen MB, BS, MD, DSc, FRCOG is a full-time consultant in reproductive medicine at Leeds Teaching Hospitals NHS Trust. In recognition of his research, the University of Leeds awarded him a personal chair in 2004 and a DSc in 2010 – the highest academic degree in medicine. Adam qualified as a doctor in 1983 and, after a few years training in obstetrics and gynaecology in London, Oxford and even a spell in Africa, he became a consultant in Leeds in 1996, helping to create one of the UK's largest and most successful IVF units, of which he is the lead clinician.

For many years Adam has had a particular interest in the causes and management of polycystic ovary syndrome (PCOS). His research covers the full spectrum of the condition including its effects during adolescence and adult life on reproductive and metabolic health, fertility, quality of life and long-term health. He is on the World Health Organization (WHO) Infertility Global Guideline Development Group and also sits on the International Federation of Gynaecology and Obstetrics (FIGO) committee for reclassifying disorders of ovulation.

Adam has had significant roles on the British Fertility Society (BFS) including Chair from 2015 to 2018. He sits on the council of the Royal College of Obstetricians and Gynaecologists (RCOG), for which he is the spokesperson on all matters relating to reproductive medicine. He also chairs the NHS England working group on funding for IVF, which aims to provide equitable funding for assisted conception throughout the UK.

He is chair of the Fertility Education Initiative, which he created to improve the provision of education to young people about all aspects of reproductive health, and has influenced the UK government to include fertility education on the national curriculum in schools.

Adam regularly features in the media on all aspects of reproductive health and is the author of over 260 peer-reviewed papers and 15 books. He is known as a charismatic speaker and communicator and lectures widely throughout the world.

Grace Dugdale BA(HONS), MA, MRSB is a reproductive biologist and nutrition scientist who has spent many years researching biological function in sex and fertility and has a number of research special interests in relation to fertility; in particular, metabolic health, the microbiome, mitochondrial function, epigenetics, fetal programming and the optimisation of embryonic development through modifiable factors in the father and mother.

Via a path of interdisciplinary research, Grace has been able to develop both extensive knowledge and a unique approach to addressing fertility issues in men and women. This research has led to the development of an evidence-based fertility and preconception care programme that considers the numerous modifiable factors that impact both male and female fertility, and also the health of the baby born. Grace now runs this fertility and preconception care clinic at the Nuffield Leeds Hospital. She also devised a fertility and preconception care course for anyone who is trying to conceive. The course was launched at Leeds Fertility and is now available online. Since lifetime health starts before conception through the impact of environmental factors on eggs and sperm, Grace is passionate about making a difference to future generations and public health through her work.

Grace is an accomplished public speaker who has made numerous TV, radio and festival appearances and is a regular contributor to media articles on fertility and reproductive health. As a member of the Fertility Education Initiative, she works to promote good-quality education in sex, relationships and fertility, as well as gender equality and healthy attitudes towards sex and reproduction in young people. She is also a member of the All-Party Parliamentary Group for Sexual and Reproductive Health.

In 2017, Grace founded Balance Fertility – a company offering online fertility services including at-home testing for hormones, nutrition and general health to optimise the preconception health of men and women who are trying to conceive.

The Fertility Book

Your definitive guide
to achieving a
healthy pregnancy

Professor ADAM BALEN
Internationally renowned fertility expert
AND GRACE DUGDALE
Reproductive biologist and nutrition scientist

Vermilion, an imprint of Ebury Publishing,
20 Vauxhall Bridge Road,
London SW1V 2SA

Vermilion is part of the Penguin Random House group of companies
whose addresses can be found at global.penguinrandomhouse.com

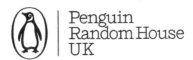

First published by Vermilion in 2021

www.penguin.co.uk

A CIP catalogue record for this book is available from the British Library

ISBN 9781785041778

Printed and bound in Great Britain by Clays Ltd, Elcograf S.p.A.

The authorised representative in the EEA is Penguin Random House Ireland,
Morrison Chambers, 32 Nassau Street, Dublin D02 YH68

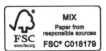

Penguin Random House is committed to a
sustainable future for our business, our readers
and our planet. This book is made from Forest
Stewardship Council® certified paper.

For Theo

Contents

Introduction

Understanding your body is truly a skill for life.

Grace writes:

My interest in reproductive science started, as these things often do, because of something personal. My older sister suffered a 'missed' miscarriage in her twenties and was distraught. Her 12-week scan failed to show a heartbeat and the baby (or fetus to use the correct medical term) had stopped growing at 9 weeks. When conventional medicine couldn't offer any explanations and with others saying it was for the best in the typical clumsy style of those who don't know what to say to someone who has experienced this devastating loss, I decided to do some research. With a background in molecular biology and genetics, I was well placed to seek answers in the scientific literature. What I discovered was to define the rest of my career.

Evidence largely from animal studies at the time showed that underlying nutrient deficiencies and under-nutrition can contribute to the risk of miscarriage. Tests on my sister showed that she had various deficiencies including zinc and iron, so I identified suitable supplements and, after a relatively short period taking them, she conceived again and went on to have a healthy pregnancy and a beautiful healthy baby boy. While I would never suggest it is always this easy and we can't be sure nutrient deficiencies caused my sister's miscarriage, she did feel immediately better that we had found a possible reason and identified something she could do to help herself. For me, it started a lifelong fascination with the creation of new life and our ability to intervene in this seemingly miraculous event.

Over the subsequent years, I've also learnt first-hand how disempowered women often are when planning and going through pregnancy. Medicine can be very paternalistic and women have typically lacked fundamental knowledge about their own bodies. This extends to everything from periods to understanding when in your cycle you are most fertile.

The needless suffering this lack of knowledge causes to countless women in differing scenarios means that I have been on a mission to support and educate women all my adult life.

For many years I not only continued to study fertility and reproductive health, but also conducted interdisciplinary research into diverse areas including the microbiome (the 'good' bacteria in our bodies), nutrition science, plant-based medicine and metabolic health. I devised a set of diagnostic tests and interventions to address what I discovered were potential contributing factors to difficulties conceiving, miscarriage, poor pregnancy outcomes and the health of the babies born. As well as being absolutely fascinating, this work has allowed me to help countless people improve their health and have the children they so desire, which is incredibly rewarding.

Understanding that one person, by herself, can't help everyone, I formed a long-standing interest in developing resources and information online to educate women about their bodies and help them improve reproductive health. In the early days, this wasn't so easy (awareness of and interest in the field has improved considerably over recent years), but there was someone else who shared my passion – Professor Adam Balen – and our paths crossed through the 'Fertility Education Initiative' that he founded. Meeting Adam in 2016 was pure serendipity and it has meant we have achieved a great deal together since. We were early deliverers of preconception care courses and clinics (most IVF clinics, whether NHS or private, still do not offer this kind of service), and we offered guidance on diverse topics including diet and nutrition, exercise, cooking and yoga, to name a few, as well as fertility screening and assessments that include at-home testing, integrating holistic interventions and medical care. As part of the Fertility Education Initiative, we have produced animations to teach young people about fertility and we give talks for patients at events including The Fertility Show, Verity's annual event for women with PCOS, and fertility events at The

Royal College of Obstetricians and Gynaecologists. We've been regular contributors to TV and radio commentary on reproductive health, including appearing in various documentaries that have covered our work. The feedback we receive from patients spurs us on to keep reaching bigger audiences to really make a difference and change the state of play when it comes to awareness of fertility and reproductive health.

The true power of this approach is the integration of the best medical care can offer with a holistic, personalised approach to optimising health and well-being. Being able to interpret scientific evidence and understand key principles of good nutrition are foundations for good health throughout adulthood. It has been an honour and a privilege to work with so many individuals and couples in this way.

Adam writes:

My story begins during my last lazy school summer holiday before starting medical school: nothing much was happening, but then came the headlines that I remember with such clarity and that, without realising, would define my life and career: 'The Miracle Baby' announcing the birth of Louise Brown, the first IVF ('test tube') baby. This was the culmination of years of painstaking research led by Bob Edwards, in whose clinic I would work some ten years later, who would only be recognised as a Nobel Laureate in the twilight of his life because of the controversies and ethical conundrums that have entangled the 'brave new world' of reproductive medicine.

Later, a brief spell in training to become a GP somehow evolved into a year working in an old mission hospital in a terribly deprived area of southern Africa. There, as one of three doctors, I found myself doing all manner of things that I wasn't trained to do, including running both the maternity and paediatric units literally single-handedly. I will never forget the heartbreaking scenes of small children dying from malnutrition, especially when measles hit and rampaged through the ward. Infertility was a big taboo and a social stigma; the witch doctors had their 'cures' and the fault was always with the woman, never even contemplated as being a male problem. I returned to London and switched from the world of general practice to a career in obstetrics and gynaecology, fired up by my African experiences, which also provided me with the confidence to push boundaries and develop new things.

Serendipity took me to work for the wonderful Professor Howard Jacobs, to this day my great mentor and true friend. Howard fused the world of hormones (endocrinology) with reproductive science led by Bob Edwards and ultrasound pioneered by Professor Stuart Campbell – all true world leaders. These were new and exciting times.

My work over the last 30 years has been devoted to the understanding of reproduction and the causes of infertility, in particular hormonal disturbances in women and polycystic ovary syndrome (PCOS). I don't believe that there is a more varied or satisfying job in the whole of medicine. The field of reproductive medicine is fascinating and has enabled me to develop skills and interests and a broad sphere, including the most advanced of scientific and laboratory technology, complex surgery and assisted conception techniques – the very creation of life. It has been an immense privilege and pleasure to serve my patients and be a part of their journeys, which are invariably 'emotional rollercoasters' and may be full of sadness and heartache, but more often than not result in great joy.

I have been privileged also to serve in key roles in national and international organisations, including the British Fertility Society, the European Society of Human Reproduction and Embryolgy (ESHRE), the International Federation of Obstetrics and Gynaecology, the Royal College of Obstetricians and Gynaecologists and chair the World Health Organization (WHO) guideline group on PCOS.

As chair of the British Fertility Society I founded the 'Fertility Education Initiative' and it was at our first meeting that I met Grace and realised that we share a passion for providing the best information and advice about reproductive health to people of all ages, whether thinking and planning for the future or currently trying to conceive.

Throughout this book we share our years of collective knowledge and experience to help guide you on your fertility journey. We have learnt over the years that reproductive health provides a window into the overall health of our patients, and enhancing health before embarking on a pregnancy is not only likely to improve the outcomes of fertility treatment but also, more importantly, the outcomes for the baby. When the functioning of our bodies at the level of individual cells starts to become impaired, these things can cause not only fertility problems, but can also affect embryonic and fetal development, leading to poorer health for the babies born. Correcting any issues that you identify is important not only to help you conceive, but also for the lifelong health of your child.

In Part 1 we describe the fertility fundamentals that apply to most couples trying to conceive and how preconception health is of paramount importance for both mother and father, and the long-term health of the child through to adulthood. Everything from the food you eat to the chemicals you are exposed to can affect the health of a child before they are even conceived due to the impact on the quality of sperm and egg cells. We will look at all of these in detail in the book. When we do this work with our patients in clinic, we see significant improvements in their general health, natural fertility and chances of having a baby following fertility treatment.

In Part 2 we provide detailed information to help you work out what may be causing your own individual fertility issues, or what may cause problems for you in the future if you are still in the early stages of planning for a pregnancy. It's important to remember that fertility isn't just about women's health – male and female fertility combine to influence the chances of having a baby, so fertility of the *couple* should be addressed to maximise the chances of pregnancy. We look at male fertility throughout the book and specifically in Chapters 10 and 13.

Finally, in Part 3 we discuss other considerations such as ethics and what to do if treatment doesn't work.

There is no better feeling than when you get that call or email with news of a positive pregnancy test and then the birth of a healthy baby. We are lucky indeed to do the work that we do. This is why we wanted to write this book, and it distils our combined knowledge into something we hope will be a game changer in your fertility journey.

PART 1

Fertility Fundamentals

If you're planning a pregnancy in the near future or trying to conceive now, it helps to understand how fertility functions in both men and women. Understanding your own body is fundamental in protecting lifelong health and at no time is this more important than when we want to create new life. Having proper knowledge of not just reproductive health but your overall health is the first step in developing a new awareness of your fertility and how you can help yourself.

Chapter 1

How Fertility Works

GOOD FERTILITY FOR men and women is a result of the genes you inherited from your parents and lifestyle factors such as diet, exercise, stress, smoking and alcohol intake. The part of this that you can control is *lifestyle*. Sometimes genetic factors will influence your fertility, but, even then, lifestyle factors can mitigate any negative effects if you know what to look for and what you need to do.

One of the most significant things that affects the fertility of a couple is their ages, in particular the age of the woman. Female fertility declines with age and a woman is at her peak fertility in her early twenties. Fertility starts to decline more quickly in the mid-thirties, though not at the same rate for all women. This can be the difficult part, as reports in the press and even discussions with doctors can make it seem like it's the same for everyone, but individual variation means that we cannot predict with accuracy when any one particular woman will become incapable of conceiving.

The age-related decline in fertility has a strong genetic component and a good indicator is your mother's fertility and age at which she reached menopause. The aim should be to complete your family before the age your mother reached the menopause, minus ten years. Given that it can take several months or more to conceive, you can start to see why fertility experts tend to advise that women should ideally try to start a family by their late twenties. The idea is that there is time to have more than one child if that is the goal and, if any problems do come up, there is time to address them before age starts to become an issue. Thirty-five is also the age at which we see *in vitro* fertilisation (IVF) success rates for women decline. Therefore, although some will go on to have children later and there are other life considerations aside from our biology, if having a family is important and you have the freedom to make these decisions, knowing that female fertility does start to decline in the thirties is something to think about.

Women are born with a fixed number of eggs that are formed during development in the mother's womb. These eggs are progressively lost over time regardless of whether you are menstruating or on the pill. As well as decreasing in number with age, egg *quality* also goes down as women get older, in line with normal cellular ageing. Interestingly, egg quality is the main thing that influences IVF success. So, although IVF can help a little when it comes to age-related fertility problems, in reality, it only really buys you a year or so. This is important to note, as one of the major misconceptions that exists is that IVF can fix everything. It can't. We still have to deal with biological reality, which is why it is so important to know what you can do over time to influence your chances of having a baby.

Lifestyle factors can impact the ageing of all cells, including eggs, and there is a rapidly evolving branch of science focused on general ageing and how to slow down the process. What is less well understood is that similar factors influence the decline of fertility with age, so the earlier in life you start to adopt healthy behaviours, the more you will be able to influence your reproductive health over time and potentially extend your fertile years.

THE SCIENCE OF FEMALE FERTILITY

Human egg cells are formed inside a female fetus during pregnancy and reach a certain point of maturity until development is halted. This doesn't change until a girl reaches puberty. Eggs sit in the ovary in a state of suspended animation, frozen at a mid-point of their development, ready to be recruited, activated and the cell division that started during ovarian development in the mother's womb completed. When a girl starts to menstruate, follicles (the fluid-filled sacs inside which egg cells are held) are 'chosen' out of the hundreds of thousands of dormant egg cells to be the ones that restart the development process in that particular egg. This takes several months from start to finish, with the completion of maturation (the 'ripening') taking about three months. The 'chosen' follicle grows to about 2cm in diameter and then releases its egg, which then passes into one of the fallopian tubes. The remnant of the follicle is now called the corpus luteum and it secretes hormones including progesterone to help maintain the uterine environment for implantation and pregnancy.

It is in the fallopian tube where the egg meets sperm and where fertilisation happens. The newly fertilised egg is now an embryo and, at this first stage of development, is called a zygote. It represents the first stage of a new genetically unique individual where the genes of the parents combine. Following fertilisation, the embryo travels down the fallopian tube into the uterus, where it implants into the lining of the uterus (endometrium) and grows as a pregnancy. If fertilisation does not happen, or if the embryo fails to implant, the corpus luteum breaks down and the endometrium falls away as a menstrual period about 14 days later.

The egg store: ovarian reserve

You are born with more eggs than you will ever need (between 1 and 2 million) and the number declines throughout childhood and the fertile years. By the time ovulation first happens and your periods start around the age of 13, there are about 400,000 eggs left. At the menopause stage, which is on average around the age of 51, there are no eggs left to be ovulated.

If you ovulate one egg each month during your fertile years, that would be equivalent to the release of only around 456 eggs, even if you ovulated each and every month, which doesn't always happen. Ovulation doesn't become regular for a year or two after puberty, for instance, and ovulation stops during pregnancy, breastfeeding and the use of certain contraceptives. Nonetheless, the number of eggs progressively and relentlessly declines, and we now know that during a woman's twenties maybe 1,000 eggs are lost each month. That's 30 every day that are simply wasted! The monthly loss of eggs goes down with age to maybe 100 per month in a woman's late

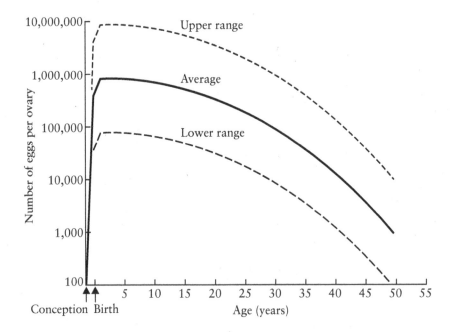

Decline of eggs with age

thirties. This steady decline is not under the influence of hormones, but instead is due to inbuilt signals in the ovaries and the eggs themselves. It's around the age of 37 years when the decline becomes more rapid until the menopause.

Hormones

Hormones, in the correct balance, are needed for conception and for a healthy pregnancy to develop. Hormones are substances that are released into the bloodstream and circulate around the body to make sure all your organs and bodily processes are working as they should. They also have a big impact on behaviour (think sex drive and testosterone). As well as producing and storing eggs, the other main purpose of the ovary is to produce hormones. The hormones from the ovary affect many different parts of the body including the brain, but especially the uterus and breasts. The hormones produced by the ovary fall into three main groups: oestrogens, androgens and progestogens (covered in more detail in Chapter 8). Women make all of these hormones, but sometimes in different proportions. Testosterone is sometimes seen as a male hormone, but it is the main androgen hormone made by the ovaries of all women. Oestrogen is actually made out of testosterone and helps the endometrium to grow.

The menstrual cycle

The menstrual cycle is divided into four main phases and each phase is significant in terms of fertility. Understanding your menstrual cycle will help you to understand when you are fertile and to interpret results of any investigations you may need (see Chapter 12).

Follicular phase

This is the phase of your cycle when the follicle that is going to release an egg that month starts to grow and produce other hormones that lead to ovulation. One important hormone involved is follicle-stimulating hormone (FSH). FSH is produced by a gland at the bottom of the brain called the pituitary gland and it stimulates the growth of the follicle, peaking between days 3 and 5 of your cycle (the days in your cycle when it should be tested). The FSH you produce naturally usually initiates the growth of just one follicle, but injections of FSH that are given during fertility treatment make it possible to stimulate the growth of others that otherwise would have died away. As a follicle grows it produces various hormones including oestrogen, and other hormones that effectively block the growth of other follicles.

Ovulation

Ovulation – the release of the egg from the follicle into the fallopian tube – is the main event of your menstrual cycle and the one that is crucial for natural conception. Ovulation happens because the growing follicle produces increasing amounts of oestrogen until it reaches a peak, where it triggers the release of a surge of another hormone called luteinising hormone (LH). LH is also produced by the pituitary gland. LH is the hormone that then starts the process of ovulation and also prepares the egg for fertilisation. Both the oestrogen peak and the LH surge are used to detect ovulation by some ovulation detection kits.

Luteal phase

After ovulation, the follicle continues to produce oestrogen and it also starts to produce another hormone that is really important for a pregnancy to be sustained if the egg is fertilised: progesterone. Progesterone usually peaks around a week before your next period (e.g. day 21 of a 28-day cycle) and is tested by GPs around this time to check you are ovulating. Measuring it on the wrong day of your cycle often happens and this can be very misleading (you can find out more about testing in Chapter 12). While oestrogen stimulates the growth of the endometrium, progesterone is the hormone that gets the endometrium ready for the implantation of the

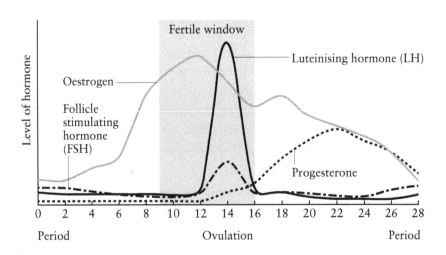

Hormone levels in an average menstrual cycle
(timings vary depending on length of cycle)

embryo. Progesterone also helps maintain the endometrium after implantation and so adequate levels are needed for a pregnancy to continue. We will cover factors that can affect the all-important balance between these two hormones in Chapter 8.

Menstrual phase

If the egg is not fertilised, it starts to break down and progesterone and oestrogen then fall. Without the hormones needed to maintain the endometrium, the lining itself starts to break down and this is your menstrual period.

Your body then enters into a new monthly cycle where the whole process starts all over again.

CREATING EGGS AND SPERM

Cells divide in two ways. One way creates a copy of the 'mother' cell resulting in the full number of chromosomes in the 'daughter' cell. This form of cell division is called mitosis and it is the way that cells making up the bulk of our bodies are produced. Cells including muscle, heart, kidney, lung, bone, hair, teeth and skin are produced in this way and are called somatic cells, which essentially means normal body cells. The other type of cell division is known as meiosis and results in half the number of chromosomes in the 'daughter' cell. Meiosis is the type of cell division that produces sperm and eggs – collectively known as gametes. Both sperm and eggs have 23 chromosomes and, when an egg is fertilised, the sperm and the egg join their genetic material together. Therefore, a healthy adult human has 46 chromosomes (22 pairs numbered 1 to 22 and then either two X chromosomes in females or an X and Y in males). (See Chapter 21 for when things work out differently and information on genetic testing.)

Eggs and the environment

The period during which eggs are awakened from their inactive state to complete the process of cell division (meiosis) and egg maturation is especially important for egg quality. The environment in which this happens, as well as maternal age, impacts how well the final processes of meiosis work. So, although our diet and lifestyle generally have an impact on our fertility throughout our life, the months leading up to conception are some of the most important in terms of our capacity to produce the best quality eggs our body is capable of producing for our age. This is one reason why the preconception period is so critical but, until recently, it has been largely overlooked by the medical profession. We will look at what you need to do in the preconception period in the next chapter.

Because egg cells or *oocytes* are as old as a woman and remain inside her throughout life until the menopause, they are subjected to the same environmental exposures as the individual woman. So, what a woman does throughout her life has an ongoing impact on her fertility and the health of her eggs. Excessive unhealthy behaviours including smoking, too much alcohol and inactivity can come together over time to provide a low-level drip-feed of damaging biochemical influences on the eggs and cells that surround them, whereas healthy habits result in healthier eggs. Everything we do to our bodies impacts the tiny structures within a cell that produce the energy for all our bodily processes, known as the mitochondria (the 'battery' of the cell), for instance. The same environmental factors also affect our genes (the bundles of DNA that provide the instructions for how our cells function) and whether or not they are 'switched on' and fulfil their intended function in the body. These two things are important for many different areas of health, not just our fertility, and we can influence some of these factors through our behaviours and habits.

It really does take two

It's important to remember that the chances of conception and a healthy pregnancy are influenced by both the male and the female partner, and it is the fertility of the *couple* that should be optimised, not just the woman. A 2019 study, for instance, demonstrated that poor sperm may contribute towards recurrent miscarriage, a fertility issue that has historically been addressed through investigations and treatments for women.[1] The study showed that the partners of women who had suffered three or more miscarriages had higher levels of damage in their sperm DNA compared to men whose partners had not suffered a miscarriage. This may not be the whole story for a particular couple, and female factors can also increase the risk of miscarriage, but certainly ignoring the male partner is not going to help achieve the best outcome. This kind of damage in sperm DNA can be improved with changes to diet and lifestyle, and this has been demonstrated in other well-conducted clinical trials. We look at male fertility in Chapter 10.

Why egg and sperm quality are important

It is a combination of good-quality eggs and sperm that together affect the chances of conceiving and going on to have a healthy baby, though egg quality is particularly important. Whereas men provide only DNA (genetic material) via their sperm to the early embryo upon fertilisation, the egg provides all the cellular machinery needed for early development, which is why oocyte quality is so important. A good-quality egg can correct defects in early embryonic development via this machinery and can compensate for poor-quality sperm, reinforcing the need for good preconception care for both parties, even where an issue has been identified with only one partner. It is also why the combined age of a couple can affect your chance of conceiving as a younger woman's eggs can compensate for potentially poor older sperm DNA in this way.

Although we are still learning about the incredible way in which diet and lifestyle can impact our health and fertility, we understand enough to know very clearly the importance of these things when it comes to creating a new life. In this way, through our eggs (and sperm too), we are laying down the foundations for the future health of our children before they are even born. So combining evidence-based dietary and lifestyle factors as part of a preconception care programme for both partners with good medical care is the best approach when planning for a pregnancy.

Chapter 2

Planning for a Healthy Pregnancy

I F YOU'RE READING this book as you start to think about trying for a baby, you have the perfect opportunity to prepare your body for a healthy pregnancy and a healthy baby in a really positive way. Learning practical steps that you can take before you conceive means that you have the potential to improve the lifelong health of your children and possibly your grandchildren, as well as your chances of getting pregnant. The ultimate preventive medicine starts before conception and can have effects that persist across generations through changes to the genetic material and cellular structures in eggs and sperm.

Many couples arrive at the point of looking at their diet, lifestyle, weight and general health after long periods of trying to conceive and not succeeding. If possible, preconception care and planning ahead can potentially avoid such delays and heartache along the way. It also gives you time to address any problems that you identify on your fertility journey and may improve your chances of conceiving naturally.

Where medical help is needed, the path for most couples who find themselves in a fertility clinic setting has often been long and difficult, and they are therefore understandably in a hurry to get on with treatment. Allowing time to address any underlying issues, however, can make a difference. If you have time pressures due to age or other circumstances, it is still worth doing what you can within whatever time you have as you wait for treatment. The advice is always to do your best within the constraints of your individual situation.

WHAT IS PRECONCEPTION CARE?

Preconception care has, until fairly recently, been a term associated only with the most basic of steps for couples including things like taking folic acid. There is, however, a huge research focus and body of evidence on environmental influences on fertility and reproduction, and there is much more you can do.[1] Given that studies demonstrate that a mother's diet and lifestyle in the year before she conceives impacts the lifelong health of the baby, and that the very immature follicles that contain eggs at the earliest stage of development take about nine months to reach maturity so that they are ready to be released via ovulation, the ideal is to create a healthy environment during that entire development period. For men, it means the sperm that is constantly being produced in the testes is as healthy as possible.

Recent papers published in *The Lancet* highlight the fact that many women enter pregnancy with low levels of key nutrients that have the potential to impact pregnancy outcomes, again an indication of the significance of the time before conception.[2] So this isn't an issue restricted to those who have fertility issues: it applies to anyone who may become pregnant. Given that around half of pregnancies are unplanned, this also emphasises the particular importance of good diet for anyone of reproductive age, especially for those who are sexually active and know they would like to have children.

Since many couples either don't start any kind of preconception care programme at all, or they leave it too late, a significant aim of this book is to change accepted practices – without adding a burden of guilt to would-be parents. We would like to encourage all couples who are planning a pregnancy now or in the future to think about optimising their general health and nutrient status as a starting point before trying to conceive. Ultimately, the aim is to feel better, physically and emotionally.

Devoting time to a period of preconception care means you can work on egg and sperm quality, which are affected primarily by age but also by diet, nutrient status and lifestyle. This helps when trying to conceive naturally (they are the 'ingredients' to make your baby!) as well as with fertility treatment. Improving egg quality can improve treatment outcomes and we have seen improvements in the number of mature eggs collected, number of eggs fertilised and number of embryos reaching a good stage of development (the five-day stage known as the blastocyst) in repeat *in vitro* fertilisation (IVF) cycles after couples improve their diet and lifestyle, for instance, and egg quality is the main thing that impacts IVF success.

Your baby's long-term health

We know that early life nutrition immediately before you conceive and during early embryogenesis (the process by which your embryo is created and develops) impacts the long-term health of your child. Genes essentially make proteins and it is these proteins that drive the activity of all cells in the body and provide an instruction manual for the development of your baby. Environmental exposures, like diet and lifestyle, can change whether genes are 'switched on' or not. These so-called epigenetic changes resulting from what we eat and do to our bodies around the time of conception impact the instructions that genes provide for particular phases of development, subtly altering the course of embryogenesis and fetal development. Pre-implantation development of the incredible early embryo is one of the most critical phases of pregnancy in terms of the future health of the child, as the way development will progress is being established. Cells divide rapidly immediately after fertilisation and then migrate first to form the basis of the embryo and the placenta, and from there to lay the foundations for the different systems of the baby's body. Key events take place that will affect the baby's heart, gut, brain and wider nervous system before a woman even knows she is pregnant.

For each of us, this means that during the time immediately before and immediately after conception (the periconception period), we have the potential to influence long-term health risks for the baby, either negatively or positively, through basic lifestyle choices. These choices can impact the risk of things like cardiovascular disease, becoming overweight and mental health disorders for our children later in life.

THE BODY KEEPS THE SCORE

Preconception care is also extremely important in order to stabilise good bodily conditions in the months leading up to conception. A newly formed embryo 'senses' the uterine environment via particular signalling pathways inside the pregnant mother, and development is directed according to prevailing conditions at the point of conception. If an embryo is 'expecting' a certain set of conditions, like either a plentiful or scarce supply of nutrients, and something changes, it can lead to what is known as developmental mismatch, which can result in various health problems in the baby.

We know from times when the population went from periods of starvation to plenty after the ravages of war that babies who were in their mother's womb during the early stages of pregnancy during the Dutch famine were twice as likely to develop heart disease in later life. The sudden switch in nutrition during early pregnancy altered the course of embryonic development such that the risk of other diseases, such as diabetes, cancer, schizophrenia and being overweight, also greatly increased for those individuals. The risk of ill health was also increased for the grandchildren of women who were in early pregnancy during times of famine.

This tells us that preconception care is important not only in ensuring both mother and father are healthy and adequately nourished before pregnancy to ensure egg and sperm cells are in optimal condition, but also to ensure that conditions are as stable as possible in the mother, so that the environment the embryo expects, the embryo gets, thus development progresses smoothly. This is why we believe that longer periods of preconception care are helpful, particularly for women who need to achieve weight changes or have other underlying issues that may affect development, including suboptimal nutrient levels. All of these factors have the potential to improve the health not only of your children, but also your grandchildren.

THE BASICS OF PRECONCEPTION CARE

The starting point for all couples who are in good health and wish to conceive is to take a series of basic steps at least six months before trying for a baby. Please don't worry if you haven't planned for this; just start whenever you can.

- **Stop smoking as early as possible.** This is important for both men (see Chapter 10) and women. Smoking can make women lose their eggs more quickly, and women who smoke are twice as likely to be infertile as non-smokers, even if they have already been pregnant before. The risks increase the more you smoke. Smoking can also affect the success rates of fertility treatment, such as IVF. Smoking during pregnancy can harm the baby, especially the lungs and brain. Smoking may also increase the risk of miscarriage.

- **Avoid drinking alcohol altogether for women.** High alcohol intake (seven or more units a week or more than three units on one occasion) is associated with heavy or irregular periods and reduced fertility. Alcohol can also affect ovulation and hormone levels (even where periods appear normal), reduce ovarian reserve and decrease the chance of success following IVF. One study found that women going through IVF who drank one or more alcoholic drinks (each drink contained 1.78 units) a day had more than twice the risk of miscarriage, with an even higher risk when drinking in the week before IVF treatment.[3] One daily drink also reduced both the number of eggs retrieved and pregnancy rates. Alcohol during pregnancy increases risks to the baby, including having a child with a fetal alcohol spectrum disorder (FASD) and lower chance of live birth. For impact on male fertility see Chapter 10 (page 141).

- **Do not use recreational drugs.** Drugs such as cannabis, cocaine, ecstasy, ketamine and amphetamines all have the potential to negatively impact fertility in men and women, including delaying conception in women. They can also cause significant harm if taken during pregnancy. Cannabis can affect hormone balance and therefore may make it more difficult to get pregnant, for instance.

- **Take the basic supplements.** Official guidance recommends taking 400mcg folic acid daily for three months before you start trying to conceive, though many benefit from taking the natural form, folate, and some need higher amounts. Most need to supplement with vitamin D, especially in the winter months. (See Chapter 4 for more on supplements.)

- **Avoid overconsumption of caffeine.** Research looking at the impact of caffeine including tea and coffee consumption on fertility is very mixed, with some studies showing it has an impact at lower levels and others not.[4] A recent analysis found coffee and caffeine consumption did not reduce the chance of getting pregnant naturally or through fertility treatment.[5] Higher levels have been shown to have an impact. Guidance from organisations including the European Food Safety Authority (EFSA) and the World Health Organization (WHO) suggest limiting intake to a maximum of two to three cups of coffee (200–300mg caffeine) or around four cups of tea per day. This advice holds for both women and men. Some studies also show an increased risk of miscarriage with increasing intake of coffee and caffeine during early pregnancy and a recent meta-analysis found there was no safe intake for pregnancy.[6] On balance, we advise our female patients to limit to no more than one cup daily as a precaution, though some choose to cut caffeine out altogether.

- **Aim for a healthy body mass index (BMI).** Being underweight or overweight is suboptimal for fertility and pregnancy, and we cover this in Chapter 6.

- **Manage pre-existing health issues.** Make sure you are assessed, managed and under the care of a suitable doctor for any health problems and discuss any medications with your doctor (see page 65).

- **Have a full screening for sexually transmitted infections (STIs) – (both men and women).** Ask your doctor for these checks before you start trying to conceive. This includes testing for chlamydia, gonorrhoea and HIV. Chlamydia and gonorrhoea are important preventable causes of pelvic inflammatory disease (PID – an infection that reaches and damages the fallopian tubes) and infertility. Chlamydia and gonorrhoea are tested by either a urine test or a cotton swab that is inserted into the vagina (women). You'll be prescribed antibiotics if you have an infection. You may also be tested for syphilis and hepatitis. Also seek advice from your doctor if you have any changes to your normal vaginal discharge, an unpleasant or fishy smell from your vagina, itching in your vagina or around your vulva, or burning when you pass urine. These can all be signs of a condition called bacterial vaginosis (BV) when there is too much of certain naturally occurring bacteria in the vagina leading to an imbalance. This can be treated with antibiotics.

- **Be up to date with smear tests and ensure your latest result was negative.** Smear tests screen for changes in the cells of the cervix (that connects the vagina and the womb) that can lead to cervical cancer if left untreated. The most common cause of these cell changes and cervical cancer is infection with the human papillomavirus (HPV). This is not always transmitted through penetrative sex and can be passed on from the hands and mouth of a sexual partner. Smear tests are recommended every three years unless you have had recent treatment for an abnormal smear or have a current HPV infection, which will show up on your smear test. Smear tests are not advised during pregnancy and so if you are due to have a test within the next year, ask your doctor to have this done before you start trying to conceive and monitor the situation if it takes time for you to conceive. Smear tests are the best way to avoid preventable death from cervical cancer, so always ensure you are checked, even if you feel apprehensive about the process.

- **Check rubella immunity via a blood test.** Rubella or German measles is a viral infection that is often mild and may not be detected. It is extremely dangerous for the unborn baby and causes birth defects if you are infected during pregnancy. Most people are vaccinated in childhood but immunity can lapse, so even if you have had the measles, mumps and rubella (MMR) vaccine, women are advised to undergo rubella immunity testing via their GP before trying to conceive. If you have not had the MMR vaccine or if testing shows you are not immune, you should be vaccinated.

THE GAME CHANGERS

There is so much more that you can do to help give yourself the best chance of conceiving and having a healthy baby beyond these basic steps. Once you have addressed the basics above, the seven steps to a healthy baby, which we will cover over the course of this book, are:

1. Improve your diet

In terms of food generally, evidence is building for the importance of diet when it comes to conceiving. For instance, a Dutch study demonstrated that patients undergoing IVF or intracytoplasmic sperm injection (ICSI) who followed basic dietary recommendations covering the intake of fruit, vegetables, meat, fish, wholewheat products and fats had a 65 per cent increased chance of having an ongoing pregnancy.[7] This is a big effect from such simple advice, so never underestimate the power of making basic changes to your diet over time. Some of our patients have conceived naturally after long struggles including failed IVF and miscarriage after following a Mediterranean diet and the important dietary principles we cover in Chapter 3.

2. Optimise your nutrient levels

In addition to the basic supplements including folic acid, it's crucial to optimise your nutrient levels including zinc, magnesium, iodine, selenium, vitamin D and omega-3. Findings from preconception care papers by *The Lancet* highlight the link between pre-pregnancy health and nutrient status of the woman and outcomes for mother and baby after birth.[8] In our clinical practice, we find these same nutrient deficiencies can also affect the chances of conceiving and we discuss what you can do about this in Chapter 4.

3. Choose a level of exercise that is right for you

Low- to moderate-intensity exercise, such as swimming, gentle jogging, brisk walking and low-intensity gym classes, three times weekly, is advised for women in addition to gentle yoga (see page 129) and moderate- to high-intensity three times weekly for men (see Chapter 10). We look more closely at tailoring exercise to you in Chapter 6.

4. Manage your oral health

Ensure you are up to date with your dental checks and that bleeding gums and other issues are treated and resolved. Gum disease is known to impact fertility and pregnancy (see Chapter 7).

5. Recognise the clues in your symptoms

Your body gives you clues as to what may be affecting your ability to conceive. Learning to interpret any symptoms you experience and understanding what you can do about them can help tip the balance in terms of your ability to conceive. We look at these factors in Chapters 3 and 7.

6. Look after your mental well-being

Preconception care is not only about physical well-being; it's important to look after your mental health and emotional well-being too. Trying to conceive can be stressful if it doesn't happen right away and it's best to manage any mental health issues before pregnancy, where possible. Poor preconception mental health has been shown to increase the chances of all types of pregnancy complication, including having a miscarriage and having a low birth weight baby after maternal age, ethnicity, marital status, education, income and number of children in the household have all been taken into consideration. Don't be afraid to ask for help and seek support from your doctor if you feel you are struggling. We look at mental well-being in Chapter 9.

7. Work on the male partner's health

Very little attention has traditionally been focused on the male partner and yet there is a significant body of evidence to demonstrate the impact of diet, lifestyle and nutrient status on male fertility, the outcome of fertility treatment and child health. Most studies looking at the role of fathers in child health have looked at preconception workplace exposures in men and their impact on the risk of major birth defects and childhood cancers, but we're learning more about the way more low-level exposures to environmental toxins and poor preconception diet in men may impact child health.[9] We'll learn more about male fertility, including the impact of paternal diet and lifestyle on child health, in Chapter 10.

Recognising that the nutritional status of both women and men before conception has such profound implications for the growth, development and long-term health of your baby gives you both an awful lot of power at a time when you may feel incredibly disempowered. And if you're a man feeling that there is nothing you can do other than provide your sperm sample, this can be a game changer.

Chapter 3

Diet and Optimising Fertility

IMPROVING YOUR DIET is the first step in your seven steps to a healthy baby as every stage of the reproductive process needs the nutrients provided by our food to function well. Because achieving a pregnancy involves the complex interaction of many different bodily systems, the balance and healthy functioning of our whole body is needed for a woman to conceive and for a man to develop healthy sperm. All of these things are fuelled by a healthy diet.

Equally, just as good nutrition is needed for our overall health and fertility, poor diet and other damaging behaviours such as excess alcohol consumption and smoking have negative effects, including on the eggs and sperm cells that will go on to develop into a baby. So eliminating things that may harm us physically, in conjunction with healthy habits, is also important.

NUTRITION IN FERTILITY AND PREGNANCY

Appropriate nutrition is essential for the growth and development of brains and bodies, and for building, maintaining, fuelling and repairing every cell in every part of your brain and body. At least 40 essential nutrients must be provided by your food (vitamins, minerals, essential amino acids and omega-3 and -6 fatty acids), and you need to eat a very varied diet in order to have a chance of ensuring sufficient intake of all of these nutrients. Diet and nutrient levels are therefore hugely important when trying to conceive and preparing for pregnancy.

In terms of specific diets, one of the most studied styles of eating when it comes to fertility is the Mediterranean diet. An important study in 2018 showed an association between how well women stuck to a Mediterranean-style diet and clinical pregnancy and live birth rates. Women who ate more vegetables, fruit, whole grains, fish, legumes, nuts and olive oil compared to other foods leading up to *in vitro* fertilisation (IVF) were more like to have a baby as a result of treatment.[1] The study accounted for things like weight, age, physical activity, calorific intake, supplement use and infertility diagnosis, so the conclusion is that following a Mediterranean diet may help women undergoing IVF increase the chances of a successful pregnancy and delivering a live baby. Studies also suggest that the Mediterranean diet can help natural fertility too. An Australian study in 2018, featuring 5,000 women, looked at pre-pregnancy fruit and fast food intake prior to conceiving.[2] A lower intake of fruit and a higher intake of fast food were both associated with a small but significant increase in the time it took to conceive.

Many other studies suggest a link between preconception diet and factors including oocyte and embryo quality, implantation and pregnancy outcomes including the live birth of a baby.[3] Preconception high-fat diets, for instance, have been shown to increase lipid (fat) content of the oocyte and affect its development potential. There is ongoing research looking at how oocytes mature within the ovary and how nutrition affects their capacity to develop into good-quality embryos, so we are likely to see more evidence to support the importance of diet for oocyte development in the future.

There is also evidence to show that particular types of food as well as specific nutrients are associated with a better chance of having a baby, and this information can guide you while trying to conceive.[4] Healthy diets that include seafood, poultry, whole grains, fruits and vegetables consistently demonstrate a link with good fertility in women and improved sperm quality in men.

Overall, there is definitely a strong association between good diet and better fertility outcomes. Add to this, if you're part of a couple and you both get involved, you really do have the capacity to make a significant difference. We often see that when two people make realistic changes across different parts of their daily routine and are able to accrue a series of marginal gains, these things can tip the balance in their favour.

DIETARY PRINCIPLES FOR FERTILITY

When it comes to diet, there is no one-size-fits-all approach (despite what you might read online) and specific variations will apply depending on individual circumstances, health issues, genetics, gut bacteria and starting points. The evolving field of nutrigenomics, where genes are tested to assess the body's ability to process particular foods and nutrients in order to personalise diet, has not become mainstream clinical practice, though this may change as evidence grows and clinical guidelines are developed.

Although the optimal dietary approach isn't necessarily the same for each and every one of you, based on the latest available evidence, we can recommend a set of dietary principles that can be used to inform your food choices as you prepare for pregnancy to support good fertility. These principles apply to both men and women, though there are certain variations and specific factors that are particularly important for male fertility and we cover these in Chapter 10.

You may find that you lose weight if you follow these principles and switch to a healthier diet. If you don't and are overweight or if you still need to lose more weight to reach the healthy range, we discuss specific weight-loss strategies in Chapter 6. If you lose weight when you don't need to, make sure you increase the amount you are eating or your specific intake of fat or carbohydrate, and also see Chapter 6 for advice.

Eat a varied diet

Dietary diversity is one of the most powerful factors under your control that can improve your well-being. Studies show that a diverse diet means that the population of bacteria in our gut (the microbiome) is also diverse, which results in better health outcomes across a range of indicators.[5] Given that optimal immune function and inflammatory status are important for things like implantation, we can start to see how the indirect effects of diet may impact on reproductive pathways and explain the association between good diet and better fertility outcomes.

Dietary diversity across all food groups and types is helpful but is especially important in terms of vegetable intake. This is because

30

vegetables are prebiotics. Prebiotics are foods that stimulate the growth of beneficial bacteria in the gut, rather than having to add them in the form of a probiotic, which is a food or supplement that already contains the bacteria. Vegetables are prebiotics as they contain the non-digestible fibre that reaches the gastrointestinal tract intact and effectively provides a source of food for the bacteria, allowing them to grow. The more variety of vegetables you eat, the better your gut microbiome (the 'good' bacteria in your gut). Current recommendations suggest we should aim to eat at least 30 different types of vegetable per week to maximise our chances of creating a diverse microbiome.[6]

A diverse diet is also important in order to ensure the spread of nutrients needed for good health. So it isn't just vegetable variety that we should aim for but also variety in terms of intake of fruit, fats, carbohydrates and protein. We should aim to vary our sources of these foods in terms of different types of fish, meat, dairy, beans, pulses, fruit and grains from day to day and week to week. One of the best ways of achieving this when life gets busy is to cook in batches and freeze individual portions (see page 37).

Eat mainly vegetables

Vegetables should make up the most sizeable portion of our diets, but vegetable intake for many is woefully inadequate. We should aim for between eight and eleven portions of fruit and vegetables daily, three of which should be fruit and the rest vegetables. Routinely having a sandwich for lunch is one of the biggest barriers to achieving the kind of vegetable intake that we should be aiming for, for our general health as well as for good fertility, because the amount of nutrient-dense food we can consume in an everyday sandwich is limited.

Lunch should include around three portions of vegetables in the form of things like salad or a vegetable-based soup, and this leaves three to five portions to be eaten throughout the rest of the day, either through breakfast (grilled tomatoes and mushrooms with your poached eggs), snacks (vegetable sticks with or without a dip like hummus) or evening meal (broccoli, cauliflower, carrots, cabbage, etc.). Depending on your starting point, this may seem like a lot, but this level of vegetable intake simply needs a change of awareness and habits, and then it becomes quite achievable. If you make this one change several months before you start trying to conceive and continue the habit through pregnancy, you will go a long way to both improving the chance of a good outcome in terms of fertility treatment and also in protecting the health of your future child. This kind of vegetable-rich diet has been shown to reduce both inflammation and oxidative stress in the body, two factors that can impact fertility and embryonic development (for more on this see page 55).

Eat a mixture of cooked and raw veg

As well as diversity and quantity of vegetable intake, the next thing to consider is combining both cooked and raw vegetables. The bioavailability of different beneficial compounds in vegetables is sometimes improved with cooking (e.g. the red antioxidant lycopene in tomatoes) or reduced (as in vitamin C content of any vegetable). Cooked vegetables can be easier to digest, so may be more beneficial for those with any gastrointestinal problems, though generally a combination of cooked and raw is best.

A HEALTHY DIET DURING PREGNANCY

Good nutrition during pregnancy itself (as well as before) also impacts your ability to have a healthy pregnancy and a healthy baby. A recent review found that the majority of studies showed that a Mediterranean diet during pregnancy had a protective effect on the health of the baby, and a recent study showed a reduced risk of gestational diabetes in the mother with this same diet.[7] The aim is to start a healthy diet and lifestyle prior to conception in a comprehensive preconception care programme and continue these habits through pregnancy to optimise your chances of both conceiving and having a healthy baby.

'Eat the rainbow'

The aim should be to have a colourful plate for each main meal. Different colours in foods indicate differing antioxidant compounds, which all have specific properties and health benefits, including for our gut bacteria. Anthocyanin in blueberries, for instance, has been shown to have various benefits for general health and studies indicate improvements to cardiovascular health, memory, energy and blood pressure with regular blueberry consumption.[8] Blueberries have also been shown to have anti-inflammatory properties. Antioxidants generally counteract what are known as free radicals (or reactive oxygen species – ROS – see page 199) in the body, which, as their name suggests, are highly reactive and therefore damaging to cells. ROS are produced as part of normal metabolism but contribute to ageing and cellular wear and tear throughout life. The body's way of neutralising the potential damage is to mobilise the antioxidants we consume in foods. Oxidative stress as a result of these free radicals can damage all cells, and there's been a particular research focus in terms of damage to sperm cells, hence the antioxidants you may see in male fertility supplements, though it is possible to overdo it with antioxidant supplements, as we will see in Chapter 4. An inability to sufficiently cope with oxidative stress in the body can also cause inflammation, which is damaging to fertility.

Eat herbs and spices

Herbs and spices have been found in numerous studies to contain compounds at a higher concentration than normal vegetables that are beneficial to health.[9] Just as colour is a marker of antioxidant content, the intense flavour of herbs and spices can be seen as an indication of their relative medicinal potential. However, we would not recommend self-medicating with herbal supplements any more than we suggest prescribing your own thyroid medication. Herbs and spices in supplement form can have significant impact, including on the liver, so always seek professional advice.

Including a range of herbs and spices as a normal part of your diet means that you can benefit from different polyphenols and other active ingredients that may have antimicrobial, neuroprotective, anti-inflammatory and antioxidant properties, or those which could improve metabolic health, without overdoing it with medicinal quantities. A 2019 review in the journal *Genes and Nutrition* found that, of the 25 herbs and spices covered in the paper, 21 had evidence of anti-inflammatory properties.[10] That's 84 per cent, with the ones most associated with anti-inflammatory properties being thyme, oregano, rosemary, sage, basil, mint, turmeric, dill, parsley, cinnamon, clove, nutmeg, lemongrass, ginger, chilli pepper, fenugreek and pepper. So a Mediterranean diet with some of the spices of the Middle and Far East thrown in is perfect!

Eat plenty of fibre

The recommended daily intake for fibre is 30g, and most people do not come close to this. High-fibre diets that feed our gut bacteria are associated with better outcomes in terms of fertility, and fibre is important for many aspects of health, including digestive and cardiovascular health. The best dietary sources of fibre are vegetables, beans, pulses and wholegrains such as brown rice. Increase your dietary fibre slowly over several weeks to reach this target in order to avoid gut discomfort and symptoms that can come with sudden increases.

Do not avoid fats

There has been greater recognition in recent years that low-fat diets are not optimal for health, but some dieting programmes still recommend this approach. We often see patients following low-fat diets in an attempt to lose weight to be eligible for IVF, but this is not the best way to prepare for pregnancy. The brain is 60 per cent fat, all cell membranes contain fats that are needed for the transport of nutrients and biochemicals into the cell for it to function, and maternal dietary fat is important for brain development of the baby. Further, dietary fat is needed for fat-soluble vitamins that are essential for health and pregnancy (vitamins A, D, E and K – think vitamin E in olive oil, nuts and avocados, and vitamin A in butter and eggs).

We would not advise high-fat diets (which can impact egg and sperm quality), but moderate daily inclusion of healthy fats and a little saturated fat is fine. Essential fatty acids (omegas -3, -6 and -9) found in foods like oily fish and seeds are also crucial for health, fertility and the development of the baby. Omega-3 fatty acid intake in oily fish is especially important to manage as most people do not get enough and would benefit from a supplement during the preconception period and pregnancy (see page 57).

Ensure an adequate intake of good-quality protein

Proteins are a source of amino acids, known as the building blocks of life, and are incredibly important when it comes to creating new life. Good protein sources include fish, meat, eggs, nuts, beans, tofu and quinoa. We would not recommend a high-protein diet, as data presented as part of a major five-year Europe-wide research programme showed that high-protein diets result in toxic compounds being produced by gut bacteria.[11] The dominance of one particular macronutrient can also be detrimental to the inclusion of other types of foods so we would always recommend balance, as with the Mediterranean diet that is consistently associated with good fertility.

Protein requirements will vary from individual to individual depending on things like exercise, and genetic variations may mean that slightly differing proportions of macronutrients suit certain people. Certain conditions can also affect the optimal relative proportion of macronutrient intake. However, an indication of an average protein consumption for a healthy preconception diet is 46g of protein per day, rising to 70g daily during pregnancy. Make sure that you eat some protein with each meal.

Eat whole grains and complex carbohydrates

In terms of carbohydrate intake, it's best to choose wholegrain versions such as brown rice and brown bread rather than the white, refined versions, most of the time.[12] Refined carbohydrate is particularly an issue if you have any metabolic problems such as diabetes or conditions with a metabolic component such as polycystic ovary syndrome (PCOS). One study found an association between a low-carbohydrate diet and improved fertility treatment outcomes for the general population and, while other studies haven't found an association, it's advisable to avoid over-consumption of carbohy-drate and choose the complex versions that haven't been stripped of the fibre-containing outer husk (and consequently the B vitamins).[13]

We do not recommend avoiding carbohydrate totally or ultra-low-carbohydrate diets like the ketogenic diet. However, there can be an over-reliance on bread and grains in the diet to the detriment of things like vegetable intake, which may explain why lower-carbohydrate diets have been associated with better fertility. High consumption of carbohydrate can also mean that the naturally occurring compounds they contain (known as phytates) can increase to a level where they block mineral absorption, including minerals important for fertility such as zinc. Advice is therefore to mostly avoid sugar and refined carbohydrates such as white bread and pasta, avoid over-consumption of bread and grains generally, and have things like biscuits only occasionally in your diet.

DARK CHOCOLATE

Dark chocolate contains some sugar but is mainly cacao, which is rich in polyphenols and also magnesium. Eating dark choc-olate in moderation during pregnancy has even been associated with reduced risk of pre-eclampsia and improved fetal growth in some studies, though some animal studies show an adverse effect on infant metabolism.[14] Again, avoid over-consumption: balance and dietary diversity are key.

Avoid highly processed foods

It's best to avoid highly processed foods, processed breakfast cere-als and ready-made meals that contain excess sugar, salt and trans and hydrogenated fats (fats that are processed), food additives and preservatives. Junk food diets and high intake of processed foods are associated with poorer outcomes, with eating fast food regu-larly being associated with almost double the risk of infertility in a recent study, for instance.[15] By junk food diets, we mean regular (rather than occasional) consumption of things like packaged pizzas, burgers, kebabs, fried foods including chips, crisps, donuts, packaged biscuits and fizzy drinks. Diets high in highly processed foods are also associated with increased levels of inflammation in the body.

If you choose processed foods too often, it has the potential to reduce your chances of conceiving. Every time you replace a healthy meal with a highly processed one, you are losing the potential for good nutrient intake and potentially health- and fertility-boosting ingredients with ones that are likely to have a negative effect. However, as we tell our patients, it is what you do the *majority* of the time that counts. An occasional takeaway (for example, once a month) won't cause harm, but having them at the level of four times per week *has* been shown to have a significant negative impact on chances of conceiving via IVF. Higher fast food intake is also associated with a longer time to pregnancy for natural conception.[16]

Eat home-cooked food

Following this one step will help you achieve all the other recommendations much more easily. Home-cooked food made from scratch is always your most nutritious option, and it doesn't have to be complicated. Cooking in batches and freezing portions for a later date helps make this more manageable if you lead a very busy life. Having some home-cooked food in the freezer ready for early pregnancy is also helpful as nausea and an increased sense of smell can make cooking extremely challenging.

Home-cooking is also associated with better weight management as ready meals and processed foods often contain a combination of high fat and high carbohydrate that significantly increases your overall calorific intake. Freshly prepared food also doesn't require the use of artificial preservatives. One important note is that frying and charred food (including barbecue cooking if overdone) increases the content of harmful chemicals known as advanced glycation end products (AGEs). These have been shown to be toxic when found in the fluid in the uterus and may affect implantation, so avoid too much frying at home.

Drink mainly water and avoid fizzy drinks

You may find a backlash against this advice online in terms of general health as some scientists argue that fizzy drinks aren't the poison that health advocates claim. However, there is evidence to show adverse effects from drinking soft drinks including colas, lemonades and energy drinks.[17] The impact of different compounds on fertility and pregnancy is also highly specific in that gametes (sperm and eggs) are very specialised cells that are extremely sensitive to environmental exposures, as is a developing baby, especially at the stage of the rapidly dividing early embryo, and there certainly isn't evidence to show there is no harm in these specific scenarios. On the contrary, there are studies indicating a negative impact on fertility, including a recent study involving 524 patients and 5,548 oocytes retrieved via IVF that concluded that soft drinks and artificial sweeteners negatively affect oocyte quality and IVF outcomes.[18]

Your main fluid intake should come from water (including sparkling), and dehydration is a common issue that can affect general health in many ways, with even minor changes in cellular water content causing changes in cell metabolism and function. We therefore recommend drinking around 1.5 litres of water daily and avoiding fizzy drinks where possible. In terms of alcohol, although an occasional glass isn't bad, it's best to wait until after your baby is born (see page 22).

Don't eat too much dairy and make it full-fat

If eating dairy works for you, don't overdo it. Studies have linked very high dietary intake of dairy with lower antral follicle counts (AFC – see page 160), but evidence to show there is a definite cause has not yet been proven and only very high levels of consumption showed an adverse effect.[19] By high levels, we mean seven or more portions per day, with a portion being the equivalent of a breakfast serving of yoghurt, rather than a splash of milk in tea. Two to three portions daily is fine.[20] Intake of low-fat dairy has been associated with poorer outcomes in some studies, so always choose the full-fat varieties.[21]

Eat organic where possible

Where possible, choose organic foods and wash non-organic fruit and vegetables thoroughly. Research has shown that pesticide content of urine declined rapidly after participants switched to an organic diet, and there are numerous studies to support the benefit of reducing pesticide exposure in both men and women.[22] Research in humans has shown improved fertility when eating an organic diet. A Harvard study found an organic diet (classified as eating organic produce three or more times per week) improved IVF outcomes – those with the highest estimated pesticide intake had an 18 per cent lower chance of conceiving via IVF than those on an organic diet, and those who did conceive had a 26 per cent higher risk of miscarriage.[23] These effects were not because the organic group was eating more fruit and vegetables, which was accounted for in the analysis. Similar adverse effects have been demonstrated for male fertility, with pesticide exposure causing epigenetic changes in sperm that can impact IVF outcomes and the chance of a live birth. We will look in more detail at environmental exposures in Chapter 8.

UNRAVELLING MISCONCEPTIONS

When it comes to diet in general and fertility nutrition in particular, online platforms are full of claims that are not always backed by research, so it's important to understand what the evidence can tell us.

Dairy

The popular narrative, especially on social media, is that dairy is bad for fertility. This isn't backed up by consistent evidence, with some studies showing a benefit from moderate intake of full-fat dairy products for women.[24] Many health and alternative practitioners still claim dairy produce is inherently inflammatory, but a 2017 systematic review of 52 clinical trials found a strong anti-inflammatory effect in those with metabolic disorders and, unsurprisingly, a strong pro-inflammatory response in those with an allergy to cow's milk.[25] Further, recent research has shown that dairy lipids (fats) specifically act against chronic inflammation in the body.[26]

However, you must always take into account your body's individual response to foods and, while most are absolutely fine with moderate consumption, you may do better by cutting out dairy. Some people may be lactose intolerant, for instance, where they don't produce lactase, the enzyme that digests lactose, the main sugar in dairy produce. This can be tested by your doctor. There is also some early evidence that A2 dairy products may be less likely to have a negative effect. The major protein in milk is casein and it has two major sub-types: A1 and A2. A2 dairy contains the latter and some studies suggest this is less likely to cause an inflammatory response, digestive discomfort and loose stools.[27] It is possible to buy both A2 cow's milk and also sheep and goat milk products, which both contain predominantly A2 casein. If you have PCOS, you may benefit from cutting out dairy products (see Chapter 15), particularly cow's milk, though we still don't have sufficient evidence on this topic.

Pay attention to how you feel after specific foods and, in the absence of testing, this will be your best clue as to how well you tolerate different aspects of your diet. Soy has also been shown in some studies to benefit women going through fertility treatment, despite getting a negative press.[28] Plant-based milks including soy, almond, coconut and oat milk can all be used as substitutes if you want to try eliminating dairy. Choose fortified varieties to replace the nutrients found in dairy like calcium and iodine. The message with all of these things is to achieve a healthy balance and avoid over-consumption of any one type of food, and with this advice you will avoid most significant pitfalls.

Wheat and gluten

Wheat deserves a special mention as it is a food that courts controversy: more specifically, the protein it contains – gluten. Again, you will find many practitioners and information online advising cutting out all gluten for everyone on the basis that it is pro-inflammatory. Evidence is mixed, with some arguing that gluten is a gastrointestinal irritant and potentially inflammatory even for those without conditions that make them sensitive to gluten.[29]

At the preconception stage, it is important to know that some people are sensitive to dietary intake of wheat and other grains containing gluten-like proteins, including barley, rye and spelt. If you experience any diarrhoea, discomfort, sensitivity or bloating in your abdomen after eating things like bread, pasta, cakes and biscuits, you may have a condition such as coeliac disease, or non-coeliac gluten sensitivity (NCGS), and it is important to see your doctor to be assessed, as these conditions can contribute to malabsorption of nutrients, delay conception and increase the risk of miscarriage, if left untreated. We cover all of these things in more detail in Chapter 7.

For those without a specific health condition, there isn't robust evidence to advise cutting out all gluten.[30] In fact, gluten-free processed foods can be less nutrient-dense, including lower levels of calcium, iron, magnesium, zinc, vitamin B_{12}, folate and vitamin D, as well as significantly less fibre than their gluten-containing wholefood counterparts. Food manufacturing processes often mean that processed foods that are gluten-free tend to be higher in hydrogenated and saturated fatty acids (more unhealthy forms of fat), as well as having a higher glycaemic index (see page 74). Naturally gluten-free wholefoods are just as healthy, but you must always take great care when eliminating foods from your diet, and ensure that you do so under professional guidance.

However, there is definitely a tendency towards overconsumption of bread and wheat in western diets. When we ask patients in our clinic what they eat from day to day, it is not uncommon to discover they eat a wheat-based cereal for breakfast, a sandwich for lunch and pasta for their evening meal, at least some days of the week. This is far too much of any one food type, whatever the food, and consequently this pattern of eating reduces dietary diversity and the spread of nutrients in the diet.

Red meat

Some studies suggest that red meat may have an adverse effect on fertility, including on the likelihood of an embryo reaching the blastocyst stage (day 5 of embryonic development) during IVF, but whether this is due to red meat or eating patterns associated with red meat consumption, including lower vegetable consumption, is hard to say.[31]

It is certainly true that eating less mass-produced meat is beneficial in environmental terms, but choosing local, seasonal foods produced using sustainable methods is the primary consideration. More people eating less mass-produced meat will also have a greater impact than a smaller number choosing a vegan diet. If we can persuade all our readers of the benefits of choosing a vegan diet on one day per week in part in order to increase your overall fibre intake, it will balance the environmental impact of those who choose to include some meat in your diet. Vegan Tuesday perhaps?

> **Note:** If you are considering reducing any food group, always seek professional guidance before making drastic changes to your diet.

VEGETARIAN AND VEGAN DIETS

Vegetarianism and veganism are becoming increasingly popular, with young people especially switching for health benefits and environmental reasons. We absolutely empathise with the environmental and ethical arguments for choosing to be vegan or vegetarian, but, in terms of health, you need to understand the implications and know how to manage the potential pitfalls. It is possible to eat a solely plant-based diet and conceive, have a healthy pregnancy and a healthy baby, but it is more challenging to get the appropriate nutrients. It is also important to cut through the noise when it comes to the evidence. A high intake of nuts, vegetables, beans and pulses is healthy, but eating highly processed plant-based foods is not necessarily the best option and the impact on health is largely untested. Human beings have also evolved eating omnivorous diets (meat and vegetables), so that is always going to suit our digestion and metabolism. Also, although strict cause and effect is difficult to firmly prove from epidemiological studies, it is possible that the main potential health risk for omnivores is not necessarily eating meat, but eating fewer vegetables and less fibre. Eating meat is an effective way to boost both zinc and iron levels that are commonly low in individuals seeking fertility treatment. Vegetarians and vegans are also at risk of deficiencies of iron, zinc, vitamin B_{12}, iodine and omega-3 fatty acids, so supplementation is usually needed, especially in the preconception stage and during pregnancy (see page 25).

Certain gene variants also lead to reduced conversion of beta-carotene (plant-based vitamin A that can't be used by the body without processing) and retinol (preformed vitamin A that can be directly used by the body), so vegans in particular need to be aware that they may be susceptible to low vitamin A if they have this gene variant.[32] Some studies show that up to 45 per cent of people may carry these variants and, given preconception and pregnancy supplements in the UK only contain plant sources of vitamin A, you can see the potential pitfalls of restrictive diets.[33]

A balanced Mediterranean-style diet with a wide variety of foods with a focus on plant-based foods will always be optimal for health, and so always think carefully about the type of diet you choose and ensure you don't deprive yourself of nutrients by focusing too much on particular types of food. Remember it is what you do the *majority* of the time that will have the biggest effect.

Chapter 4

Nutrients and Supplements

ALONGSIDE A GOOD diet, you should also ensure you have sufficient levels of vitamins and minerals, firstly for your own health in preparation for conception and pregnancy, but also for the health of the baby. If you have problems with your gut and digestion, you may have problems with your nutrient levels, so you can only address your nutrient status if you have first addressed any gastrointestinal problems (see Chapter 7).

Good nutrition is essential for reproductive pathways to work well for both men and women (we cover the nutrients that are especially important for men in Chapter 10). Minerals in particular are the vital foundation for the effective working of our hormones, and mineral *balance* as well as sufficiency is needed. Overall, the science clearly shows an association between nutrition and reproductive health, as well as the interdependent relationship between vitamins and minerals.

Because western diets have low dietary intake of numerous vitamins and minerals, many women enter pregnancy with low levels of key nutrients including iron, zinc, iodine, vitamin D and magnesium. A cumulative effect of poor diet from teenage years into adulthood can build up over time, meaning the body stores of these nutrients that are crucial in pregnancy are running low. This means that a tipping point of different deficiencies can come together to impact the ability to conceive, as well as embryonic development.

The annual National Diet and Nutrition Surveys (NDNS) in the UK repeatedly highlight this poor dietary intake, including the latest study published in 2020 with a significant percentage of the population consuming below the Lower Reference Nutrient Intake (LRNI – the minimum intake we should be aiming for) value for the 11 nutrients surveyed and a *decrease* compared with previous surveys including lower folate and vitamin A levels and much lower blood folate.[1] Findings from the NDNS are also reinforced by conclusions of preconception care papers by *The Lancet*, which highlight that young women are particularly at risk of mineral deficiency and most women of reproductive age are not nutritionally prepared for pregnancy.[2] Poor dietary intake of nutrients is equally reported in men.

Dieting and intense exercise can also reduce nutrient levels, so all of these things should help you start to recognise some of the root causes of any fertility issues, or the areas to focus on if you're just starting out.

Given pregnancy can also be very depleting on the body, with nutrients diverted to the fetus before a woman's own body's needs are met (in biological terms, the embryo can be termed a parasite!), starting with good nutrient levels before you conceive is crucial for your own health and well-being, especially in preparation for the early stages of motherhood when you are likely to be sleep-deprived and tired. Good preconception health also sets you up well for breastfeeding, which confers significant health benefits on mother and baby. Low nutrient levels after having a baby can also be a factor in problems conceiving a second or subsequent child. Some of our patients conceive naturally after fairly simple correction of nutrient deficiencies, sometimes after long struggles to conceive.

For women, ensuring good body stores of vitamins and minerals is crucial in order to meet the demands of pregnancy. It's much better to work on this before you conceive rather than trying to 'catch up' by topping up low levels of specific nutrients *after* conception. This is partly because the embryonic development that occurs before implantation is such a crucial stage of pregnancy and many of the events in these early days determine the outcome for the baby.

Do you need supplements?

For all of us, the aim is for the main sources of nutrients to be from food, hence the dietary principles we outlined in the previous chapter. This doesn't always happen, however, and if you have had low nutrient intake for many years, especially where there is a history of digestive issues or restrictive diets, you will usually need to take supplements, at least in the short term. If you know you ate lots of junk food as a teen and through your early twenties, for instance, or that you have only just started eating your five a day (only to discover after reading the last chapter that should be more like ten!) *and* if you experience symptoms such as fatigue, frequent infections, poor exercise tolerance, skin or period problems, or a general lack of well-being, then the chances are you will have some nutrient deficiencies.

We haven't tested a single patient yet in our clinics who hasn't had either an outright deficiency or suboptimal levels of certain nutrients, despite most taking a preconception multivitamin and mineral and often eating relatively healthy diets. (You can see examples of nutrients that we find are commonly low and the associated symptoms and effect on reproductive outcomes in the table on page 364.) Supplements tend to contain the recommended daily allowance (RDA) for a particular nutrient, but this may not be enough to bring levels back up to normal from a place of deficiency. Also, different minerals in particular often need differing conditions to help with absorption. One example is zinc, which is best taken on an empty stomach just before protein and away from fat and carbohydrates. Further, dairy, caffeine and polyphenols can inhibit iron absorption, with high levels of tea drinking in particular often implicated in low ferritin (iron store) levels. This means that taking everything together isn't always the best way to boost your levels of different minerals.

Getting all our nutrients from food means they are in a natural, bioavailable form with the cofactors needed for their absorption and functioning in the body. When this doesn't happen, deficiencies develop and so testing also gives us information about how best to change our diets to meet the needs of the body. We should never address gaps and deficiencies through supplementation alone – we should always aim to improve and modify diet where needed to correct the underlying causes of the deficiency, alongside any supplementation required to correct the deficiency.

If you have certain symptoms, it can be beneficial to take specific supplements (see page 364).

The importance of getting tested

If you don't have digestive symptoms that point towards issues with absorption (which need resolving first), we recommend starting your preconception programme by having your levels of key nutrients tested (see table on page 364). We would be cautious about offering fixed advice for standardised supplementation for everybody, as individual needs vary and you can also overdo things (see our website – Resources, page 371 – for some preliminary guidance, which includes taking a good-quality preconception multivitamin as a starting point).

KEY VITAMINS

Folic acid

The current advice for pregnant women and those trying to conceive is to take 400mg (4mg) folic acid and 10mg (400iu – international units) of vitamin D, and nothing more, with recommendations to take higher doses of folic acid (500mg or 5mg) for some, including those with high body mass index (BMI – >30), diabetes, coeliac disease, taking medication including metformin, anti-epilepsy drugs and anti-retroviral drugs, or if either parent has a neural tube defect or family history of neural tube defects. Men may also benefit from supplementation.

Although the standard NHS advice is to supplement with folic acid in the preconception stage and through the first trimester in pregnancy to avoid neural tube defects in the baby such as spina bifida, what is actually protective is adequate maternal levels of folate (vitamin B_9), which is the natural form of folic acid used by the body. Sufficient levels of blood folate are important for egg quality and maturation, as well as fertilisation and implantation. Supplementing with folic acid is also associated with improved outcomes including reduced levels of infertility and miscarriage, and improved chance of conceiving via IVF. There are certain gene variants, however, that reduce the body's ability to convert folic acid into its bioavailable form. If you have been supplementing with folic acid for some time and your blood folate levels are low on testing, it may be that you have such a gene. Methylenetetrahydrofolate reductase (MTHFR) mutations are variants of a particular gene responsible for metabolising folate and we discuss these in Chapter 7. There is therefore an argument for all couples planning a pregnancy to supplement with folate rather than folic acid, either as part of a B complex supplement or preconception multivitamin supplement. The B vitamins work with each other in the body so they are best taken together.

There are two forms of folate that you can try: methyl folate or folinic acid. Some people may experience side effects with methyl folate, so build up slowly to the 400µg daily (or more if this is indicated for you), or substitute with folinic acid if you notice a reaction to methyl folate that does not go away. Use of folinic acid requires professional supervision. Sufficient levels of serum folate are needed for healthy development of the placenta, as well as neural tube development, so it is vital to avoid deficiency. There is some evidence to suggest very high levels in the blood may not be a good thing, so if you have been trying to conceive and supplementing for a long time, you can ask your GP to test your folate levels.[3] Reduce your intake under supervision if your result is above the normal range.

Vitamins D and K

Adequate levels of vitamin D are important for both men and women. Deficiency of maternal vitamin D has been associated with reduced chance of *in vitro* fertilisation (IVF) success in some studies.[4] A recent study also showed reduced chance of having a baby naturally in women with low vitamin D, but when researchers looked at overall diet quality and other nutrients such as iron and folate, low vitamin D on its own wasn't found to reduce the chance of pregnancy, reinforcing the need for a healthy diet generally and good levels of all nutrients.[5] Once your levels get into the normal reference range much higher amounts have not been shown to offer further benefit and may even impact your egg quality (possibly by lowering vitamin A).

Magnesium is needed to produce vitamin D from sunlight or to process vitamin D taken in supplements and most people don't get enough magnesium. Vitamin K is also needed for vitamin D to work well, and growing evidence suggests you should supplement vitamin D with vitamin K_2.[6]

Vitamin D mobilises free calcium in the blood (a potential cause of vitamin D toxicity at high doses), which may lead to calcium being laid down in soft tissue such as arteries (a cause of cardiovascular disease). Vitamin K directs free calcium into bone and, in the MK4 form especially, is protective for bone and teeth. Vitamin K_2 is important during pregnancy for skeletal development of the baby and studies in rats indicate it may be important for sperm health.[7] Vitamin K_2 is a fat-soluble vitamin and dietary sources include butter, cheese and egg yolks, so vegetarians and those who have been following low-fat diets or restricted diets may be at risk of deficiency. High calcium supplementation can also lead to calcification of arteries and other soft tissue, so vitamin K_2 may also be beneficial when supplementing with calcium, as is needed for coeliac disease.

Ideally, the aim is to supplement with vitamin D and aim for optimal serum levels rather than particular doses (in other words, you need to have blood tests to monitor the levels). If you find that your vitamin D level does not improve after tablets, there are some effective oral sprays on the market. A vitamin K_2 supplement comprising two forms – MK4 and MK7 – may be beneficial alongside vitamin D, and doses up to 1mg daily are likely to be safe, unless contraindicated for you, which is mostly for those on blood thinners that work through their action on vitamin K. We recommend discussing this with your doctor or nutritionist.

Vitamin A

Vitamin A works alongside vitamin D, with the body not able to properly utilise vitamin D without sufficient levels of vitamin A. Vitamin A is also important for egg quality and the formation of the blastocyst (day 5 embryo). Both deficiency and excess vitamin A can cause problems for fertility and embryonic development, with extremely high levels of preformed retinol (the animal-sourced form of vitamin A) having the potential to cause birth defects. Standard advice in the UK is therefore to avoid supplements containing retinol and not to eat organ meats such as liver and kidneys (which contain high levels of preformed vitamin A). However, vitamin A is important for fertility. Low dietary intake is common and pregnancy supplements in the UK only contain plant-based sources that are the precursor of vitamin A and need to be taken in much higher quantities to convert to adequate quantities of vitamin A.

Gene variants that limit conversion of beta-carotene to retinol are also common so vegans and anyone avoiding eggs and dairy may be at risk. In the UK, it is likely to be safe to take 750μg of preformed vitamin A daily for a short period before conception, with outright deficiency less likely to be an issue, though always seek professional advice to avoid the risk of birth defects.[8] Synthetic versions of vitamin A (etretinate and isotretinoin) can cause birth defects and should be avoided altogether.

Deficiency of vitamin A can also lead to fetal growth restriction and developmental problems, with a recent study showing that malformations in the baby were associated with nutrient deficiencies, including vitamin A.[9] Vitamin A deficiency can also impact egg quality and may cause infertility. Because your body cannot use vitamin D properly if you are deficient in vitamin A, and both are needed for conception and pregnancy, it is important to include vitamin A-rich foods such as butter and eggs in your diet, along with plant-based sources such as sweet potato and butternut squash.

Your need for vitamin A increases in the third trimester of pregnancy, so you may benefit from increasing preformed vitamin A in the diet during this stage, especially if you are predicted to have a preterm delivery or in the case of fetal growth restriction. If you are suffering from secondary infertility (see page 104) and experienced any of these things in previous pregnancies, seek advice from your treating doctor regarding preconception supplementation.

CAN YOU TAKE TOO MANY SUPPLEMENTS?

As we've outlined above, both poor dietary intake of minerals and mineral deficiencies are common. Conversely, some patients come to see us who are taking a combination of different supplements that takes them above the RDA for particular nutrients.

Selenium is often included in male fertility supplements, for instance, and if taken either alongside other (say) selenium-containing antioxidant supplements as well as dietary intake of Brazil nuts, which are high in selenium, it can be easy to push intake above recommended levels. We see this scenario reflected in test results, sometimes even after patients have followed professional advice from others. Good levels of selenium are important for thyroid function, sperm health in men and for pathways involved in DNA repair generally, but selenium can be toxic if levels rise significantly above the normal reference range. This can be especially important for couples who have been trying to conceive for a long time and may have been supplementing at quite high levels throughout without any assessment.

MINERALS

Often, the balance between different minerals is as important for both male and female fertility as making sure you have enough of each one.

Zinc and copper

For women, numerous studies demonstrate the importance of zinc for oocyte development and ovulation, for instance, as well as for the production of DNA, and synthesis and metabolism (production and processing) of hormones in the body.[10]

For fertility, zinc levels should be higher than copper, but this is usually turned on its head in our patients. Both zinc and copper are needed for good fertility, but when copper is too high and zinc is too low, this can be a cause of inflammation. Inflammation can have a negative effect on your health (see page 98). Studies have also shown that an imbalance between zinc and copper is associated with poor cognitive development in childhood and later educational attainment in adult life.[11] Copper needs to be just right: not too low or too high, the latter being toxic. Interestingly, what is healthy in terms of a good balance of zinc and copper changes during pregnancy, with copper levels rising steeply through the early stages and peaking in the second trimester. Unlike with high copper in the preconception stage, however, this is associated with healthy pregnancies, though the reason why this is the case is not fully understood. High-copper diets, including vegetarian and vegan diets, can worsen an impaired balance between zinc and copper. In particular, vegetarians who have been on the pill for a long time without supplementing are at risk of low iodine, low zinc, impaired zinc–copper balance and low iron, which can wreak havoc with the menstrual cycle and also thyroid function. Therefore, the earlier you put the pieces together and start taking action, the better the outlook for your general health and fertility. We will cover thyroid function and hormones in Chapter 8. We discuss minerals for men in Chapter 10.

The impact of previous oral contraceptive use

The majority of women start trying to conceive following a period on oral contraceptives, which have been associated with reduced levels of several nutrients including vitamins A, B_1, B_2, B_6, B_{12}, C, and E, folate, magnesium, zinc, selenium and co-enzyme Q10.[12] Anything that contains or raises oestrogen in the body increases the absorption and retention of copper in the body. This includes pregnancy, oral contraceptives and being overweight, as fat tissue is metabolically active and produces different hormones, including oestrogen. High copper levels can inhibit zinc absorption (and vice versa). Given that zinc is needed for egg development, hormone balance and many reproductive processes, you can start to see why problems with periods are common among women who have recently stopped taking the pill.

If you are able to come off the pill at least three months before you start trying to conceive, this will give your body time to rebalance ready for pregnancy. You are also likely to benefit from taking extra magnesium (200–300mg magnesium glycinate daily) and zinc (15–20mg zinc picolinate daily) in addition to a multivitamin. We cover this in more detail on page 115.

Iodine

Iodine is a vital mineral for thyroid function (see Chapter 8) and also for the baby's brain development during pregnancy. A significant percentage of women do not have sufficient dietary intake; even minor deficiencies can affect things like IQ in the baby. Excess can also be damaging, especially during pregnancy, so never exceed the recommended allowances. It can be difficult to test for iodine levels, as it is not routinely available on the NHS, so the standard advice is to take 150mg daily for at least three months prior to conception. You may benefit from taking slightly higher amounts under medical supervision if you have certain symptoms including breast issues such as cysts (see page 119). Requirements increase during pregnancy to 220mg daily. If you are taking thyroxine medication, this will supply adequate levels of iodine.

TESTING NUTRIENTS

If you think you may have nutrient deficiencies, especially when it comes to minerals, it's best to seek professional help. You need to get tested, supplement as needed, and then be retested until all your nutrient levels are normal. However, testing blood doesn't tell the whole story. Some minerals, such as magnesium, are under what is known as homeostatic control and you have to be in a state of quite extreme lack before a magnesium deficiency will show up in a standard blood test, for example. Dietary intake of magnesium also tends to be low and many people have what is known as subclinical magnesium deficiency.

Blood levels generally also give a snapshot of a particular day and can change depending on the food you've eaten and supplements you've taken, so blood testing alone does not always give us enough information. Nutrient levels can also vary through the menstrual cycle. Hair testing can indicate mineral status over the last three months, but hasn't been adopted by mainstream medicine, partly because it hasn't been through accepted approval and validation processes. What can be useful is to compare blood, hair, diet, medical history and clinical symptoms including digestive health when assessing individual need for nutrients. Hair testing can provide an indication of heavy metal load in the body, including lead and mercury, which can have adverse effects on fertility. Testing red blood cells (rather than plasma or serum – the fluid component of blood) for nutrients including magnesium can be another way of assessing body stores and nutrient status for a particular mineral, and is something to explore if you continue to experience problems.

You can usually request the following nutrient tests via your GP: ferritin, folate, vitamin B_{12}, vitamin D, zinc, copper, selenium, serum magnesium and calcium. This is helpful for both men and women. Some GPs also offer vitamin A and omega-3. Results that fall into the normal reference range for general health may not be optimal for fertility and pregnancy. Ferritin is one of the most important as it has a very broad reference range but good levels of iron are crucial for pregnancy and development of the baby's brain. We like to see preconception ferritin levels between 50-80µg/L. Always ask to see a copy of your results and seek additional advice where needed.

Next steps

We find that when we work with patients to restore optimal nutrient levels, they experience significant improvements in well-being and symptoms, regularisation of the menstrual cycle and, often, either natural conception or improved outcomes of fertility treatment. We also see subtle shifts like longer cycles or earlier ovulation in cycles that have previously had a short luteal phase. It is also worth noting that work to assess and improve your individual health based on test results will always trump following generic advice or taking off-the-shelf supplements in the hope of improving egg quality or improving your chances of conceiving.

You will read a great deal of information on this both off- and online, and it is easy to be lured by the idea of the wonder supplement(s) that are good for fertility or egg quality. The reality is that you need to consider your own individual health as the foundation for getting pregnant (check the box below to see which level of testing is right for you).

WHICH TESTING IS RIGHT FOR YOU?

Do you have:

☐ A history of or recent unhealthy diet?

☐ A history of or recent restrictive or weight loss diet?

☐ Symptoms such as premenstrual syndrome (PMS), irregular periods, headache, fatigue, depression, anxiety, digestive symptoms?

☐ A history of being on the contraceptive pill?

☐ A history of or recent intense exercise?

☐ A history of or recent high alcohol intake (>12 units per week)?

☐ Difficulties conceiving?

☐ A history of or recent significant stress?

If you have ticked one or more of the above boxes, consider extended testing and start with your GP.

If you are healthy, symptom-free and none of the above apply, you can start with the supplement suggestions on our website (Resources, page 371) and request basic tests via your GP: vitamin D and ferritin as a minimum.

ANTIOXIDANT SUPPLEMENTS

Oxidative stress occurs in the body when reactive oxygen species (ROS) produced during normal metabolism or external factors cannot be balanced by the body's supply of antioxidants, a situation that can affect fertility through the impact on sperm, oocytes and/or the mitochondria (the 'batteries' of the cell responsible for energy production). Oxidative stress can be caused by things like smoking, excess alcohol, being over- or underweight, exposure to environmental toxins and older age, as well as with conditions such as polycystic ovary syndrome (PCOS) and endometriosis.

The natural conclusion, therefore, is that antioxidant supplements have the potential to improve fertility. However, the exact roles of different antioxidants have not yet been fully worked out and it can be difficult to know from the research what is best for you as it depends on many different individual factors. Also, it is possible to have too high an intake of antioxidants, depending on your starting point. Assessing the level of oxidative stress in your body isn't easy and it's important to know that minerals, including zinc and selenium, and vitamins, including vitamins C and E, are also antioxidants. A recent review concluded that only very low-quality evidence suggests that antioxidants generally may improve the chances of a woman conceiving and going on to have a baby.[13]

Antioxidant supplements include carnitines, alpha lipoic acid, resveratrol and co-enzyme Q10, among others, and you should only take these supplements during the preconception phase if indicated for you. There is evidence to suggest that supplementing with antioxidants during early pregnancy can affect development of the placenta, so always be careful when trying to conceive naturally and consider avoiding antioxidants in the second half of your cycle when you may be pregnant.[14] If you have an underactive thyroid, you should not supplement with carnitines.

Co-enzyme Q10

Co-enzyme Q10 is perhaps one of the most studied antioxidant supplements, but also perhaps the most difficult to get right given the raft of conflicting information you may come across from various different sources. Co-enzyme Q10 is a naturally occurring antioxidant that declines with age and also with certain medications such as statins, something that is more relevant today with many delaying parenthood. Co-enzyme Q10 has an important role to play in fertility and preconception care, with numerous human and animal studies indicating benefit including for egg quality, but you must use it appropriately based on your personal circumstances.[15]

There is good evidence to support the use of co-enzyme Q10, as long as you consider all the factors relevant to you and are not simply blindly following advice for universal doses that you may find online. If you are older than 35, are overweight, have premature ovarian insufficiency (POI) or have an underlying condition such as endometriosis or PCOS, you can consider doses of up to 600mg daily. If these do not apply, consider doses of up to 100mg initially.

Omega-3 and omega-6

Omega-3 fatty acids are polyunsaturated fatty acids (PUFAs). The two main omega-3s needed for fertility and pregnancy are docosahexaenoic acid (DHA) and eicosapentaenoic acid (EPA) and are mainly found in fish. DHA is needed for the baby's brain development and EPA is needed for DHA to cross the placenta. Alpha-linolenic acid (ALA) is another type of omega-3 fatty acid found in vegetable oils, nuts and flaxseeds, but is not a form the body can easily use. Algae is a better vegetarian source of omega-3, but shouldn't be used if you have thyroid problems. Dietary sources of DHA are almost exclusively from fish and, given DHA is needed for the baby's brain development, supplements are usually needed if you are vegetarian. Healthy sources of omega-6 include walnuts, avocado oil, sunflower seeds, almonds, chicken and eggs, and these are good foods to include in your diet.

We usually measure the ratio of omega-6 to omega-3 in the blood with a ratio of between 1:1 and 3:1 considered healthy. Modern diets typically throw out this balance and every single patient we have tested has had an impaired ratio, so testing and supplementing based on individual results can be helpful in the preconception period.

Although the implications of an impaired ratio for general health are now contested, one study from the University of Southampton found that higher maternal levels of omega-6 during pregnancy were associated with higher levels of body fat in the child at four and six years, while higher levels of omega-3 were associated with greater muscle and bone mass.[16] This suggests that both changes in the diet to reduce omega-6 and supplementation with omega-3 may be beneficial. As well as foods containing omega 6, high carbohydrate intake can also increase levels of this fatty acid. We have found that the best approach if you have a significantly impaired ratio is to supplement at a higher level of EPA for around three months (preferably longer), alongside 560mg DHA daily, before fertility treatment. Then reduce to a maintenance dose of EPA along with 560mg of DHA in the two months before.

We would also suggest asking your doctor to check that your triglycerides are within the normal range when trying to conceive. This is helpful to check heart health before pregnancy and also because some people see an increase in triglycerides after supplementing with omega-3. If you have unexplained high triglycerides, you can try stopping omega-3 supplements to see if they come down and should then stop supplements permanently if this is the case.

Overall, the evidence supports ensuring adequate levels of all the key nutrients to ensure you are nutritionally prepared for pregnancy. Learning to recognise your individual needs can help you avoid potential negative effects of low levels of particular vitamins and minerals and may help improve your fertility.

Chapter 5

Trying to Conceive Naturally

I F YOU ARE trying to conceive naturally, we recommend following a preconception care programme that includes a healthy diet and the other steps we've so far outlined for at least three months, as this is important for the health of the pregnancy and the health of your baby. You should then start to have unprotected intercourse. If you don't conceive straight away, you can continue trying for a total of 12 months before consulting a doctor for fertility investigations. There are certain circumstances in which you should seek medical help sooner, for example if you have any indication of something that may be affecting your fertility including irregular periods, painful intercourse, severe period pain, you have a known medical condition that affects your fertility or if you are over 35. If your partner has had any operations on his testes or any chronic illness that he thinks may affect his fertility, it is also worth getting checked out sooner. We will cover these areas in more detail over the course of this book.

It's worth noting that you can request routine preconception blood tests for vitamin D, ferritin, folate, B_{12}, zinc and copper, as well as for things like rubella immunity immediately before you start having unprotected sex.

TIMING OF INTERCOURSE

Having sex every two to three days after the end of your menstrual period through until the week before your next period means that

59

you will have a chance of conceiving that month. However, this can be easier said than done as the stresses of trying to get pregnant can make sex seem like a chore. The use of fertility monitors or apps that can help pinpoint the timing of ovulation is not always a good thing as again this can take the focus off what is best and natural. You may find this approach creates tension around sex, puts pressure on your relationship and often simply isn't needed. If you are having reasonably regular cycles and reasonably regular sex, you are likely to have sperm waiting in the fallopian tube for when the egg is released at ovulation.

Frequent ejaculation is good for sperm health, as sperm sitting in testes once produced will die off and release toxic compounds that impact healthy sperm cells. So spontaneous sex that doesn't feel pressured is the best approach for many different reasons.

The fertile window

Ideally, sperm should be waiting for the egg when it is released to reach your egg in optimal condition. An egg can survive for around 24 hours once it is released before it starts to break down. Sperm can survive for up to five days inside a woman's body, so this gives a total of around six days when you are fertile and capable of conceiving. This is known as the fertile window and it's best to have sex at least every couple of days during this time. The rest (indeed the majority!) of the time, the purpose of sex is pure pleasure and bonding with a sexual partner.

Ovulation

For women, there are bodily signs that ovulation is about to occur and these can be monitored to indicate whether you are ovulating and also the timing of ovulation. This includes cervical mucus that acquires a typical 'egg white' consistency; in other words it is clear and will stretch into strings if pulled apart. Other signs you may notice around ovulation are pain in your ovary or breast tenderness. An increase in body temperature also occurs immediately after the release of the egg. It will remain slightly higher rather than falling around the time your period is due if you conceive.

Body temperature needs to be monitored over several months to be a reliable indicator as, once the temperature increases, ovulation has already happened, so you need to understand the range of days of your cycle during which you ovulate, and this can vary from month to month. Having said this, if you have a regular cycle, we don't recommend routine measurement of body temperature when starting trying to conceive as it can add tension early on, which can be unhelpful.

A typical cycle is often described as 28 days with ovulation occurring on day 14, but in reality this is for illustrative purposes only and occurs for only 13 per cent of women. A healthy menstrual cycle for good fertility is usually between 25 and 30 days (29 days on average) and the day of ovulation can vary, though women experience wider variations in reality. Menstrual cycles also tend to shorten very slightly with age. Shorter cycles at a younger age are associated with lower ovarian reserve and cycles less than 25 days can make it harder to get pregnant, as we cover in Chapter 8. Learning to interpret these clues in your body can really help when trying to conceive.

Given that you ovulate on average 12–14 days before the expected date of your next period, your egg will be fertile up to around 11 days before your next period. You can work out the end of your fertile window by subtracting 11 from the total length of your cycle. So for a 28-day cycle, expect ovulation on days 14–16, with the fertile window starting on day 9 (5 days of sperm viability) and ending on days 15–17 (1 day after ovulation). You can work out the start of your fertile window by subtracting 19 days before the expected date of your next period. So, if you have variable cycles, take away 11 days from the longest and 19 days from the shortest to calculate your fertile window.

It can be helpful to have an idea of when you are likely to ovulate, either through monitoring bodily signs like cervical mucus or the more mathematical approach, to make sure you are having sex at the right time of the month. If you have a very long cycle (that is, more than 35 days), this is a sign you may not be ovulating, and you are likely to need to seek medical advice.

First day of period

28 day cycle

| 1 | 2 | 3 | 4 | 5 | 6 | 7 | 8 | 9 | 10 | 11 | 12 | 13 | 14 | 15 | 16 | 17 | 18 | 19 | 20 | 21 | 22 | 23 | 24 | 25 | 26 | 27 | **28** |

First day of period

32 day cycle

| 1 | 2 | 3 | 4 | 5 | 6 | 7 | 8 | 9 | 10 | 11 | 12 | 13 | 14 | 15 | 16 | 17 | 18 | 19 | 20 | 21 | 22 | 23 | 24 | 25 | 26 | 27 | 28 | 29 | 30 | 31 | **32** |

Ovulation

Fertile window

End of cycle

Days in menstrual cycle

Cycle length (days)	Fertile window (days)
23	Day 4 – 12
24	Day 5 – 13
25	Day 6 – 14
26	Day 7 – 15
27	Day 8 – 16
28	Day 9 – 17
29	Day 10 – 18
30	Day 11 – 19
31	Day 12 – 20
32	Day 13 – 21
33	Day 14 – 22
34	Day 15 – 23
35	Day 16 – 24

(If you have a variable cycle length, subtract 19 days off your shortest cycle and 11 days off your longest cycle to get the first and final days of your fertile window.)

How to determine your fertile window

WHEN SEX IS DIFFICULT

Sex is important if you're trying to get pregnant. While this may seem obvious, it's not always that simple. Some couples find sex difficult, uncomfortable or even painful. These problems usually pre-date trying to conceive, but can also lead to people seeing fertility specialists for assistance.

Physical factors

If you're having problems with sex, it is essential to see if there may be a physical problem. For example, some women are born with a septum, or barrier of skin, that may restrict the size of the vaginal opening or its internal capacity. A fairly common problem is when the hymen, which comprises thin skin within the opening of the vagina, either doesn't stretch properly when sexual activity begins or is thicker than usual. This can quite easily be corrected by a small, simple operation. After surgery it may be necessary to use vaginal dilators, which are designed to be used by the patient herself to gently stretch the vagina and ensure that the problem doesn't recur.

Sometimes there can be problems within the pelvis such as endometriosis, ovarian cysts or scarring from previous infection (see pages 243, 245 and 250), which can lead to pain during or after intercourse. These problems can be investigated and often treated by a combination of a pelvic ultrasound scan and then a laparoscopy (see page 177).

Psychological factors

Sometimes difficulties with sexual intercourse may result from psychological concerns, and this can be the case for either partner. First it is important to know that anything you discuss with your GP, fertility specialist or counsellor will always be strictly confidential. While we encourage couples to attend together, we appreciate that sometimes there may be issues from the past that you may not wish your partner to know and so you can always ask to be seen alone. This may include a past history of having been abused or difficult relationships. Overall we do encourage openness so that you can work together with your partner to achieve a resolution, but this can take time.

You may be referred to a psychosexual counsellor for advice and assistance. This is likely to involve several sessions over a period of time. The aim will always be to help you to achieve a normal sex life. This, however, isn't always possible and sometimes it is necessary to seek the help of a fertility clinic to help overcome the barriers by artificially assisting conception using techniques such as directly inserting sperm into the womb (intrauterine insemination, IUI – see page 204) or even *in vitro* fertilisation (IVF), both of which can even be done with sedation if required.

For women, psychological factors may lead to increased sensitivity in the vagina and a spasm of the muscles around the vagina. This is often termed 'vaginismus'.

Some men may have problems with impotence and find it difficult to either achieve or maintain an erection. This can sometimes be due to underlying medical conditions, such as diabetes, vascular or neurological problems, or can be due to psychological difficulties. Again seeking the help of a psychosexual counsellor is important and can help overcome the difficulties. Some men are able to masturbate and produce a sample of sperm, even if they cannot ejaculate during sexual intercourse, and this can then be used for IUI or IVF treatment.

Sometimes medication can help with erections, either taken orally (such as sildenafil or tadalafil) or occasionally applied into the urethra (penile opening) or injected into the penis (such as alprostadil). Some men with severe neurological problems or spinal cord injury may require the use of an external vibrator or even electroejaculation methods to help produce sperm for IUI or IVF – these procedures carry certain risks and must be performed in a specialist centre.

MEDICAL CONDITIONS AND FERTILITY

Many conditions, and sometimes the drugs used to treat them, may not only reduce fertility but also lead to increased risks during pregnancy. It is therefore essential to ensure that you receive the advice of your doctor before starting to try to conceive in order to optimise any long-term health problems.

It is important to check that you are not taking any medication that could either interfere with the chance of conceiving or increase the risks of developmental anomalies in the baby (teratogenicity). Sometimes medications need to be changed or modified or additional supplements advised – for example, the dose of folic acid that you should be taking needs to be increased in certain situations, such as epilepsy.

COVID-19 AND PREGNANCY

We have been writing this book during the evolution of the Covid-19 pandemic and at the time of publication the situation is still evolving. There are still many unknowns about the effects of the virus on fertility and pregnancy or the safety of the various vaccines that have been developed.

It appears that pregnant women may become very seriously unwell with Covid-19 and have an increased risk of preterm birth.[1] It is therefore it is important to try to get vaccinated before pregnancy, especially if you have polycystic ovary syndrome (PCOS), as emerging evidence suggests that women with the condition may be more at risk.[2] Taking steps to mitigate disease severity by ensuing that you are healthy is important. The large majority of women who get Covid-19 while pregnant, however, will experience only mild or moderate cold-/flu-like symptoms, though there is increased risk of hospitalisation in the third trimester. To date, there is no evidence to suggest that the virus causes any serious harm to the developing baby or an increased risk of miscarriage, although there have been cases of transmission from a mother to her baby during pregnancy or birth. In the majority of cases of newborn babies developing coronavirus very soon after birth, the babies have been well. Some babies have been born prematurely to women who were very unwell with Covid-19. A high fever can lead to miscarriage, premature labour and also potentially to developmental anomalies very early in pregnancy (even before a pregnancy test is positive). There is no evidence at the time of writing that Covid-19 has caused developmental anomalies.

The virus has been found in semen samples of men affected by Covid-19. There is some evidence to suggest that Covid-19 may persist in the testes, raising the possibility the virus may affect male fertility and could even be sexually transmitted, although to date this has not been found to be the case. There have been early individual case reports of men who were infected with Covid-19 and subsequently died who were found to have damage in the testes including to the seminiferous tubules where sperm is produced. It is possible, therefore, that the virus may cause damage without entering the cells. As it is a new virus, there is much that we do not know, including whether there will be lasting effects, but we do advise caution and taking all the necessary steps to avoid infection. However, there is no hard evidence to date that the infection itself is either sexually transmitted or has caused infertility. Any debilitating illness or fever, however, may have an effect on male fertility for at least three months, which is the time that it takes to make sperm.

Although we do not know if specific foods, vitamins and minerals will be protective given the very recent emergence of the virus, early research suggests the potential importance of sufficiency of certain nutrients for avoiding serious illness with Covid-19, including vitamin D, magnesium, zinc, selenium, iodine and vitamin K.[3] One recent study investigated international dietary patterns in relation to risk from the virus and found an association between lower Covid-19 mortality rates in countries where consumption of fermented foods was greatest.[4] Research from Harvard and King's College London also discovered that eating a high-quality diet rich in plant foods can protect against Covid-19, with those eating the highest quality diet found to be ten per cent less likely to develop Covid-19 than people eating the lowest quality diet and forty per cent less likely to become severely ill. Other studies have concluded that the gut microbiota may be an important factor in risk from Covid-19.[5] Although more research is needed to confirm some of these hypotheses and findings of early studies, eating a healthy diet and maintaining sufficiency of all nutrients is a sensible approach that supports good immune function, will benefit general health and fertility and will not cause harm.

Vaccines have now been developed using different methods. None contain the live virus and so they appear to be safe if given during pregnancy, although at the time of writing data is limited to vaccinations given in the second and third trimesters.[6] The current advice in the UK is that it is safe to be vaccinated if you are planning a pregnancy and while pregnant, but recommends women discuss the benefits and risks with their doctor. The recommended vaccines for pregnant women are the RNA vaccines. Fever is a potential side effect of all the vaccines. The very early developing embryo is undergoing dramatic changes even before a pregnancy test is positive, and a high fever may have an impact on organ development and even cause miscarriage. So perhaps the safest approach would be to receive the vaccine in the first ten days of your cycle, so that there is no chance of an early pregnancy. Or, if you find yourself pregnant before being vaccinated, wait to be vaccinated until after twelve weeks of pregnancy (usually two months after a positive pregnancy test).

These are our views and the situation is continually evolving. The most up-to-date information for the UK can be found on the websites of the Royal College of Obstetricians and Gynaecologists (RCOG) and the British Fertility Society (BFS).

Whether or not there are any underlying issues relating to sex or medical conditions, or concerns regarding Covid-19, getting pregnant often isn't straightforward for many. Because schools have historically taught unprotected sex inevitably leads to pregnancy, it can come as a bit of a shock if it doesn't happen straight away. Understanding your body and when you're most fertile can make all the difference, especially if your periods are irregular, so ensuring you are getting the basics right and knowing when to seek help can go a long way in helping you avoid unnecessary problems.

Chapter 6

Fertility, Weight and Metabolism

CREATING ANOTHER HUMAN being is an energetic process. From the swimming of sperm cells through the uterus and into the fallopian tubes, and an egg cell forming the foundation of a baby, to actually growing a new human during pregnancy, reproduction requires lots of energy. This means that in order to conceive and progress through a pregnancy, especially when there have been difficulties conceiving, our bodies must be able to convert the energy from food into a form of energy our cells can use efficiently – in other words, we need good metabolic health. Part of this is paying attention to our weight, though you can be slim and have a metabolic disorder and you can be overweight and malnourished in terms of micro-nutrients (vitamins and minerals), so the scales don't tell the whole story.

Our bodies need a range of nutrients to function and produce energy from food including B vitamins, sulphur, magnesium, zinc, selenium and co-enzyme Q10, so ensuring we are adequately nour-ished, as we discussed in Chapter 4, is vital. The dietary guidance covered in Chapter 3 is an important starting point for everyone when trying to conceive. Some people find they lose weight when they switch to a much healthier style of eating without having to actively 'diet'. For those who would still like to lose weight after making these changes, or indeed want to gain weight, there are other strategies you can try in order to help you do so in a healthy way. We cover these further steps in this chapter. Leaving behind some of the ideas you may have developed from society's obsession with weight is key to helping you achieve optimal health and prepare yourself for pregnancy.

FERTILITY AND METABOLISM

Your fertility depends on energy metabolism in many ways and good metabolic health supports egg and sperm quality, whatever your body weight. This includes a good supply of energy from food to the ovaries and oocytes. The cells that surround your eggs work together to process the carbohydrates, amino acids and fats that you eat to provide the energy needed by your eggs for maturation, fertilisation and embryonic development. Nurturing your body in all the ways we describe in this chapter supports all of these processes.

These processes can be affected if you are overweight or have recently gained weight, or if you have a poor diet, an eating disorder such as anorexia nervosa, or impaired blood sugar control such as diabetes. These things in turn can impact your reproductive health and fertility.

Another condition that has a big impact on metabolic health is polycystic ovary syndrome (PCOS) – a common hormonal disorder that can come with weight gain, irregular periods and a high number of developing follicles (incorrectly termed 'cysts') in the ovary (see Chapter 15). PCOS can impact fertility as disturbances to these metabolic processes affect egg quality, so diet is especially important if you have it. Regardless of whether you have PCOS, high-fat diets, and poor metabolism generally, affect the development potential of the oocyte, and being overweight for any woman can damage mitochondria in the oocyte. Damaged mitochondria can be passed on to the baby, which increases the chance of metabolic problems in the child. Being overweight as well as metabolic disorders in either parent can also have an impact on the baby through epigenetic mechanisms – that is, changes to whether genes are switched on or off according to environmental exposures like diet and lifestyle. So, as we observe time and again, the same mechanisms that can impact fertility can also affect the health of the child in many different ways.

FERTILITY AND WEIGHT

A healthy weight is important for fertility and being either under- or overweight can cause problems. Regardless of how we weigh in, the same principle applies to each one of us: the aim is to be healthy and develop sustainable, lifelong habits that will help nourish you and your baby, and maintain or achieve a stable weight that is normal for you. If you need to gain or lose weight, this approach is far preferable to potentially damaging diets and eternally fluctuating weight, especially for reproductive health.

If you need to gain or lose weight, and for metabolic health and fertility generally, it's helpful to think about the following:

- **Identify your 'why'**: Changing habits takes perseverance and motivation, so the likelihood of achieving any goal is improved when you have a clear purpose; a reason why you would like to achieve something. Wanting to have a baby and be a healthy parent provides a perfect sense of motivation.

- **Ensure you have optimal levels of micronutrients (vitamins and minerals)**: Being adequately nourished is vital in maintaining a healthy weight in the long term and avoiding yo-yo dieting, whether you want to gain or lose weight (see Chapter 3).

- **Optimise digestive health**: Seek professional advice if you have gastrointestinal symptoms such as bloating, loose bowel movements or discomfort after eating – a healthy digestion and a healthy microbiome support weight management (see Chapter 7).

- **Reduce stress**: Elevated cortisol levels can result in difficulty gaining as well as losing weight. We cover strategies to manage stress in Chapter 9.

- **Check your thyroid function**: An underactive thyroid can contribute to weight gain, so having a full thyroid screen and managing thyroid function appropriately is an important component of any weight-loss strategy, especially when trying to conceive. An underactive thyroid can also be associated with an intolerance of cold, constipation and increased hair coarseness. An overactive thyroid causes weight loss, and accompanying symptoms can include a racing heart, anxiety and insomnia, so it is worth getting tested if you struggle to maintain weight in the absence of vigorous exercise even with high energy intake.

- **Seek professional support:** If you sense you struggle to lose or put on weight for psychological reasons that you find hard to change, including binge eating or conversely over-exercising or undereating, then it's important to ask for help to improve things. It is much better to seek support before you conceive as pregnancy then becomes much easier, especially if you find the prospect of pregnancy weight gain daunting.

How being overweight can affect fertility

Being overweight can impact fertility in many ways, including affecting egg quality, the uterine fluid that creates the environment in the womb, and the lining of the uterus (endometrium) that is important for implantation, as well as *in vitro* fertilisation (IVF) success rates. Fat tissue also produces hormones, and being overweight can lead to increased oestrogen production, which can cause symptoms such as premenstrual syndrome (PMS), heavy periods and tender breasts. (We will learn more about hormone balance in Chapter 8.)

Being overweight causes inflammation in the body and increases the risk of problems during pregnancy including gestational diabetes, as well as hypertension and problems during childbirth, often because the baby is too big. Miscarriage rates also seem to rise with increasing maternal weight. Fetal development can also be affected, with increased rates of congenital anomalies in the babies of overweight mothers, particularly defects affecting the spine (spina bifida and other neural tube defects), gut and heart.

Being overweight has become stigmatised and even the word obesity can be difficult to come to terms with if attached to us personally, but it does have clinical significance and it is important to understand the risk factors. The more overweight we are, the bigger the risks in terms of fertility and pregnancy. However, the concept of health at any size is important as we can improve things by focusing on metabolic health and nourishing ourselves well for pregnancy rather than only thinking about weight.

Body mass index (BMI) is a measure of weight in proportion to your height and is calculated by dividing your weight by the square of your height, and is expressed in units of kg/m². A healthy weight usually means you will have a normal BMI (19–24.9kg/m²). A BMI of more than 25kg/m² is considered overweight and a BMI of more than 30kg/m² obese. If you have a lot of muscle (usually athletes or those weight-training), your BMI does not always reflect whether you are a healthy weight.

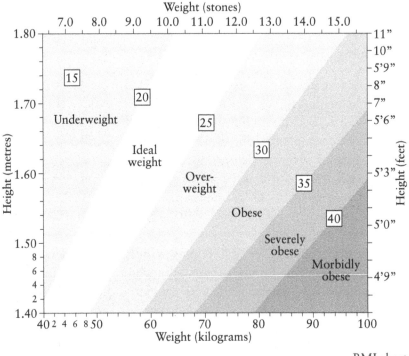

BMI chart

If you still need to lose weight after following the steps above and dietary guidance in Chapter 3, there are certain principles that you can apply:

- **Assess your relationship with food:** If your food patterns include emotional eating, binge eating or overeating, seek support from your GP, who will be able to refer you to local groups or individual counselling where appropriate.

- **Change one habit at a time:** If you have big changes to make, make things more achievable by, say, first increasing your vegetable intake and then working from there.

- **Focus on eating nutrient-dense, home-cooked foods:** Cook regular, healthy meals that you enjoy at home rather than low-calorie processed foods.

- **Eat enough protein:** Controlling hunger is important when it comes to weight loss, so aim for foods that boost satiation (the feeling of being full and satisfied after a meal). Studies show that diets rich in protein are very satiating.[1] Eating some protein of varied sources at each meal and aiming for approximately 0.8g of protein per kg of body weight per day for adults allows dietary balance. Choosing a good proportion of vegetable protein (such as soy, beans and pulses) can be helpful in managing negative effects of excessive meat consumption. Combining protein and fat together is also highly satiating, so a little cheese can be a good thing if dairy is right for you and you don't overdo it.

- **Watch your portion size:** Eat until you're satisfied but don't overeat. Ensure your portion size is sufficient to leave you feeling full rather than stuffed, and adjust your portion size and meal intervals so that you feel true hunger (as opposed to just your stomach feeling a little less full) by your next meal. Try skipping one meal to become reacquainted with that stomach-rumbling feeling of hunger that regular overeating can make us forget.

- **Watch your shopping trolley:** Don't buy junk foods that you know lead to overeating. It may be crisps, a particular brand of biscuits or chocolate; whatever it is for you, if you can't stop eating it if it's in front of you, simply don't buy it.

- **Chew your food properly and eat slowly:** Digestion starts in the mouth and inadequate chewing means we can't maximise the nutrient potential of food. Eating slowly also allows time for the body to sense that our stomach is filling.

- **Avoid excess alcohol consumption**: Alcohol has a high calorific value without contributing nutrients and will increase weight gain, so avoid overindulging to help weight control as well as fertility. Alcohol also increases the tendency to snack on unhealthy foods, indulge in fast food and unhealthy hangover remedies, and over time these have an effect. Beware of calorific fizzy drinks as mixers too.

- **Avoid high-glycaemic index foods**: High-glycaemic index (GI) foods rapidly convert into sugar and cause spikes and then troughs in blood sugar, which doesn't help hunger management. These include some breakfast cereals, white bread and pasta, fruit juice and many snacks. Aim for low-GI foods most of the time: foods that are low in sugar and high in fibre. These include whole grains and non-starchy vegetables, such as broccoli, courgette, onions, mushrooms and peppers. Fruit juice that has the fibre removed has a higher GI than whole fruit, and overconsumption should be avoided.

HAVE SOME POTATO-FREE DAYS

Potatoes are not bad depending on how you cook them and if you don't eat too many. Boiled new potatoes with the skin on or jacket potatoes (choose small ones) contain nutrients including vitamin C and fibre and are satiating, so potato consumption is actually associated with better weight management. Mashed potatoes have a high GI and therefore should be an occasional rather than regular inclusion. Fried potatoes have a lower GI, but are higher in fat. Having some potato-free days leaves room for the range of other vegetables and complex carbohydrate such as organic brown rice that are beneficial to include. You can create a good, tasty substitute for deep-fried chips by lightly parboiling skin-on potatoes cut into chunky chips, then baking them with a little olive oil in the oven for up to an hour. If you're following a low-GI diet for health reasons, such as diabetes, or a low-carbohydrate diet for weight loss, you will need to avoid potatoes.

- **Avoid fizzy drinks:** This is helpful for weight loss as well as fertility as the sugared versions are high in calories and contain refined sugar that causes sharp peaks followed by crashes in blood glucose, without contributing any nutrients. Studies have shown that fizzy drinks contribute to a greater proportion of weight gain than can be attributed to the same calories coming from normal food.[2] Some may assert that low intake is acceptable as long as you remain in calorific deficit (an approach that can be problematic in reality anyway and usually fails in the long term – see page 37), but in our personal view these drinks have no redeeming features and should be avoided where possible. Sparkling mineral water is fine.

YOUR BODY SHAPE

Getting to know your body shape is really helpful in understanding your metabolic health and the degree to which it might affect fertility. Where you carry weight is significant even if you are not actually overweight:

- Abdominal fat (around the tummy) is linked to poor metabolism, whereas fat around the hips, thighs and bottom is less problematic.
- Fat in the lower back area is more associated with insulin sensitivity.
- Fat at the bottom of the neck and a double chin means you are more likely to have metabolic dysfunction.
- Waist circumference should ideally be less than 79cm in women, while a measurement that is greater than 87cm carries a significant risk of health problems such as diabetes.

Though genetically determined, fat distribution does tell us about risks in terms of weight and helps us understand where to focus our attention in terms of diet and lifestyle, and the importance of improving factors associated with metabolic risks where we can. Exercise has a significant effect on reducing visceral fat and reducing cardiovascular risk, for instance.

Do you need to lose weight?

Focusing purely on weight, even when you want to lose weight as your primary goal, is short-sighted if the approach isn't sustainable. Long-term health is key, and losing weight in an unhealthy way simply trades one problem for another. This is why many people fail to stabilise weight loss and get caught up in an endless cycle of weight loss followed by weight gain. Furthermore, the health benefits of eating a wholefood nutritious diet apply regardless of BMI, and studies show improvement to cardiovascular risk for participants on a Mediterranean diet even when they do not lose weight.[3]

In practical terms, an important thing to consider is your relationship with food. What we eat can become so entangled with emotions, including judgement, shame, poor self-esteem and the need for control, that starting any kind of eating programme before addressing these things if they apply is setting ourselves up to fail. If you have a regular comfort food, then that is an indication you are using food to soothe emotions and, if you do this too often, this is what you must address in order to lose weight. Some people are more predisposed to comfort eating, and recognising this from the outset will help you find a solution that works for you. This may mean distracting your attention away from food and choosing substitutes for snacks when you are looking for comfort: it could be a relaxing bath, a chat with a friend, a hug or a hobby that absorbs your attention. It may also be that there are deeper issues that need your attention, including self-esteem, shame that you may have picked up in childhood or unresolved trauma that needs some work. We will cover this in more detail in Chapter 9.

Abandoning the focus on weight loss for a time can be a huge relief. Learning to enjoy food again in a guilt-free way as a starting point for weight loss may seem counter-intuitive, but it is something that people often lose in the challenge to manage weight.

How being underweight can affect fertility

Being underweight can have a negative impact on fertility in various ways including stopping ovulation. Having low levels of nutrients from undereating can also affect egg quality and the ability to provide for embryonic and fetal development. Allowing time to build up sufficient body stores of key nutrients following a deficiency will help minimise the impact on the developing baby and reduce the risk of maternal depletion that can arise after pregnancy.

Some people eat well and are naturally slim without a low BMI having an effect on fertility. If you have regular periods, this usually means your fertility is not affected by your weight, but you still need to be eating sufficient quantities of food during regular meals and not over-exercising. Sometimes, gaining a little weight if you have a low BMI (18–$19kg/m^2$) can still be helpful even if these things apply to you but you are not conceiving.

If you need to gain weight and you have followed the steps on page 70 including getting your thyroid checked, important principles include:

- **Eat more nutrient-dense foods:** Try eating more nutrient-dense foods that will help you to put on weight in a healthy way, including fat and protein.

- **Get tested for coeliac disease:** Coeliac disease can manifest as low BMI. A simple blood test is the first step, so it is always worth excluding this as a cause, even where you don't have classic digestive symptoms such as diarrhoea or a noticeable reaction to eating wheat (see page 40).

- **Increase your portion size:** Try to increase your portion size a little at each meal and build this up slowly over time.

- **Don't skip meals:** Regularly skipping meals for any reason will reduce your overall calorific intake and make it harder to gain weight. Ensure you eat three regular meals of adequate portion size daily.

- **Don't over-exercise:** If you are exercising daily for extended periods or undertaking very vigorous exercise, you can reduce this down to help gain weight.

- **Reduce fidgeting:** Be conscious of burning nervous energy through hyper-activity and fidgeting: these constant movements contribute to elevated metabolism. Address the underlying stress and aim for a more relaxed state.

SUPPLEMENTS

Seek professional advice to adjust supplement dosage according to your weight (folate should be increased to 5mg for those with higher BMIs, for instance). (See Chapter 4 for more on supplements.)

Striking a balance

When it comes to weight and fertility, balance is key. If you eat low-calorie foods that do not meet your nutrient requirements, you may damage your health and compromise your ability to meet the nutritional needs of your baby during pregnancy. One study showed that micronutrient levels were inadequate in a number of weight-loss diets and researchers concluded that these diets could result in 'clinically relevant nutritional deficiencies'.[4] This is very much what we observe in our patients who have been attempting to lose weight over many years – they often have multiple deficiencies that compromise their health and ability to conceive. Interestingly, the weight-loss diet that was shown to provide the best micronutrient intake was through reduction of refined carbohydrate, as this type of food provides a relatively poor contribution to overall nutrients. This may be one reason why diets lower in carbohydrates have been associated with improved fertility outcomes in some studies.[5]

Despite these findings, the popular mantra in terms of weight management is focused mostly on calorie reduction and the principle of 'energy in equals energy out'. If we eat more than we need, excess 'energy' is stored as fat. However, there are various problems with this focus on calories. Firstly, the calorific content of food is often difficult to accurately assess, and estimates as to calorie count for differing foods may not be correct. The calorific content of food changes depending on various things that impact the availability of its energy content. As a general rule, the more processed a food, the more accessible the calories will be to the body. Secondly, focusing only on calories can mean unhealthy, processed low-calorie food is prioritised over healthy, nutrient-rich food. Finally, it can cause hypervigilance, which can lead to disordered eating and eating disorders.

Our metabolic rates vary too, and some burn calories more easily than others. So dieting is sadly not equal for everyone, and understanding this in an era of Instagram influencers telling you that your genes are not stopping you losing weight can be helpful! There is also some evidence to suggest that the total amount of fat in our bodies remains stable over time (due to genetic and other factors) and any weight lost returns when you start eating normally again – the so-called 'set point' for our bodies.[6]

Some people have genes that are associated with higher BMIs and may cause an increased tendency to binge eat. You are more likely to have one of these if you have PCOS, for instance. There are other genes that mean we are less likely to burn calories for keeping us warm, which leads to an increase in calories laid down as fat. Finally, there are other variables that impact our tendency to gain weight, including things like thyroid function, which we will discuss in Chapter 7, which again may respond to improved diet and nutrient status.

THE 80/20 PRINCIPLE

Aim for a healthy '80/20' balance where you eat healthy foods most of the time (around 80 per cent) and foods you consider unhealthy occasionally (around 20 per cent of the time). Balance, eating food you enjoy and a healthy relationship with food are the keys to long-term weight management.

METABOLIC HORMONES

Metabolic hormones are the ones that control hunger, satiety and the conversion of food into energy in your body. They are also important when it comes to fertility and managing weight.

Insulin

Insulin is the hormone that allows you to use sugar from food for energy or to store as fat. It is the main hormone released from the pancreas (a large gland in your abdomen) after eating and it helps blood sugar (glucose) enter cells around your body. Overweight people develop resistance to insulin so that it works less efficiently and the pancreas produces higher amounts in order to overcome this 'insulin resistance'. Levels of insulin and glucose increase in the blood with higher body weights and, when glucose levels reach a critical point, diabetes occurs. There are two main types of diabetes:

- Type 2 or late-onset diabetes is where glucose levels rise in the presence of high levels of ineffective insulin.

- Type 1 diabetes occurs when the pancreas has stopped producing insulin and is more common in younger people.

The risk of impaired glucose tolerance is also higher if you have PCOS (see Chapter 15). Although women with PCOS may develop insulin resistance irrespective of BMI, both having PCOS and being overweight result in a worsened combined effect on your body's ability to control blood sugar and can exacerbate the hormonal and fertility problems that are associated with the syndrome. Metabolic disorders are significant for everyone, however, and there is an increased rate of insulin resistance seen in women with recurrent miscarriage.

If these issues apply to you, the dietary guidelines above are particularly important. Your GP can also test how well you control glucose by measuring glycosylated haemoglobin (HbA1c) or sometimes oral glucose tolerance, and you can be retested to check for improvements after making changes to your diet and lifestyle if they are outside the normal range.

Ghrelin

Ghrelin is the hormone that signals hunger and is produced mainly by the stomach in order to encourage us to eat. Ghrelin is also secreted at our usual mealtimes, and studies show that the ghrelin response can be 'trained' so that our bodies anticipate a meal at certain times.[7] This may be helpful in developing a routine and managing hunger during weight loss. Skipping a meal can help put you in touch with the feeling ghrelin gives you and is key to maintaining a healthy weight. Though it isn't tested, getting acquainted with hunger pangs that come from increased ghrelin can be helpful to keep overeating in check and ensure we only eat in response to true hunger.

Leptin

Leptin has traditionally been known as the hormone that signals to your brain that you are full, but recent studies show that what it actually does is signal how much fat you have.[8] The more fat you have, the more leptin you will produce, which allows your body to detect whether you are starving or not by sensing lowered fat levels. The end result is that you want to eat as levels of leptin decrease. The same mechanism is at play if you're starving or if you lose weight – lower leptin tells your body to send nutrients to areas of the body essential for survival, like brain function, and away from the high demands of reproduction. This is why low body weight can be bad for fertility – in the extreme, ovulation and the menstrual cycle tend to stop.

Interestingly, for women of reproductive age leptin levels vary across the menstrual cycle, but for men they remain stable over a 28-day period. A recent study suggested a possible relationship between serum leptin levels and enhanced fertility, with another study finding that higher leptin levels in women with higher BMIs were associated with unexplained infertility.[9] Leptin can even affect your egg quality as it regulates processes needed for the oocyte to develop and mature into a form that is capable of forming a healthy embryo after fertilisation. Working with your body to try to normalise your response to hunger and fat detection hormones can help with weight management.

SLEEP, ROUTINE AND EATING HABITS

If you want to maintain a healthy weight, sleep and routine are key. Having enough sleep is important as short sleep duration is associated with increased risk of type 2 diabetes. Studies indicate seven to eight hours is best, and fewer than six may be harmful for overall health and fertility.[10] Research also shows various adverse effects on metabolism following disturbed sleep.[11] If you sleep badly, your metabolic response to a meal is impaired the next day. This can be made worse by poor food choices to compensate for the energy slump, in the same way you might eat unhealthy 'hangover food' following a night of heavy drinking. As a general rule, eating more calories earlier in the day helps your body use energy better and your body clock work better. Similarly, try not to eat your main meal too late – aim to eat by 7pm. Eating meals late into the evening tends to lead to a tendency to higher body weights and may also disrupt sleep, as reduced energy intake is one of the environmental cues that makes us sleepy. For many, therefore, the old maxim 'breakfast like a king, lunch like a prince and dine like a pauper' may be helpful.

EAT BREAKFAST IF IT IS RIGHT FOR YOU

Old advice that breakfast is the most important meal of the day for everyone has been somewhat debunked. Breakfast eaters tend to lose weight and maintain a healthy weight better than non-breakfast eaters, but studies on breakfast-eating indicate this is due to the increased involuntary movements resulting from higher energy derived from eating breakfast, rather than the breakfast itself.[12] These small increased movements burn energy and improve the metabolic response to the next meal. Further research has shown that some people are in fact genetically pre-disposed to skip breakfast.[13] For those who have this genotype, it may be more beneficial to skip breakfast if you are a healthy weight. Skipping breakfast can also extend your overnight fasting hours, which has physiological benefits. The message is to listen to your body, then build a regular routine based on what is right for you as an individual.

Our daily routine including mealtimes and timing of exercise can impact how our body works via what is known as the circadian clock, and vice versa. The circadian or body clock is controlled in the brain via a set of genes and hormones that respond to environmental cues such as light, energy intake and temperature. Melatonin is the hormone that sends you to sleep as daylight fades and temperatures cool, whereas cortisol is the hormone that wakes you up in response to increasing light and warmth. Our behaviours can either disrupt or support the workings of these hormones. Poor-quality sleep can lead to bad eating habits, which can affect general health and fertility. Shift work, irregular sleep patterns, irregular mealtimes and disrupted sleep will all impact on your circadian clock. There is growing evidence to show the circadian clock is involved in regulation of nearly every part of the female reproductive pathway including areas of the brain involved in hormone balance, the menstrual cycle and pregnancy.[14] Disordered circadian rhythms may contribute to altered menstrual cycles, worsened period pain and, some scientists believe, changes to the follicular phase of the menstrual cycle (see page 13), changes in hormone levels and increased miscarriage rates.[15] Male fertility is also affected, with shift work being a known risk factor for male factor infertility and poor sleep known to affect testosterone levels.

ESTABLISH A GOOD SLEEP ROUTINE

- Aim for eight hours' sleep – though some have genes that make them need less.
- Have a set bedtime and waking time.
- Try to get natural daylight exposure early in the day.
- Reduce activity and mental stimulation in the two hours before bed.
- In the evening avoid screen time which delivers high-frequency light at the blue end of the spectrum that stimulates the waking part of the brain.
- A warm bath can relax you, but beware of overheating in excessively hot baths, as this can work against melatonin (the 'sleep hormone') production.
- A cool, dark room is important to maximise melatonin production and allows you to fall asleep easily and stay asleep. Blackout blinds to minimise light pollution and a room at 17°C optimise the ambient conditions for deep sleep.
- You may also want to try a daylight lamp that slowly increases light emission as an alarm to further support your circadian clock.
- Avoid caffeine after midday.
- Minimising partner disturbances such as snoring are other strategies if you know that sleep and routine are problematic for you.

EXERCISE

Exercise has so many benefits for the body and mind, from relaxation and stress reduction, to improvements in metabolic markers and general health, so exercise should always form part of our daily routine.

Being physically active is also important for fertility and pregnancy, but people tend to overestimate what is good for them for fertility and underestimate what is best for pregnancy. However, remaining physically active during pregnancy improves outcomes, maternal health and the health of the baby. Staying physically active is also associated with better mental health, and this is vital for pregnancy and after the birth to protect against the possibility of postnatal depression. Exercise has been shown to improve underlying features and symptoms of PCOS. So we advise starting a programme of exercise while trying to conceive that you can safely sustain during pregnancy. Studies indicate that mild to moderate exercise that includes a mixture of low- or medium-intensity cardio with weight-bearing exercise is best for women trying to conceive.[16]

Spending too long sitting down is also associated with adverse health outcomes and poor metabolic function, including type 2 diabetes, being overweight, coronary heart disease, some cancers and even premature death. Studies looking at workplace exposures and male fertility also show an association between jobs that involve long periods sitting down and reduced male fertility.[17]

Short bouts of exercise do not compensate for a sedentary lifestyle, so don't let sessions at the gym become the only active part of your day. Aim to get up from your desk at least every 15 minutes (drinking enough water can help with this!), take the stairs, walk to work where possible (taking a route that minimises exposure to air pollution) and move your body as you wait for the kettle to boil. Walking is an excellent antidote to excess sitting, so even short, regular walks will make a difference. If you have a very inactive day, these small habits can help to mitigate the negative effects of all that sitting, and will have a positive impact on metabolism and, as a consequence, fertility.

A level of exercise that is good for you is personal. If you are used to being fit and active you can usually do more and maintain good fertility. Over-exercising during a preconception phase, even when very overweight, however, may be unhelpful if you overeat to compensate. As with everything, balance is key, especially when trying to improve your fertility.

Exercise for weight loss and metabolic health

Exercise is extremely important for general and metabolic health, but actually contributes much less to weight loss than changes to diet. This is because our bodies and behaviour tend to adapt in order to compensate for the additional exercise, so there is a tendency to eat more when undertaking more vigorous exercise. However, exercise has been shown to contribute more to weight maintenance after weight loss than diet, so aiming for an individualised, balanced, long-term weight-loss strategy that includes exercise is important.

Interval training

In terms of aerobic exercise, interval training is more effective than fixed-pace. 'Scout's pace' while walking or jogging is a good example. This can be simply 30 minutes of brisk walking, and breaking into a run that raises the heart rate one minute out of every ten, so your total running time is three minutes during a thirty-minute walk. Interval training can also be varying the gradient and intensity on a treadmill or cross trainer in the gym across the duration of your session.

Weight-bearing exercise

Weight-bearing exercises help build muscle tone, improve metabolic health and aid weight loss. Yoga, resistance training (including squats, lunges and stairs at home) and weight-training are all good forms of weight-bearing exercise. Muscle cells have a higher metabolic rate than fat cells (they are working harder and so use more energy) and so weight-bearing exercise is helpful for losing fat and improving metabolic health. Keeping physically active through aerobic exercise is also important, so always include some cardio.

EXERCISE IN THE MORNING

Some studies show that exercising in the morning results in greater weight loss than exercising after 3pm, so aim to do at least some exercise at the start of the day.[18] One study showed that those who exercised in the morning were generally more active throughout the day than afternoon or evening exercisers, taking more steps in total, and also ate slightly less, and consequently lost more weight.[19]

WEIGHT-LOSS STRATEGIES

Firstly, it's important to stress that you should only try to lose weight before trying to conceive and not while pregnant. Our experience is that most people lose weight in a sustainable way that is good for fertility by following the tips that we have outlined above and in Chapter 3. So start with a healthy eating programme, consider the other principles we've discussed and then follow an exercise programme that is tailored to you.

If you still need to lose weight, other options to consider include:

- **Fasting diets** can be beneficial for weight loss and potentially other metabolic indicators such as cholesterol and inflammatory markers. You should not attempt a fasting diet if you have an underlying health condition, including eating disorders, if you lack energy, have recently been on a different kind of diet or you are experiencing chronic stress. You can consider the 5:2 diet where calorific intake is significantly reduced on 2 days per week (to 500 calories for women, 600 calories for men); time-restricted feeding where you restrict eating each day to an 8-hour window (e.g. 7am–3pm or 12pm–8pm); or fortnightly intermittent fasting where there are two weeks of reduced calorific intake followed by two weeks of normal (not excessive) eating. One potential benefit of this model is that you may avoid the metabolic adaptation that comes with dieting. In other words, your metabolism slows once you start to lose weight in order to preserve body fat as a survival mechanism, and having shorter periods of intermittent rather than constant fasting may prevent this kicking in. The jury is still out on this with proponents of each method producing evidence to support their preferred approach. The definite benefit of fasting diets is that you are not constantly counting calories, and it may reduce the risk of disordered eating.

- **Counting calories** day to day is another way to try to lose weight, but it often fails and can result in unhealthy food choices, lead to poor nutrient intake and impact on enjoyment of daily life. However, it can work for some.

- **Preconception bariatric surgery** to reduce the size of the stomach that results in significant weight loss is the most extreme solution. Note this may increase the risk of adverse effects for the baby if you conceive too quickly afterwards, and there is a lack of research in this area. We recommend that you have this surgery as early as possible if you are planning a pregnancy and ideally allow a year for your body to adjust under the supervision of a specialist dietician.

You need to find an approach that works for you, but it is best to seek professional advice when it comes to any kind of weight-loss strategy. It is also important to stabilise weight preferably three months before you conceive (see Chapter 2).

THE MENSTRUAL CYCLE AND WEIGHT

The fluctuation of hormones across the menstrual cycle results in measurable changes in metabolism, physical response to exercise and eating patterns. Oestrogen tends to improve physical performance and exercise recovery, so phases of the cycle when this hormone is at its highest are the best times to maximise exercise levels, though more research is needed and a personalised approach is best.[20] Data is mixed on progesterone but some studies show that high progesterone levels around the time of ovulation cause metabolic changes that indicate this time may be the best for weight-bearing exercise to build lean muscle.[21]

In terms of eating, other studies show that binge eating is more likely both during your period and in the week following ovulation, as progesterone can induce food cravings, possibly in combination with falling oestrogen.[22] Although energy expenditure increases slightly during the luteal phase, so does appetite, so it's important to avoid overeating in response to hunger during the second half of the cycle. You can keep a diary to monitor how your appetite, energy levels and exercise change across your cycle to help personalise your approach.

A plan for your cycle

- Menstruation: rest more and forgive yourself lapses in eating without letting go of any control altogether.

- Follicular phase (early cycle after your period but before ovulation): focus on exercise and healthy eating during this time. This is the time to push your fitness a little harder if you are trying to be more active and focus on weight-bearing exercise.

- Ovulation: continue with healthy eating and exercise.

- Luteal phase: be aware of overeating in the second half of your cycle (but allow yourself a little extra) and maintain light exercise.

It's easy to feel disheartened if you're experiencing fertility challenges or finding it hard to lose weight, but we hold incredible power if we know what to do. Understanding how we can change what we do to our bodies for our general well-being as well as our fertility means we have power that previous generations have not had; power that we can use to protect the lifelong health of our children.

Chapter 7

Other Factors that Affect Fertility

I F YOU'VE BEEN working on your diet and lifestyle but haven't yet conceived, there are other aspects of your health that can be looked into. Fertility investigations are usually very focused on reproductive health, but there are many bodily processes and systems that need to work well to achieve a pregnancy. When things start to go wrong with some of these processes, problems can build up such that you aren't able to sustain a pregnancy.

Therefore, if you do not have a medical condition and you haven't conceived, there are likely to be underlying issues that may contribute to difficulty conceiving aside from a known diagnosis. Fertility issues in men and women are often a red flag for other health concerns and can be an early warning sign of potential problems later in life that share common areas of biological dysfunction. Addressing underlying health issues when trying to conceive may therefore offer significant protection against future illnesses for both parents as well as your child and during pregnancy.

We have already described how diet, nutrients, exercise, weight and metabolism can impact reproductive health, and we will look at hormone balance in the next chapter. This chapter focuses on other things that can impact fertility and pregnancy such as gut health, inflammation and oral health; factors that are often overlooked in typical medical investigations.

The clues from your body

Many people tolerate ongoing symptoms including headaches, digestive complaints, fatigue or low mood, and accept them as normal aspects of modern living. It's also common for patients to experience these concerns with general health and well-being being dismissed by doctors, and find conventional medicine often has little to offer. When you start to understand the underlying causes, however, these symptoms provide important clues as to what we need to work on to improve fertility.

The aim with fertility treatments should be to understand *why* you are not conceiving, not simply to artificially engineer a pregnancy through *in vitro* fertilisation (IVF).

GUT HEALTH

We looked at how a balanced diet can help with good gut health in Chapter 3, which includes the gut microbiome (the 'good' bacteria essential for health). The microbiome is the population of micro-organisms that live in your body (including bacteria, viruses and fungi) that support the digestive system and other bodily functions. Different parts of the body have their own microbiome including the gut, lungs, skin, vagina, nose and mouth. Diet, lifestyle and environmental exposures have the potential to impact the microbiome in all parts of the body, but especially the gut. The gut microbiome affects all aspects of health – immune function, mental health, hormones, weight and metabolism, and fertility – so this is a crucial aspect of health over which we have some control. A healthy gut microbiome is also important for pregnancy, childbirth and the future health of a child.

The gut microbiome can impact fertility because it affects so many bodily processes that can impact reproductive health. In fact, growing research suggests many diseases start in the gut, and evidence is building that the microbiome is one of the most significant modifiable factors that can affect human health.[1] The preconception health of the maternal gut microbiome is particularly important because it 'seeds' the microbiome of the baby during childbirth. This lays the foundations for lifelong health and immune function,

Maternal factors that influence baby's microbiome

Maternal gut microbiome
Maternal vaginal microbiome
Delivery: vaginal / caesarean
Feeding: breast / bottle

Mother's microbiome lays foundation for baby's microbiome

Microbiome develops, influencing baby's immune system

Preconception microbiome

Microbiome continues to evolve

The adult microbiome is influenced by age, genetics, diet, medication and geography

Modifiable factors affecting gut microbiome

Positive influences

Strong evidence for:
• Diverse Mediterranean diet
• High fibre intake
• High vegetable intake
• Polyphenols
• Fermented foods

Some evidence for:
• Gardening
• Pets
• Coffee

Negative influences

Strong evidence for:
• Antibiotics
• Processed foods
• High animal fat intake
• High alcohol intake

Some evidence for:
• Soft drinks
• Sugar
• Artificial sweeteners
• Poor sleep

The development of the gut microbiome

as the immune system develops in the infant gut based on this early colonisation of bacteria from the mother. How a baby is fed and early environmental exposures add to this founding population of bacteria to build a child's microbiome, health and immune function as they grow. Diet and lifestyle factors then continue to shape the gut microbiome throughout life.

THE MICROBIOME AND WEIGHT

The gut microbiome (the 'good' bacteria in your body that are essential for health) can impact fertility in many ways. This includes an impact on weight and metabolism. Certain species of bacteria are associated with lean bodies and others with overweight ones. There is ongoing research looking at the microbiome to help with weight management with some probiotic supplements showing promise, but it is an incredibly complex area.[2] In the meantime, it's important to know that what you eat affects the bacteria in the gut (the dietary principles in Chapter 3, including eating probiotic foods, all help). Significant recent research has shown that it is the proportion of carbohydrate, fat and protein that is particularly important in terms of your individual microbiome's response to food.[3] This means that finding a balance of macronutrients that is suited to you is probably more important than following trends for eliminating particular foods. The best advice we can give while this research is underway is to pay attention to your body: people often report that they gain weight if they overdo the carbohydrates, or feel worse after sugar, or have more energy with more protein or feel better on less fat, for instance.

Research also suggests that the bacteria in your gut can affect food choices via the gut–brain axis (the vagus nerve links the gut and brain).[4] While we do not have clear evidence of how we can harness this type of response to our benefit, it is plausible that the more you move towards healthier food choices, the better the make-up of your microbiome will be, and the less you will crave sugary, fatty foods.

How do you know if you have a problem that might impact your fertility?

In order to work out if you have a problem with your gut health, it's useful to understand what is normal. Generally, a healthy gut will produce normal bowel movements one to three times per day most days of the week. This means stools that are neither too loose nor too hard. Signs of an unhappy gut include bloating, excessive gas, cramping, constipation, diarrhoea, sensitivities to particular foods or bowel movements fewer than three times per week and more than three times per day. Very foul-smelling stools can be a sign of nutrient malabsorption. If you regularly go more than two days without a bowel movement, have difficulty passing stools, or if you can't hold on once you get the urge to go, these can all indicate problems. Mucus in faeces can indicate problems including infection or Crohn's disease and blood in faeces can be a sign of inflammatory bowel disease (IBD) or bowel cancer. Very pale or very dark faeces can also signal problems.

A history of antibiotic use for any previous infection, food poisoning, excess alcohol and junk food diets can all have negative effects on the microbiota, so pay attention to your history as well as your current symptoms.

Conditions such as irritable bowel syndrome (IBS), coeliac disease, Crohn's disease and ulcerative colitis can impact digestion, and these conditions all require medical testing and intervention. If you are diagnosed with IBS, there are certain types of foods that are known to worsen symptoms, and your doctor or dietician may recommend eliminating FODMAPs (fermentable oligosaccharides, disaccharides, monosaccharides and polyols). FODMAPs are poorly absorbed carbohydrates that can trigger symptoms in some and include fructans contained in wheat, rye, onions, garlic and beans, lactose in dairy, fructose in fruit (which when eaten in excess can cause problems) and polyols in certain fruit and vegetables and some artificial sweeteners.

Coeliac disease

One condition that is known to reduce the chances of conceiving and increase the chance of miscarriage is coeliac disease, which causes significant problems when left undiagnosed. Coeliac disease is an autoimmune disease (not a food allergy) triggered by eating the gluten contained in wheat, barley and rye (see page 40) and it is very commonly misdiagnosed as IBS. Around 50 per cent of people who go on to be diagnosed with coeliac disease do not experience digestive symptoms or a noticeable reaction to wheat.

Coeliac disease is more common among people experiencing fertility problems and, if you have not been able to conceive and especially if you have suffered miscarriage, you should ask to be tested. The first stage of testing is a simple blood test and you need to be eating wheat every day for a period of six weeks to ensure you do not get a false negative. Other symptoms of coeliac disease include fatigue, nutrient malabsorption including anaemia, hair loss, anxiety, poor mental focus, late puberty and tooth enamel defects including discolouration.

A combination of inflammation, a triggered immune system and nutrient deficiencies are thought to cause the fertility-related complications that come with coeliac disease. If you have coeliac disease and follow a strictly gluten-free diet, however, your risk falls to almost the same level as those who do not have the disease. Having a diagnosis is extremely important as treatment requires strict and lifelong dietary changes, including the need to avoid cross-contamination of foods, and it is of an entirely different order to a gluten-free lifestyle choice that some choose to make.

Food sensitivities and other triggers

If you have ruled out a medical condition but still have symptoms without a known cause, including abdominal discomfort, bloating, constipation and diarrhoea, there are other aspects to consider. Each symptom such as bloating could have multiple potential causes, so it is important to go through a process under professional supervision to work out what the problem may be. As well as specific conditions, some people find that stress, exercise or specific foods trigger digestive symptoms. In addition to consulting your GP, it's helpful to identify for yourself any particular patterns of symptoms. There is a specific process to follow that involves recording *all* food and drink you consume (including sauces, supplements and snacks) as well as exercise, stress, sleep and general circumstances, along with symptoms over a period of several weeks. If you notice patterns to your symptoms or reactions to specific foods, you can restrict individual foods you identify one by one for a time to see if you notice improvements, and then reintroduce the food to confirm it does indeed cause you a problem.

THE VAGINAL MICROBIOME

The vaginal microbiome has become a significant focus of fertility research, especially in an IVF setting where the process of conception is highly controlled. Certain species of bacteria have been shown to be associated with better outcomes, notably *Lactobacillus* species. In the vagina, low diversity has shown to be beneficial, in contrast to the gut, and higher diversity is associated with worse outcomes in fertility treatment. A high percentage of *Lactobacillus* species in the vagina along with the presence of one particular species – *Lactobacillus crispatus* – are associated with increased rates of pregnancy following embryo transfer in IVF treatment.

Specific microbes are also associated with conditions such as bacterial vaginosis (BV) and thrush, and can signal underlying vaginal microbiome problems. BV is a common cause of adverse outcomes including spontaneous preterm birth and endometritis (inflammation of the lining of the womb).

However, we advise caution when it comes to vaginal microbiome testing unless you are under the care of a teaching hospital or an academic research programme. Unless you test daily for a prolonged period, it is very difficult to gain an insight into your unique microbial make-up and there is no clinically validated intervention to address an impaired vaginal microbiome, though this is the focus of intense research.

There are studies to indicate benefit of probiotic supplements, for instance, many of which are available commercially.[5] The most commonly researched probiotics for modulating the vaginal microbiome in fertility studies are *Lactobacillus fermentum*, *Lactobacillus salivarius*, *Lactobacillus casei*, *Lactobacillus reuteri* RC-14, *Lactobacillus gasseri*, *Lactobacillus rhamnosus*, *Lactobacillus acidophilus* and *Lactobacillus crispatus*. Evidence from these studies has demonstrated changes to the vaginal microbiome and improvements in IVF outcomes but, again, there isn't sufficient evidence from large-scale trials to make universal recommendations at this stage and we don't fully understand the long-term implications of these interventions.

If you have repeated infections such as thrush or BV, or any symptoms that may indicate you have an infection, such as strong-smelling discharge, itchiness or discomfort during sex, see your GP for advice or speak to your fertility specialist. You may benefit from an oral probiotic supplement.

There is some evidence to suggest that high intake of certain vitamins (A, C, D, E, folate and beta-carotene) and minerals (calcium, iron and zinc) support the growth of healthy *Lactobacillus* species in the vagina, while diets high in fat encourage the growth of unhealthy microbial species.[6] Other factors including stress, vaginal douching, use of tampons, antibiotic intake, a high number of different sexual partners and anal sex preceding vaginal sex can all negatively impact the vaginal microbiota.

ORAL HEALTH

In terms of fertility, gum disease is associated with both a delay to natural conception and reduced IVF success. There are various mechanisms at play. One is through inflammation in the mouth causing inflammation throughout the body that ultimately impacts reproductive pathways. Another possible mechanism is through an imbalance in the oral microbiome resulting in dysbiosis in the gut.

Women can also be more susceptible to the effects of dental plaque at certain times due to fluctuating sex hormones, which are known to influence oral bacteria. This results in an exaggerated inflammatory response during pregnancy and in women taking oral contraceptives, so these are important times for women to take care of oral health.

Mineral deficiency is also a significant cause of tooth decay, and fat-soluble vitamins A, D and K are also important to build and maintain healthy teeth and for the development of the fetal teeth, face and jaw bones. Mineral malabsorption can lead to problems with the teeth (as with coeliac disease), so problems in the mouth often signal other health issues.

Having a healthy diet to promote healthy teeth, being up to date with dental health checks and aiming to resolve any issues, including bleeding gums, prior to conceiving is a vital component of preconception care that many overlook.

THE IMMUNE SYSTEM

Good immune function is needed to achieve a successful pregnancy and is especially important for normal implantation and placentation (development of the placenta). Research shows that a deficiency of particular immune cells known as T regulatory cells is associated with unexplained infertility and recurrent miscarriage, for instance.[7] Balanced immunity is also important for an embryo to implant – you can learn more about this on our website (see Resources, page 371).

Immune response is affected by numerous factors including nutrition, obesity, stress, infection, smoking, alcohol and environmental toxins, so optimising all of these factors at the very least eliminates the potential for negative consequences of lifestyle habits on implantation. Medical conditions that can trigger an overreactive immune response and rejection of the embryo include infection, autoimmune conditions, diabetes, glucose intolerance, endometriosis and micronutrient deficiency.

Inflammation

Inflammation is the body's natural, first-line response to infection or injury. Acute inflammation is a necessary component of immune function and healing that involves a complex biological response to harmful invaders, such as bacteria, viruses, damaged cells or irritants.

Chronic inflammation occurs when the immune system gets a faulty distress signal and mobilises its defence by triggering the release of white blood cells as though you were sick or injured, but because there's no infection to attack or injury to repair, they end up causing damage to healthy bodily tissues and processes. This kind of inflammation is associated with increased risk of various diseases, including cardiovascular disease, cancer and Alzheimer's, and may even reduce life expectancy overall.

CAUSES OF CHRONIC INFLAMMATION

- poor diet and lifestyle
- stress
- being overweight
- excessive exercise
- exposure to environmental toxins
- poor blood sugar control
- free radical damage
- autoimmune diseases
- endometriosis and polycystic ovary syndrome (PCOS)

HOW INFLAMMATION AFFECTS FERTILITY

- delayed natural conception
- reduced chance of success with IVF
- impaired menstrual cycle regularity
- impaired sex hormone production and ovulation
- reduced egg quality and developmental competence after fertilisation

The link between immunity, inflammation and nutrition

Immune cells are present throughout the intestine and food can act as a trigger for these cells. For instance, research shows that eating a high-calorie western-style breakfast can stimulate production by gut immune cells of a particular inflammatory molecule (a cytokine), interleukin-17 (IL-17).[8] The high IL-17 that follows can be detected in the blood as the effects of eating poor-quality food can spread throughout the body, leading to systemic inflammation. In comparison, a fruit-based breakfast did not cause the same inflammatory response as the 'fry-up' breakfast group in the same study. However, our inflammatory response to food is personal to each one of us, and recent research shows that individuals can have unique responses to eating fat and sugar, for instance, meaning that the same amounts of these foods may be unhealthy in one person but not in another.[9] Being overweight or having higher body fat percentages means a greater inflammatory response after eating is more likely. These responses are all linked to the bacteria in our guts with certain species associated with healthier responses to eating and others showing the opposite. Even though there is individual variation, the principles we covered in Chapter 3 provide the best guidance for an 'anti-inflammatory diet' based on the latest evidence.[10]

BIOLOGICAL FUNCTION

As well as things like immune function and the microbiome that affect the functioning of our whole bodies, there are processes taking place in individual cells that can affect sperm and egg quality. These things are relevant because they are also affected by diet and lifestyle so we can do something about them.

Mitochondria

Mitochondria (the 'batteries' of the cell) produce the energy needed for the body to function. They essentially convert energy from the calories in food to a form of energy that cells need to fuel biochemical processes – ATP (adenosine triphosphate) – in the same way we need to convert crude oil into petrol to fuel a car's engine.

Mitochondria are important for egg and sperm quality (see page 17) as both cells need lots of energy. The egg is the largest cell in the body and it provides the energy that fuels development of the early embryo. Sperm have a long way to swim so need energy for this journey. The more mitochondria that work well within each egg, the better the oocyte quality and the more energy the embryo it forms after fertilisation will have for early development, so the more 'competent' it will be. Poor mitochondrial function in the oocyte and embryo can therefore contribute to infertility and developmental abnormalities because a damaged mitochondrion produces less energy. As well as worsening with age (a torch light fades as the batteries start to wear out), mitochondrial function can be affected by damaging lifestyle habits, toxic environmental exposures, high-fat diets, being overweight and nutrient deficiencies – factors that can all lead to increased oxidative stress. Conversely, mitochondrial function may be protected through dietary restriction, so optimising weight and avoiding overeating and too much fat can help. Mitochondria need various nutrients to function including B-vitamins, sulphur and antioxidants (including co-enzyme Q10 – see Chapter 4). Organ meats such as liver and kidney contain high levels of co-enzyme Q10, but avoid consumption during pregnancy as they are high in preformed vitamin A, which can be toxic and cause birth defects if taken in very high quantities. Men can include these meats for sperm health.

Epigenetics

Epigenetics is the study of how your behaviours and environment can cause changes that affect the way your genes work. Having a faulty gene is one way for disease or health problems to arise; the other is for a healthy gene to stop working effectively. This can be caused by anything you put in or do to your body: from diet and exercise to the pesticides in food and smoking. There is growing evidence to show that epigenetic changes can impact reproductive health, including egg and sperm quality.[11] One study found that certain phthalates (preservatives commonly used in toiletries and cosmetics) caused changes to the genes in sperm that resulted in worse outcomes from IVF treatment for the couple.[12] Another found that what a woman eats around the time of conception can change the genes that control development in a newly formed embryo.[13]

Telomeres

Telomeres are the caps at the end of strands of DNA. In the same way caps on the end of shoelaces prevent fraying, telomeres protect DNA as it replicates by helping to ensure that an exact copy of DNA is made when it replicates (e.g. during cell division) so that mutations do not arise. Telomeres shorten with age and with damaging lifestyle factors and, as they shorten, mutations in DNA become more likely during replication.

This increased tendency towards DNA mutation has a direct impact on fertility and is another mechanism through which age impacts both male and female fertility. Mutations in sperm DNA cause poor morphology and motility, while telomere length in combination with mitochondrial function is important for egg quality.

The common factors that impact biological processes

There is overwhelming evidence to show the principles of good diet, nutrient status and other lifestyle factors that we describe can help support these biological processes that underpin good fertility.[14] Each individual component of the advice we give has the potential to impact on many levels, and when a number of different changes are made over time, marginal gains really can accumulate to help people conceive. We see this in our patients who make these changes.

Here are some of the key steps we suggest:

- Follow the Mediterranean diet (as outlined in Chapter 3), which is linked to anti-inflammatory effects, and avoid pro-inflammatory foods (such as junk foods and trans fats in snacks like crisps).

- Start by eating anti-inflammatory foods and introduce supplements, such as n-acetyl cysteine and curcumin, later if needed to avoid excess antioxidant intake.

- Optimise weight where possible as higher BMIs are associated with increased inflammation (see Chapter 6). Avoiding overeating, reaching a healthy weight and intermittent fasting are all strategies that may make a difference to mitochondrial function.

- Identify any food sensitivities or allergies by testing and/or following an elimination process (see page 95 and our website for further information).

- Take steps to manage stress (see Chapter 9).

- Aim to improve sleep quality as poor sleep can trigger inflammation, and melatonin produced during sleep is anti-inflammatory (see page 84).

MTHFR MUTATIONS

The MTHFR (methylenetetrahydrofolate reductase) enzyme is critical for folate metabolism in the body and is needed to convert the supplemental form, folic acid, into its bioavailable form used by the body, folate. Folate is important for fertility and pregnancy, with deficiencies causing neural tube defects (such as spina bifida) in the baby. MTHFR gene variants are recognised as having the potential to impact both male and female fertility including the risk of miscarriage.

In simple terms, having an MTHFR mutation means that if you supplement with folic acid, although easily absorbed, it will be harder for your body to convert folic acid into folate. The data is mixed in terms of exactly how this may impact fertility, and routine testing is not currently recommended by guidelines from the National Institute for Health and Care Excellence (NICE) for fertility.

From our observations, it seems some are more affected than others. If you have been taking folic acid or a multivitamin containing folic acid for at least three months and your folate is low on testing, you can request a homocysteine test via your GP. If your homocysteine is high, it may be worth being tested for MTHFR mutations. Elevated homocysteine is a risk factor for miscarriage and, when combined with low folate, it is more likely this will impact your fertility. MTHFR mutations can also be accompanied by gall bladder dysfunction and, if you have suffered from gallstones before middle age, this can also be an indicator.

Eleanor and Matt: Underlying health issues

Eleanor (33) was suffering from primary infertility after trying unsuccessfully to conceive naturally for two years. She had a very irregular menstrual cycle caused by PCOS and wasn't ovulating. She also had significant gut issues at the time, including diarrhoea, bloating and IBS-type symptoms, which escalated into severe abdominal pain just before her first consultation with Grace. Eleanor was also overweight and suffered from anxiety and had a history of depression, for which she took antidepressants. Matt (35) was generally healthy with a normal BMI.

Test results confirmed that Eleanor had two MTHFR variants that needed to be considered in her treatment. She also had a significantly impaired omega-3 ratio, suboptimal ferritin (iron), B12, vitamin D and dysbiosis in the gut, including yeast and clostridium difficile bacteria. Eleanor also had elevated serum alanine aminotransferase (a marker of liver function). The results for Matt showed normal semen analysis, a deficiency in vitamin D and impaired zinc–copper ratio.

After initially attending our preconception care course, Eleanor and Matt started dietary changes over a period of several months following a personalised dietary and lifestyle programme including appropriate supplements to address symptoms and correct deficiencies.

After 12 weeks, Eleanor had lost a significant amount of weight by following a healthy diet (without calorie counting), her periods had regularised, she was getting positive ovulation results with at-home tests, her digestive symptoms had improved, and she reported increased cervical mucus and significantly enhanced well-being. On retesting we found that Eleanor had improved vitamin D, zinc, ferritin, B12 and omega-3, and Matt had improved vitamin D and zinc.

Two weeks after testing Eleanor emailed to let us know she had had a positive pregnancy test! She was so shocked after so long trying and expecting to need IVF. Three weeks later an early pregnancy scan showed a heartbeat and, nine months later, following a normal, full-term pregnancy, a healthy baby boy was born.

SECONDARY INFERTILITY

If you already have at least one child and you are struggling to conceive again, it is possible that previous pregnancies may be contributing. Pregnancy is very depleting on the body, with nutrients preferentially diverted to the fetus over the mother, and it can easily lead to postnatal deficiencies. If you then add breastfeeding into the equation, which is also very demanding on the body, it is easy for a woman to slip into a state of multiple deficiencies.

Poor sleep that often comes with a new baby and the stress related to new parenthood can also have an impact. This once again highlights the importance of preconception care as ensuring body stores of nutrients are adequate prior to pregnancy helps protect against depletion and also prepares you for breastfeeding. Where this is a factor in subsequent infertility, it often can be corrected through a sufficient preconception period of testing, supplementation and suitable focus on a healthy, nutrient-rich diet. Seeking advice and support if your child is not sleeping in order to improve your own sleep can also be helpful in addressing secondary infertility.

We have many success stories from couples who had faced lengthy struggles to conceive, often experiencing miscarriages and failed IVF along the way, only to conceive naturally and go on to have healthy pregnancies and healthy babies by making some of these changes. We can't offer guarantees that you will be able to conceive naturally, but we can tell you this work will get you in the best possible health for pregnancy and parenthood, improve the health of any babies you go on to have and put you in the best place for a successful outcome of any fertility treatment you may need.

Chapter 8

Hormone Balance

ROM THE USHERING of girls into womanhood to the creation of life itself, hormones have a profound effect on the lives of women throughout adulthood, from puberty to menopause and beyond. Hormones define some of life's most important moments and impact how we feel day to day, minute to minute. Understanding them and the foundation on which they are built – the menstrual cycle – is fundamental for good health and well-being.

You may be wondering therefore why we have left focusing on such an important and seemingly obvious aspect of fertility until this point in the book. It's because we find that when the other areas of health that we have covered so far are optimised, hormone levels improve.

When we refer to hormones generally in this chapter, we actually mean sex or reproductive hormones. We have covered the main metabolic hormones including insulin and leptin in Chapter 5, and we will cover adrenal hormones involved in the stress response in Chapter 9.

It is essential to work on the foundations of your good health before you consider taking pills to address hormone issues. We often find, for instance, that menstrual cycles regularise and symptoms improve once our patients have addressed the underlying factors of nutrient deficiencies, high or low body weight, and gastrointestinal issues. Standardised advice aimed at all women with the catch-all aim of 'balancing your hormones' is unlikely to be effective without addressing the underlying causes that are personal to you.

Testing your hormones

Your first opportunity to check your hormones if you are experiencing difficulties conceiving is a hormone 'panel' of blood tests, organised by your GP. This will assess your levels of follicle-stimulating hormone (FSH), luteinising hormone (LH), oestrogen, progesterone, and sometimes testosterone (see page 153 for more details). If the timing of each test is correct (in relation to where you are in your menstrual cycle), results should indicate whether or not you have normal ovarian function and are ovulating. This is helpful to identify medical conditions such as polycystic ovary syndrome (PCOS) or rule out other problems.

It is important to ensure that any tests and advice on hormones that you may come across online are provided by professionals who have the clinical experience and expertise to underpin their service. Always seek the advice of your doctor.

What is not usually scrutinised during initial investigations is the relative balance between the different hormones, whether hormones are high or low in the range and whether your symptoms and cycle interval are indicative of any particular problems. For instance, if you've had a scan to check your uterus and ovaries, and the endometrium (lining of the womb) looks thin, then you may have a problem with suboptimal oestrogen. If you experience spotting before your period and you have a short luteal phase of the menstrual cycle (the second half of the menstrual cycle after ovulation), then you may have an issue with progesterone and difficulty sustaining a pregnancy. If you have PCOS, elevated androgens can lead to irregular periods and difficulties conceiving and, although lifestyle is the first-line treatment recommended for PCOS, clinical practice generally is still playing catch-up in terms of nutrition and lifestyle medicine and lags behind the scientific evidence, though much work is being done to change this.

Holistic approaches such as diet, lifestyle, correction of deficiencies and certain supplements can be effective, but there is a significant level of unreliable information online that lacks a substantive evidence base and more research is needed. There is also a point at which professional supervision is needed in order to understand which approaches are suitable for you as an individual as the underlying science is complex – as is the human body – and it takes skill, knowledge and clinical experience to tailor interventions to your unique circumstances.

The effort is worth it though, not least because hormones also affect our brains. Both pregnancy and perimenopause alter brain function and can increase brain fog, forgetfulness and anxiety. Oestrogen is protective and the loss of this hormone at menopause starts the changes in the brain that put women at increased risk of Alzheimer's compared to men.[1] However, knowledge is power as dietary and lifestyle factors make up a big proportion of your risk of developing this disease and affect mental health and cognition generally. So, making changes to improve your fertility will also help protect your brain now and as you age.

FACTORS THAT CAN AFFECT HORMONE LEVELS

- diet and nutrient status
- body fat percentage and metabolic health
- stress
- exercise
- the microbiome
- thyroid function
- endocrine disruptors
- supplements

HOW TO TELL IF YOUR HORMONES ARE CAUSING PROBLEMS

Before we look in detail at factors that can affect hormones in the body, it's helpful to understand whether or not you have symptoms that may indicate a problem. Since a healthy menstrual cycle is the foundation for good fertility, this is your starting point for assessing what may be happening in your body. It is always important to seek medical advice rather than rely on self-diagnosis. Being informed and empowered to play your part in your own healthcare rather than being a passive recipient, however, is an important feature of progressive medicine.

What does a healthy menstrual cycle look like?

When it comes to fertility, a healthy menstrual cycle is a regular cycle typically between 25 and 35 days in length, with mostly continuous moderate bleeding that is mainly bright red in colour of 2–5 days' duration with a definite start. If you have spotting in the days leading up to your period, you need to consistently use more than one sanitary product every four hours, there are large clots in the blood, you suffer pain that cannot be managed with over-the-counter painkillers and a hot water bottle, you experience a very irregular cycle or have abdominal pain that persists throughout your cycle, these are all signs that something may need addressing. Cycles shorter than 25 days mean that you may have a short luteal phase, which may contribute to difficulties conceiving and may indicate low levels of the progesterone needed to sustain a pregnancy.

While some of these symptoms can be common, it does not mean they are necessarily normal, and you should not accept them as such without trying to get to the bottom of what may be causing the issue. It is common for patients with endometriosis to report that their severe pain was described as normal period pain when they first sought medical help, leading to a delay in diagnosis, for instance. We have also seen incidences of premature ovarian insufficiency (POI) being missed as skipping a period is seen as normal, with sometimes not even the red flag of a very high FSH blood test result recognised as serious (see Chapter 24 for more on POI).

Delays in diagnosing underlying conditions mean at best that suffering and infertility is unnecessarily prolonged and, at worst, can cost you your ability to have your own biological children. Historically, of course, many aspects of female reproductive health and fertility have not been taught fully in schools. As a result, a lack of fundamental knowledge among women of the workings of their own bodies remains a significant source of disempowerment and we are passionate about educating girls and women to correct this. If you started your periods late, this could be a sign that you were underweight as a teenager (see page 44) or suffer from an underlying condition such as coeliac disease (see page 94), for example. The importance of understanding these issues comes into very sharp focus when trying to conceive, but they are vital for the well-being of all women at any life stage.

A summary of common problems

The table below shows symptoms that may point to underlying hormonal disturbances and have the potential to impact fertility.

SYMPTOM	POSSIBLE CAUSES	THINK ABOUT . . .
Acne or skin changes across the menstrual cycle	· Hormone imbalances including excess oestrogen · High BMI · PCOS	· Diet and lifestyle to support hormone metabolism · Weight loss if BMI is 25+, or higher than normal for you · Zinc supplements
Irregular or missed periods	· PCOS · Hormone imbalances · Low body weight · Undereating · Over-exercising · POI · Stress · Thyroid conditions · Coeliac disease	· See GP for investigations including PCOS, coeliac, thyroid · Test for pregnancy · Eat more/gain weight · Nutrient testing · Consider chaste berry under professional supervision after addressing the above
Spotting for more than two days before your period	· Low progesterone · Fibroids · Endometriosis · Thyroid disease	· Check for ovulation via tests, basal body temperature monitoring · See GP for investigations including hormone tests including progesterone

PMS	· High oestrogen · Low progesterone · Stress · Inflammation	· Diet and lifestyle to support hormone metabolism and reduce inflammation · Strategies to deal with stress (see Chapter 9) · Vitamin B_6, zinc, magnesium, evening primrose oil
Tender breasts	· High oestrogen	· Diet and lifestyle to support hormone metabolism and reduce inflammation · Sufficient iodine intake and/or supplements
Heavy periods	· High oestrogen · Anovulation · High BMI · Fibroids	· Diet and lifestyle to support hormone metabolism and reduce inflammation · Consider weight loss if needed, as above
Regularly seeing clots larger than 2cm in menstrual blood	· High oestrogen/ impaired oestrobolome (see page 117) · Thyroid problems · Clotting disorders · Endometriosis · Adenomyosis	· Diet and lifestyle to support hormone metabolism and reduce inflammation · Consider weight loss if needed, as above · See GP for investigations
Light periods	· Low oestrogen · Low BMI · Smoking · Undereating	· Diet and lifestyle to support hormone metabolism and reduce inflammation · Consider weight gain if needed · Stop smoking · Vitamin E if endometrium also thin

Short luteal phase	· Low progesterone · Stress	· Check for ovulation/ test progesterone · Strategies to reduce stress (see Chapter 9) · Vitamin B_6, zinc, magnesium, vitamin C
Bloating	· Dysbiosis in the gut · Impaired oestrobolome (see page 117) · Hormone imbalances	· Diet and lifestyle to support hormone metabolism and reduce inflammation · Focus on gut microbiome – seek professional advice · Consider probiotic foods and supplements
Headaches	· High oestrogen · Low magnesium · Stress · Poor sleep	· Diet and lifestyle to support hormone metabolism and reduce inflammation · Magnesium glycinate supplementation starting at 200mg and increasing to 300mg if needed · Strategies to tackle stress (see Chapter 9) · Sleep hygiene routine (see page 84)

HOW DIET AFFECTS HORMONES

Nutrient status, weight and exercise can all impact hormone levels, as we've seen in previous chapters. Undereating and low body weight are both potential threats to optimal hormone levels and a healthy menstrual cycle, for instance. It is also believed that inadequate levels of certain nutrients may contribute to menstrual cycle dysfunction as studies indicate that supplementation can help improve symptoms.[2] This is not surprising because, of course, your body needs sufficient levels of raw materials to fuel all biochemical processes. For example, for a woman to have a period, the endometrium needs to thicken during the early part of the cycle before being lost during menstruation in a cyclical monthly pattern. Numerous nutrients are needed for this to happen:

- Iron is essential for the blood formation needed for building the endometrium.

- Vitamin C enhances iron absorption and copper is needed to maintain adequate iron levels.

- Folate is needed for cell growth and survival.

- Vitamins B_6 and B_{12} are needed for red blood cell formation.

- Magnesium regulates numerous biological processes including those involved in maintaining cell membranes – vital for the transport of nutrients into the cell.

Nutrient requirements and metabolism change with hormone fluctuations during the menstrual cycle. It therefore follows that if you are deficient in one or more nutrients, this could impact on the finely balanced systems that underpin ovulation and hormone production.

Nutrients can affect hormones both directly and indirectly. To produce hormones, you need cholesterol, for instance, which is found in every cell in the body and is also important for production of vitamin D and bile acids in the liver.

Hormones do not work in isolation, however, so if ovulation is important for sufficient progesterone production, the DNA synthesis needed for ooctyes to complete cell division to form an ovulation-ready egg becomes an important part of your hormone balance, and this requires nutrients including zinc and B vitamins. Studies also suggest that inadequate selenium levels increase the risk of a short luteal phase, which is caused by suboptimal progesterone produced by the corpus luteum and means the endometrium is less receptive to implantation.[3] And, of course, vitamin D receptors are found in all reproductive tissues, pointing towards the pivotal role of vitamin D for fertility that is observed clinically.

Many pre-existing underlying health conditions, including diabetes and inflammatory bowel disease (IBD), get worse during the second half of the cycle if a woman hasn't conceived that month, when oestrogen and progesterone levels start to fall again. This worsening coincides with lower levels of certain nutrients such as amino acids, which suggests that the body uses more of these nutrients during ovulation and the luteal phase, possibly in anticipation of a possible pregnancy. These lower nutrient levels are thought to contribute to symptoms of premenstrual syndrome (PMS) and, the more serious form, premenstrual dysphoric disorder (PMDD), which include premenstrual low mood and anxiety. It is no surprise therefore that PMS also brings increased appetite, food cravings and higher calorific intake. Levels of neurotransmitters associated with good mood (including serotonin) also fall in line with nutrient levels during the second half of the period. It makes sense therefore that a good diet can help improve symptoms and, although further research is needed, these studies certainly point towards an important role for nutrition in the health of the menstrual cycle.

HOW MINERALS CAN IMPACT HORMONES

Minerals that are commonly low that also have an impact on hormones and the menstrual cycle are zinc and magnesium. Many people find they benefit from supplementing with these minerals over and above levels found in a standard preconception multivitamin, though be aware that taking individual minerals can drive other minerals down and too much of anything can be toxic. Too much zinc can cause a copper deficiency, for instance, so don't exceed more than 40mg daily or continue zinc supplementation for more than three months without ensuring you have enough copper through diet, supplements or a pre-existing high level on testing. Magnesium is never included in sufficient quantities in standard multivitamins as it makes pills too bulky for a one-a-day, so this is one mineral we routinely recommend, though don't take more than 300mg daily.

Research indicates that minerals are important for hormone metabolism either directly or indirectly:[4]

- Correcting a zinc deficiency has been shown to increase testosterone levels in men and may help balance androgens in women.

- Magnesium plays an essential role in many functions of the body and is needed for the body to produce vitamin D from sunlight and process vitamin D from supplements. It is therefore an important cofactor for this vitamin that is crucial for reproductive function.

- Manganese is important for cholesterol metabolism, which is the starting point for sex hormone production. The US-based BioCycle Study also found that low manganese intake was associated with increased risk of anovulation.[5]

- Studies indicate adequate intake of boron improved a range of reproductive functions including levels of sex hormones for those with previously low boron levels, reduced menstrual pain, increased the half-life (the length of time the substance persists in the body) and bioavailability of both oestrogen and vitamin D, and improved response to vitamin D supplementation and magnesium absorption.[6] Note that too much boron can be toxic, especially for the thyroid.

Finally, interaction between hormones and nutrients works both ways, with hormones including oestrogen helping to keep levels of ceruloplasmin in balance, for instance. Ceruloplasmin is important in the regulation of copper, iron and zinc. Start by taking a multivitamin and mineral, aim to have some basic tests via your GP where possible, and pay attention to signs and symptoms you experience. It can be quite complicated, so the take-home message is to be aware of this complexity and seek appropriate advice from your doctors.

GUT HEALTH AND HORMONES

One surprising aspect of our health important for hormone metabolism is gut health. In fact, some animal studies show a direct impact of diet on fertility via gut bacteria.[7] As we've seen, a healthy gut microbiome is important for a healthy pregnancy, and many of our patients come to us with digestive symptoms. Some studies have shown that oestrogen metabolism by the gut can impact menstrual symptoms and may have a role in fertility.[8]

Sex hormones are predominantly produced in the gonads (ovaries and testes) and have an effect both locally and around the body. Once hormones have done their job, they need to be neutralised and expelled by the body. For example, oestrogen is produced from testosterone by the ovaries, thickens the lining of the womb ready for ovulation and then travels to the liver and on to the gut to be processed before it is passed out of the body. There are three different potential pathways for the first phase of oestrogen detoxification in the liver, and the relative balance between these pathways is important in terms of things like breast cancer risk.[9] One pathway is associated with heavy periods with large clots and breast tenderness, so these symptoms indicate your oestrogen metabolism could be improved. All three pathways direct oestrogen from the liver into the gut for it to be processed by the oestrobolome (more on this below) and excreted in stools. Various nutrients including vitamin B_{12}, folate and magnesium are all important cofactors in this process, highlighting once again the need for sufficiency of all nutrients for optimal reproductive function. Magnesium in particular helps to ensure more oestrogen is metabolised along the healthiest pathway, which is another reason why magnesium is likely to be important for hormone balance.

Problems can arise if the processing of hormones becomes faulty, and hormones that should be excreted re-enter the circulation and raise overall levels of that particular hormone. The liver and the gut therefore both need to be working well for optimal hormone balance. Eliminating environmental toxins and limiting alcohol can support the processing oestrogens in the body, and alcohol is a known risk factor for breast cancer because of this.

The oestrobolome

The oestrobolome is the group of gut bacteria responsible for processing and eliminating oestrogen from the body. When gut bacteria get out of balance, oestrogen that has already been used in the body that should be expelled is reactivated and returns to the general circulation.[10] This adds extra oestrogen to the body pool. When slightly raised, oestrogen can cause constipation, reduced sex drive and depression. Higher levels still can be associated with infertility, weight gain and serious illnesses such as breast cancer. Excess oestrogen produced in this way is also thought to contribute to symptoms of endometriosis. Studies indicate that altering the composition of the gut microbiome improves many symptoms associated with excess oestrogen.[11] In our patients, we do often see that when digestive symptoms improve, menstrual symptoms improve too. Other signs that you may have an impaired oestrobolome include bloating before your period, emotional symptoms of PMS, including irritability and tearfulness, heavy periods and headaches, especially around your period. Problems with the oestrobolome can also cause low levels of oestrogen.

What can you do?

Though research is ongoing, anything that disrupts the gut microbiome has the potential to affect the oestrobolome, including medication and supplements. All the things we covered in Chapter 7 in terms of microbiota health may have the potential to impact oestrogen metabolism, including poor diet and antibiotic use.[12] Some claim certain foods may be particularly beneficial when it comes to hormone metabolism, including cruciferous vegetables such as broccoli, cabbage and cauliflower, though this hasn't been proven in well-conducted studies. There is also no evidence whatsoever that seed cycling (where certain seeds are eaten at different stages of the menstrual cycle) has an impact on hormones. Popular supplements targeting the oestrobolome include various plant extracts and herbal supplements such as resveratrol, dong quai and Diindolylmethane (DIM), which have some evidence to show benefit for hormone levels and oestrogen metabolism but have not been tested in fertility studies, so be cautious about what you take as the impact on fertility and pregnancy is largely unknown.

THYROID

We will cover more on thyroid function in Chapter 12, but there are some important dietary and lifestyle considerations when considering hormone balance.

The thyroid is a small gland in the front of the neck and it plays a major role in endocrine (hormone) function affecting almost every cell of the body. Good thyroid function is an essential component of good health, energy levels and hormone regulation; therefore optimising thyroid function when trying to conceive and for a healthy pregnancy is vital.

Thyroid problems are much more common in women than in men (though some men are affected) and can contribute to weight gain or loss and irregular periods, with menstrual cycle disturbances being three times more common in women with an underactive thyroid. Women experiencing an irregular cycle, sudden changes in weight or difficulties in either maintaining or losing weight should always be investigated for thyroid problems.

In terms of diet and lifestyle, you will come across a huge amount on the impact of diet and nutrients in terms of thyroid function and this is one of the worst areas for unsubstantiated claims, with relatively little scientific evidence to support specific diets for thyroid function or autoimmunity, including that dairy is bad for thyroid function. There are currently no human trials to support this assertion. Evidence is mixed in terms of soy, so we would always advise caution in terms of excessive intake and aim for no more than a once-weekly inclusion if you suffer from thyroid autoimmunity. Similarly, there is no substantive evidence to suggest that adopting a gluten-free diet is beneficial for thyroid autoimmunity in the absence of coeliac disease, though if you have one of these conditions, you are more likely to have the other and it is always important to be tested for both. If you have a noticeable adverse reaction to these foods, however, we recommend seeking professional advice or trying a properly conducted dietary exclusion process, as outlined on page 95, to see if symptoms, including thyroid function, improve. There is one small study that suggested a potential benefit of what is known as the 'autoimmune protocol'.[13] The autoimmune protocol has traditionally been viewed with scepticism by scientists and, since it is a very restrictive diet, extreme caution should be advised before embarking on it because of this, especially in the preconception period. There isn't sufficient evidence to support widespread adoption, though research on diet and autoimmunity is ongoing so this may change.[14]

Foods that do have an evidence base that warrants avoidance if you have thyroid problems are excess or raw cruciferous vegetables, sea plants including dulse, seaweed or kelp (the high iodine content may cause or worsen hypothyroidism), and millet, which may suppress thyroid function even when iodine levels are adequate.

We do observe clinically in our patients that improving diet quality and correcting nutrient deficiencies often improves and stabilises thyroid function and it is recognised that nutrient deficiencies (or excess) may have a negative impact. Adequate levels of ferritin, zinc, selenium, iodine, vitamin A and vitamin D are all important for thyroid function. There are some studies that show a benefit of selenium supplementation in those with thyroid autoimmunity, but test first and seek professional supervision.[15] Sufficient iodine is extremely important for thyroid function and many women enter pregnancy with low levels. Even mild deficiency can impact fetal brain development, and countries with low iodine intake have higher incidences of goitre (a swelling of the neck caused by an enlarged thyroid gland). Low iodine has also been shown to reduce *in vitro* fertilisation (IVF) success rates. Excessive iodine intake can worsen thyroid problems and is not recommended, however, and the medical profession consistently advises 150mcg of supplemental iodine daily in the preconception period. Some may benefit from additional intake and if you still have breast tenderness or issues such as benign cysts in the breast after optimising all the factors we have covered in the book so far and you do not have thyroid autoimmunity, you could discuss with your doctor whether it may be beneficial to increase iodine intake as studies do indicate this may be beneficial for these symptoms.[16]

ENVIRONMENTAL TOXINS AND ENDOCRINE DISRUPTORS

A final factor to consider in terms of hormones is the potential for environmental toxins in the form of air pollution, pesticides in foods and preservatives in personal care products to impair normal function. Endocrine disruptors are chemicals (endocrine disrupting chemicals or EDCs) that negatively impact the endocrine system because of their similarity to the sex hormones we produce naturally. They often have oestrogen-like effects in the body and have many potential negative effects on biological function, including on the menstrual cycle, production of sex hormones in the ovary, the proper workings of hormone receptors, progression of endometriosis, PCOS and also fertility. EDCs can also impact hormone metabolism by increasing or decreasing the breakdown or clearance of hormones, which ultimately has the potential to cause reduced thyroid hormone levels and increased oestrogen. As well as effects on hormones, environmental toxins can contribute to infertility by damaging female and male reproductive function, impacting egg and sperm quality and reducing embryonic and fetal competence.

Avoiding environmental toxins including exposures to plastics, heavy metals and air pollution where possible is therefore important. (See Chapter 10 for recommendations that apply to both women and men, and there is more information on our website – see Resources, page 371.) Remember, though, that we don't live in a bubble and we simply cannot avoid these exposures altogether: sadly, the planet has been seriously contaminated by human activity, but the global population continues to rise. While we advise minimising exposures where possible, this shouldn't become a source of stress and there is a balance to be struck with this approach. We look at how to keep stress to a minimum in the next chapter.

Chapter 9

Stress, the Mind and Fertility

ONE OF THE most common experiences of men and women who face difficulties conceiving is stress. Anyone who has dreaded the first sight of menstrual blood every month, experienced the two-week wait following an embryo transfer during *in vitro* fertilisation (IVF) treatment or willed the line signalling a pregnancy to appear on a test stick – and any partner who has shared in these events – will know only too well how heartbreaking this journey can be.

For those who have suffered the added burden of miscarriage or stillbirth, the profound sense of loss and grief for the life once nurtured inside you can be overwhelming. Feelings that your body has failed you, that you are less of a person because you aren't able to do this fundamental thing that everyone around you seems able to do, the longing to hold your own baby in your arms, and the guilt over the peaks of pain, anger, jealousy or even hatred with each passing pregnancy announcement are all things we hear from our patients.

The fertility journey can be a uniquely lonely and isolating experience because these feelings are not easy to share given the intensely private nature of what you face. It can be especially difficult knowing that many aren't able to truly understand this kind of pain. We know that the well-meaning but often thoughtless comments from those around you when it comes to the question of children or even passing a pregnant woman in the street can sometimes feel too much.

When these feelings become overwhelming, many worry the stress will impact their fertility. It's important not to deny or diminish these feelings, but having strategies to cope can help. Understanding how stress may affect you and then looking at practical things you can do to help yourself is important, and this is what we'll look at in this chapter.

YOU ARE NOT ALONE

Being aware of these emotions as they pass through and seeking help where needed can make a difference, and there are many national and regional infertility groups (see Resources, page 371) that can signpost you to support locally. Remember you are not alone. All the emotions you are experiencing are completely understandable and shared by many.

DOES STRESS IMPACT FERTILITY?

It's natural to worry that all this stress will impact your chances of conceiving, and this is an area that has been the subject of intense debate over recent years. Though there is still controversy, one popular narrative in the fertility sector at the moment is that stress does not lead to difficulties conceiving either naturally or via IVF, rather that infertility causes stress.

This is based on high-quality research by psychologists who have not found an association between self-reported stress and IVF outcomes. One such meta-analysis of 14 studies concluded that emotional distress does not reduce the chances of pregnancy.[1] A conflicting meta-analysis, however, found a small but significant association between stress and reduced chance of conceiving.[2] Psychology-based studies do have limitations, however, so this isn't conclusive evidence as there are biological consequences of stress that do have the potential to affect reproductive pathways.

One indicator of stress in the body is the hormone cortisol. Recent research from the University of Nottingham investigated cortisol levels laid down in hair grown in the three months prior to fertility treatment.[3] Cortisol is secreted from the adrenal glands, which sit just above your kidneys and produce hormones that help regulate key bodily functions such as the stress response, metabolism, immune function, blood pressure and healthy gastrointestinal function. Cortisol production is stimulated by signals from the pituitary, which in turn is controlled by the hypothalamus in the base of the brain – the hypothalamic-pituitary-adrenal (HPA) axis. The HPA axis acts as a kind of master switch of the body's stress response and is very sensitive to stress. Researchers in Nottingham found that increased cortisol was indeed associated with reduced IVF success. It is also well known that the increase in cortisol levels triggered by stress can negatively affect many different aspects of health, including sleep quality.

The physical manifestations of stress can be explained by the evolutionary 'fight or flight' response to threat. In other words, human beings evolved in a world where they faced much greater physical threat from predators and, like other animals, they would have had to either fight the predator or run away in order to survive. When faced with threat, a number of changes are triggered in the body that are designed to maximise survival. A cascade of stress hormones initiates well-orchestrated physiological changes in response to a stressful incident. These include increases in breathing and heart rate, and blood flow directed to muscles and away from other organs (including reproductive ones) to maximise energy supply to power the escape, or to fight to defeat the threat.

The Nottingham research suggests that more long-term stress may impact fertility, perhaps contrasting to the more short-term stress reported around the time of IVF treatment in many studies conducted by psychologists. Again, conclusions from these studies are debated and other studies looking at more short-term measures of cortisol have yielded mixed results.[4] We discuss the evidence in more detail on our website (see Resources, page 371).

While the jury is still out on this, it's important to remember that the effects of stress are temporary. Stress is part of everyday life and we can't avoid it entirely and insulate ourselves from each and every source of worry and anxiety. We don't need to eliminate *all* stress from our lives in order to improve our well-being. Remember it is likely that short-term stress around the time of IVF treatment does not have a significant effect. Whatever the reality, however, it's helpful to devote time to things that can counter the effects of stress and focus on your well-being rather than being falsely reassured that you don't need to do anything at all. This is important for a healthy pregnancy and your well-being as a new mother, too.

NAVIGATING YOUR FERTILITY JOURNEY

Having a positive, proactive strategy to cope with your emotions and manage stress at what can be a very stressful time can make a big difference. There are some important steps we recommend to our patients that help.

Manage life's stresses

While the impact of stress on fertility is debated, you will feel better if you take steps to mitigate against the effects of stress:

- Minimise avoidable or very significant stressors where possible. For example, if there is serious conflict in your wider family or friendships and contact depletes you emotionally, recognise the source of this stress and try to manage boundaries and contact so that you don't feel this as a constant.

- Recognise the impact that chronic ongoing stress is having on your life. This is essential in protecting the long-term health of both men and women. This may be a career where you routinely have to work excessive hours in a high-pressure environment and travel to different time zones, throwing out your body clock.

- Allow more time to recover emotionally if you have experienced more than two or three significantly stressful events in the last year (e.g. moving house or serious illness of you or a close family member) or one major trauma (e.g. bereavement or serious accident). Trauma leaves a lasting impression physically as well as emotionally, so taking a mind–body approach is most effective. Many people are keen to have IVF treatment as soon as possible after being referred for treatment, but often pausing and giving yourself this time where needed can make all the difference.

Look after your mental health

Infertility can affect mental health and be a cause of depression and anxiety. A previous termination can rear its head psychologically, for instance, or a nagging anxiety, when explored, can point towards unresolved childhood trauma, perhaps revealing a lack of safety and security in a person's upbringing such that they either consciously or subconsciously fear they will not be able to provide an emotionally safe environment for their own child.

It's helpful to at least understand your own emotional landscape in order to be able to help yourself and prepare for the future that is so desired. That isn't to say we should strive to be perfect or 'fixed' – nobody goes through life sanitised from pain and suffering – but that we should seek to heal what we can in preparation for pregnancy and parenthood.

Below are some of the signs that you can look out for that give an idea that you may benefit from more support:

- Are there issues from your childhood or your past that you haven't processed through therapy or some other structured process? This may be a factor that is causing unhealthy behaviours or unhappiness.

- Overachievement or a lack of achievement, or shared coping mechanisms among siblings, can all point towards underlying emotional factors that need additional support.

- Sometimes mess is a sign of emotional turmoil, while in other people very strict tidiness and perfectionism is a sign of a need to create external order to prop up a vulnerable inner world.

By looking at these things, you can use the preconception period to think proactively about your mental and emotional well-being. Given one in three of us will suffer from mental health issues at some point in our lives, this is something we should all be taught from a young age but, in the absence of that, preparing for parenthood is an excellent opportunity and a way of laying the foundation for this work with your children. Support is always available (see Resources, page 371).

Deal with negative emotions and overthinking

Feeling your feelings is an essential part of coping with them. However, a tendency to 'ruminate' on worries and negative thinking without processing feelings in a healthy way is a significant contributor to anxiety and poor mental health. Recognising a tendency to ruminate without repressing emotions is an important first step. Other helpful techniques include:

- Have a set time to discuss difficult thoughts and feelings with your partner (try to end this positively with a hug!).

- See a counsellor or therapist. Ask your doctor to be referred or see the British Association for Counselling and Psychotherapy (BACP) website (see Resources, page 371). Every country will have its equivalent.

- Be aware of negative thoughts and don't allow them to spiral into rumination.

- Keep a worry journal: have a dedicated slot to write down any negative thoughts and emotions at the end of the day to get them out before you sleep.

- Tame your mind: discipline yourself not to think about what's worrying you outside of these set activities – find ways of dealing with thoughts and emotions by processing them but not dwelling on them constantly. Meditation can help.

- Take time to process uncomfortable feelings: close your eyes and sit with the emotion. Try to feel rather than think. Breathe in deeply through your nose, and exhale through your mouth, making your out-breath longer than your in-breath, and repeat a word in your head (e.g. 'calm'), focus on the breath or count to avoid thinking about what's bothering you.

- Have an imaginary safe, happy place in your head: it could be a cottage by the sea replete with a puppy . . . whatever works for you. Furnish this place with everything that you want and need to feel happy, safe and loved, and take time to go to this place in your head when you feel stressed or upset. This will allow you to return to a state of calm and help to self-soothe and regulate your emotions.

- Take regular exercise such as brisk walking, cycling, gentle jogging or swimming.

- Get out in nature and sunshine, have a bird feeder, take up gardening or have plants visible from your window (even if it's a window box) – all of these things have been shown to boost mood.

Be aware of addictions

Many people believe addictions are restricted to alcohol, smoking, drugs and damaging behaviours like excess gambling. But we can use a whole range of things to soothe emotional pain, escape day-to-day reality or distract from confronting unwanted feelings. As well as drugs and alcohol, this can include addiction to work, money, status, power, sex, shopping, cosmetic procedures and cleaning. Also be aware of unhealthy habits and attitudes to foods: emotional eating, binge eating, starving, control or eating disorders. Food (or its restriction) can be used to soothe emotional pain.

Work on a healthy mindset

Working on the way you think about your experiences can help you cope with your emotions as you navigate your fertility journey.

- Focus on what you can control. There is a paradoxical state of being happy and hopeful yet remaining detached from the outcome as much as possible. Do your best with all that you have under your control and trust the rest will work itself out somehow.

- Let go a little. It's so easy to allow tension to creep in and end up feeling knotted up inside with all that you are trying to manage. It's also common to clench on so tightly to the desire to have children that it becomes an overwhelming and urgent need. Often people aren't aware of the tension they are holding in their bodies as they grasp tightly to what they want. Relax your jaw, unclench your fists, let your shoulders relax and breathe. Then notice the difference. We find if you loosen your grip just a little and believe that everything will work out in the end, you are more likely to get what you want.

- Use the power of your mind. In a professional environment, mentors would advise using a vision board. You could use a vision or mood board to help you to focus and bring about the desired outcome. Visualising is a technique widely used in sports and you could try visualising yourself acting on some of the healthy behaviours we discuss that have the potential to increase your chance of success.

- Keep a gratitude journal and remember each day the things you are grateful for.

- Consider other ways to bring joy into your life – some of our patients have bought a dog or a cat, for instance. Just make sure it's right for you. All the things we cover in this chapter have the capacity to boost your health and well-being, and looking after these areas of life helps shift the intense focus away from fertility.

Practise yoga and meditation

There are numerous studies demonstrating the physical benefits of yoga and meditation, including on inflammatory markers and stress hormones like cortisol, all things that may impact the ability to conceive.[5] Meditation has been shown in various studies to impact inflammatory pathways in the body and affect expression of genes controlling inflammatory processes.[6]

Yoga and meditation reverse the pro-inflammatory effects of psychological stress in the body. Yoga also has benefits for general health through reducing stress and promoting good-quality sleep.

Though more research is needed, there is evidence that regular yoga is associated with better fertility outcomes.[7] A recent review of 87 different studies concluded that yoga can help couples overcome infertility and increase IVF success rate through improved physical and psychological health of men and women.[8] We therefore always advise including yoga in your weekly routine. Kundalini, yin and hatha yoga are good for general fertility and Iyengar yoga is best for muscle tone and weight loss. We don't recommend ashtanga yoga for female fertility.

Protect your relationships

Another area that can come under strain when trying to conceive is our relationships. Infertility and IVF can be emotional and stressful, and this can spill over into how we relate to partners, friends and family.

These can be difficult times for your most intimate relationship, with your partner, and it may affect each of you differently and at different times. Remember that simple kindness to yourself and each other will help you get through what is often a challenging time. Communication is key and will help you to recognise the emotion underlying someone else's behaviour – and your own. It is often when you feel most annoyed with a partner that they most need your love and support. Being supportive of each other also helps to maximise benefits of a preconception care period and turns it into a positive experience. One study showed that making lifestyle changes with a partner improved weight-loss outcomes, for instance.[9]

Facing fertility problems can also impact sex and intimacy, especially when sex is scheduled month in and month out to coincide with ovulation, so it's important to be aware of this. Making a conscious effort to maintain sex and intimacy will not only help in trying to conceive, it will help to de-stress, and remain happy and hopeful. Sex and intimacy are beneficial for emotional well-being, and sex also produces a bonding effect due to the release of coital oxytocin, the 'cuddle' hormone. Having spontaneous sex in the second half of your cycle when you are past the fertile window (for heterosexual women) can help avoid intimacy becoming a chore intended only for procreation (see also page 60).

Relationships with wider family and friends, including parents, siblings and work colleagues, can all be put under strain and vary according to how open you choose to be with them about your circumstances. Some people find it easier to keep everything very private, which can mean those around you won't always be as sympathetic as you would like when you're struggling. Choosing to tell others about what you are going through can mean you have more support, but they will often say the wrong thing, hit a nerve when you don't feel like talking about it or not ask how you are enough because they simply don't know what to say. Be aware of all of these things and try to be forgiving of yourself and those closest to you.

Keep socialising

When facing fertility problems, it's common to stop doing the things you enjoy as fertility treatment can be all-consuming. Some couples stop socialising and avoid occasions where they are likely to meet children or pregnant women. All of these things are completely understandable and you certainly don't have to go to baby showers if they make you feel terrible. However, we always encourage our patients to try to enjoy and make the most of what they have now. Life has its phases and the things that you may take for granted now, you will miss later.

Know that for most of you reading this book, it is a time that will pass, and the majority will go on to conceive.

Make a plan for better self-care

Recognising the importance of self-care and proactively fostering good emotional well-being is the first step. The second is knowing what to do about it. In its simplest form, self-care is about being kind to ourselves and accepting ourselves as imperfect human beings.

You can make a plan by writing down these headings:

- Emotions

- Mind

- Body

- Relationships

- Work

- Finances

- Spiritual (anything that gives a sense of a bigger world outside of your own experience – this could be the natural world or meaningful travel)

Under each heading, make a note of what is working well in that area, problems to solve and opportunities for improvement. Write down any areas that are not under your control and write: 'I accept that this is not under my control and I let go of any stress this is causing me.' Try some of the suggestions from this chapter that you think will work for you. Use what is working well as positive motivation and a reason for gratitude and write down ideas for tackling anything else. Focusing on your own happiness is never selfish, and in this case it also helps prepare for parenthood in a sensible, balanced way.

Keep going

When you're in the middle of challenging circumstances, it can often feel like you're stuck, but the simple capacity to keep putting one foot in front of the other and reminding yourself to just keep going can help spur you on. Don't forget the strategies we've covered and to nurture yourself along the way. We are rooting for you.

Chapter 10

Male Fertility

FOR A SINGLE sperm to make it to an egg is the rough equivalent of a human being swimming around two kilometres through a shark-infested thick soup with the currents of a swirling ocean to finally reach a treasure chest (that needs unlocking!) in an underwater cave – all without prior fitness training. It's quite an incredible feat.

Sperm cells measure on average around 50µm in length (0.0000005cm – tiny!) and they have to swim over a thousand times their own body length to reach an egg. Most don't make it that far. Of the millions of sperm in a normal ejaculate, only a few hundred reach the fallopian tube. They swim at speed first through the cervix, then up the uterus and, finally (for some), into the fallopian tube, enduring the changing environments of different parts of the female reproductive tract along the way.

They first encounter the hostile, acidic pH of the vagina before passing through the cervix, where they face the cervical mucus challenge – a day or two late and the oestrogen-induced slippery fertile mucus that allows the passage of sperm is gone, to be replaced by a thicker mucus brought on by increasing progesterone following ovulation, a mucus that is difficult for sperm to penetrate.

If timing is right and they do progress, the sperm cells then enter the uterus to face the biochemical army of an immune response and varying 'currents' of the uterine fluid. Once inside the uterus they have to find their way through the two tiny openings (ostia) that allow passage from the uterus into the fallopian tubes, where, all being well, one should find and fertilise the egg.

It's no wonder, then, that sperm quality is needed for good fertility: it's survival of the fittest. Sperm are also the only cells that are 'designed' to function outside the human body, and the success of these unique cells involves a number of tightly controlled regulatory processes that all need to work well in order to produce a high number of cells with the right shape that can also swim well and fast. It is the swimming ability of sperm that allows an embryologist to select a sperm for intracytoplasmic sperm injection (ICSI – see Chapter 18) when needed for male factor fertility issues.

An incredible synchrony between man and woman is also needed. Recent research shows that the egg releases chemical signals that attract particular sperm over others.[1] These chemicals come from the follicular fluid that is released along with the oocyte at the time of ovulation and they increase the chance of fertilisation occurring. What is interesting is that it seems eggs may select sperm that is more genetically compatible, meaning that partner compatibility at a genetic level may be a factor in the fertility of a heterosexual couple.

How common is male infertility?

Given the level of performance needed for a sperm cell to successfully reach an egg, it isn't surprising that male factor contribution to difficulty conceiving is significant. In terms of the burden of infertility, data suggests that around one in three cases of subfertility is solely male factor.[2] Approximately one in three is a combination of male and female factor. This means that up to two-thirds of cases involve male factor that is currently untreated.

These days, the only medical treatment for male factor infertility is *in vitro* fertilisation (IVF) or ICSI, meaning that women have to undergo invasive medical treatment that carries a degree of risk and side effects, sometimes for reasons that have nothing to do with their own health. There is also growing evidence that paternal diet and other environmental factors impact not only sperm quality, but also early embryonic development, overall pregnancy outcomes and the health of the baby through into adulthood.[3] It is therefore vital to understand what can be done to address the underlying causes of male as well as female fertility issues in order to optimise sperm health even for healthy men.

If the fertility of the couple is thoroughly assessed in this way, it may reduce the need for medical intervention, increase the prospect of treatment success where needed and protect the health of the baby. Of course, there are medical conditions that need treatment and underlying genetic factors that can't be changed, so it is vital for all men to have a thorough medical investigation, but for all cases where a male partner is providing the sperm (rather than donor sperm), it is worth optimising diet, nutrient status and underlying health to put you in the best place possible for a successful outcome.

Sperm production

Sperm is continually formed in the testes in a process called spermatogenesis, which lasts approximately three months. Unlike women's eggs, men's sperm are not as old as the man and newly produced sperm is only ever three months old. However, male fertility does also decline with age but to a lesser degree. The decline is also much less clear with men but includes a longer time to conceive generally, more losses due to things like miscarriage, greater need for ICSI during fertility treatment and lower chance of success with IVF for men older than 50. It also depends on the age of the female partner or egg donor as a younger woman's eggs can correct sperm defects during early embryonic development.

Semen analysis

If you haven't conceived after regular intercourse for a year, one of the important early investigations for a heterosexual couple is a semen analysis via your GP (for details see Chapter 13). This will tell you whether male factors are contributing to this delay. It is important for both of you to be investigated to ensure your fertility as a couple is assessed. Knowing there are problems with female fertility, for instance, should not mean you do not have the appropriate male investigations.

WHAT HAS AN IMPACT ON MALE FERTILITY?

Because sperm is constantly being turned over in the testes, it is very responsive to lifestyle factors such as diet, exercise, excess alcohol and smoking (see page 141). Even stress has been shown to impact semen quality, though it's not clear if this has a meaningful effect on male fertility.[4] All of these things can affect the parameters that are tested in a semen analysis and a good score does not guarantee overall sperm health and likelihood of conception.

Other factors that are actually more associated with IVF success that are not routinely tested include DNA damage, epigenetic changes and oxidative stress. Equally, a poor score on a semen analysis does not preclude getting pregnant, but does mean it's likely it will be more difficult and indicates that there are underlying problems. It only takes one good sperm from an ejaculate of millions to fertilise an oocyte, so the link between male fertility and sperm quality and quantity is not well understood. Sperm factors that impact IVF success can, however, be improved by dietary and lifestyle factors, and while this certainly isn't the only story when it comes to male infertility, we always recommend working together as a couple to achieve the best outcome (see Chapters 2 through to 7).

Let's now go through the main factors that influence sperm quality.

Oxidative stress

Oxidative stress arises as a result of normal functioning of the body, but causes problems when there is an excess of the reactive oxygen species (ROS) produced (see page 199). Oxidative stress may be caused by smoking, alcohol, being overweight, environmental pollutants, infection, chronic disease, autoimmunity and possibly also the presence of a varicocele (an enlargement of the veins within the testes). Protective antioxidants and certain supplements have been used to combat the effects of ROS, including co-enzyme Q10, folate, vitamins B_6, B_{12}, C, E, zinc and selenium. We will look at these later in the chapter.

Exercise

Sedentary lifestyles negatively impact sperm quality. One study showed that 30 minutes of moderate- to high-intensity exercise improved sperm parameters in previously sedentary men.[5] Sperm quality declined again about a week after exercise stopped; therefore it is important to maintain a programme of exercise in the long term.

Extreme exercise can have a negative effect due to increased oxidative stress in the testes, so triathletes and professional sportsmen may find their sperm is in need of some TLC. Furthermore, tight-fitting Lycra shorts may also have a detrimental effect so loose-fitting shorts or jogging bottoms are better.

Nutrition

Appropriate nutrition is essential for good sperm production. Junk food diets have been shown to negatively affect sperm health and a poor diet during adolescence can have lasting effects. The same dietary guidance applies to men in terms of the Mediterranean diet and the other principles outlined in Chapter 3.

The two main differences for men are:

1. Low-fat dairy seems to be better for male fertility.

2. Soy may have a negative effect, so vegans need to be careful not to overconsume foods such as tofu.

Foods that have evidence to suggest benefits for sperm health include:

- olive oil (a good natural source of vitamin E)

- nuts including walnuts, almonds, hazelnuts and brazil nuts

- tomato juice and cooked tomatoes (high in the antioxidant lycopene)

- carrots (high in beta-carotene)

- avocados (high in vitamins and essential fatty acids)

- fruit for its vitamin C content (especially berries)

- dark chocolate or raw cacao (high in antioxidants)

- coconut water

- pomegranate juice to reduce oxidative stress and increase sperm count, and pomegranate oil to increase mobility

- beetroot juice: while there isn't direct evidence that beetroot juice improves erectile dysfunction, given the wider benefits for general health including increased blood flow, this is one glass of red that you can share safe in the knowledge the overall result is likely to be a small boost to general health – without the hangover the next day

It is also important to keep well-hydrated. The bulk of daily fluid intake should come from water, with excess caffeine and fizzy drinks not recommended.

EATING NUTS

A well-conducted trial found that daily consumption of 60g of nuts (a mixture of almonds, hazelnuts and walnuts) for 12 weeks improved the DNA fragmentation (damage) in sperm compared with a control group not eating nuts.[6]

A recent study found that the male partners of women who had experienced three or more miscarriages were significantly more likely to have greater levels of sperm DNA fragmentation than the partners of women who had not had a miscarriage.[7] We are not suggesting that eating nuts will cure cases of recurrent miscarriage, but it is certainly significant if there is an easy, natural and healthy option that may improve one factor that is contributing to what is a very distressing medical problem.

Do you need to supplement?

There is a growing body of evidence to support the potential benefit of certain supplements to improve semen, though with mixed results. Some research does suggest that supplements may improve fertilisation and pregnancy rates during IVF treatment, especially where there is a male factor fertility issue or previous failed IVF cycles.[8] However, there is considerable variability between studies in terms of supplements used, the outcomes measured and the men included in the trials. Overall, it's important to ensure sufficiency of all micronutrients to optimise reproductive function. Some of the nutrients that are especially important for men are vitamin D, folate, selenium, manganese, copper and zinc. However, we advise caution so as not to take excessive amounts or supplements that are not needed. It is much better to start with diet and lifestyle before trying different supplements. This means eliminating sources of oxidative stress in terms of junk food and excess weight (see Chapters 3 and 6) before you try to use supplements as a sticking plaster.

We strongly recommend that you get nutrient levels tested prior to taking supplements and that you seek professional advice to ensure you are following the most appropriate regimen for you. We often see male partners mirroring the deficiencies of their female partner, especially for vitamin D, as couples often have similar diets and lifestyles, including sun exposure, so always pay attention where one of you shows as being low in a particular nutrient on testing, as it is likely your other half will be similarly depleted.

In terms of antioxidants, given that sperm is so sensitive to oxidative stress and numerous studies show a benefit in healthy volunteers, it is likely to be safe for most men to take a low-level combined antioxidant supplement.[9] The danger lies with young, healthy men taking very high amounts of different compounds. For men who are overweight, older than 40, have a diagnosed sperm problem (see Chapter 13) or previous failed IVF or IVF with ICSI treatment, it is likely to be safe to take higher amounts of antioxidant supplements. We do not have sufficient evidence to make universal recommendations in terms of amounts, however, as more research is needed. Protective antioxidants include the enzymes superoxide dismutase, catalase and glutathione peroxidase together with ascorbic acid (vitamin C), alpha-tocopherol (vitamin E), glutathione, albumin, carnitine, carotenoids, flavonoids, urate, proteasome modulators and the amino acids taurine and hypotaurine. Certain supplements have been used to combat the effects of ROS, including co-enzyme Q10, folate, vitamins B_6, B_{12}, C, E, zinc and selenium.

A recent review of the evidence found that 26 studies reported a benefit from taking antioxidant supplements on semen parameters, the outcomes of fertility treatments and the numbers going on to have a healthy baby.[10] The most commonly studied supplements were vitamin E, vitamin C, carnitines, co-enzyme Q10, N-acetyl cysteine, lycopene, folic acid, selenium and zinc. These are not our recommendations, however, and other reviews highlight the need for further research. We therefore advise seeking professional advice before taking supplements and take a personalised rather than generic approach.

A NOTE ON CAFFEINE

Evidence looking at the impact of caffeine on male fertility is very mixed with some studies showing no effect on IVF outcomes, but some showing a longer time to pregnancy associated with male caffeine intake.[11] Some studies indicate that caffeinated fizzy drinks are more harmful to male fertility than tea and coffee.[12] However, one study also showed that moderate caffeine intake from tea and coffee (slightly less than three cups per day) was associated with more DNA damage in sperm.[13] Therefore, we recommend limiting tea and coffee to no more than two cups daily for men. For the rest of the day, try herbal teas and hot water with lemon juice for your hot drinks.

Oestrogens

An increase in oestrogen levels caused by the typical Western diet, which is high in animal fats, proteins and refined carbohydrates, can also have an impact on male sexual development. Cow's milk contains substantial amounts of oestrogens, indeed more than half of British cows that are farmed for their milk are pregnant. A number of plant foods (e.g. soy and seeds) also contain weak oestrogens (phyto-oestrogens). Synthetic oestrogens (found in the contraceptive pill) have not only been ingested by women but may also find their way into drinking water.

Weight

Being overweight has been shown in numerous studies to have an impact on male reproductive health and spermatogenesis.[14] Having an elevated body mass index (BMI) lowers testosterone levels, for instance, which has many adverse health effects in men, including reducing sperm quality. Men who are significantly overweight may also have problems with sexual function due to lower testosterone. Despite these effects, scrutiny of the available evidence has failed to demonstrate clear associations between male BMI and standard semen parameters and much more research is needed.

Gut health, sperm and the microbiome

Although this is an understudied area in terms of male fertility, the impact of the gut microbiota on general health is just as relevant for men as it is for women. Good digestion is important for the absorption of nutrients from food, metabolic health and avoiding inflammation.

Men with coeliac disease have been found to have sperm with poor morphology and motility, so testing in cases of male as well as female subfertility is also warranted. We therefore recommend any digestive symptoms are investigated and you follow the principles to support a healthy gut microbiota outlined in Chapter 7.

There is also growing research on the importance of the seminal microbiome and this has shown that men had improved sperm health after taking probiotic supplements.[15]

Sleep

Sleep is important for male general health and fertility. Testosterone levels are affected by sleep, which in turn affects semen production.

Studies have shown that men falling asleep after midnight have higher sperm antibodies than men who slept earlier.[16] Poor-quality and insufficient sleep have been shown to affect sperm quality and reduce testicle size. A Danish study found that men who had late nights, woke frequently in the night or struggled to get off to sleep had a 25 per cent lower sperm count than men who experienced good-quality sleep.[17] Shift work is also associated with poorer sperm quality.

Alcohol

Men may be a little dismayed to learn that even low levels of alcohol consumption can damage sperm production. A Danish study of 1,200 men found just 5 units reduced sperm quality, with the more alcohol consumed, the worse the sperm count and morphology.[18] A very strongly negative effect was observed in men who drank 25 units or more in a week, which equates to 2.5 bottles of wine or 12.5 pints of beer. This may sound a lot, but it's surprising how alcohol consumption can creep up. It's very easy for a regular beer or glass of wine to build up to the point that it exceeds a healthy level.

Relatively low levels of male alcohol consumption is associated with reduced success of IVF, with one study showing a daily beer reduced chances of having a baby after treatment.[19] Excessive alcohol also lowers testosterone and exacerbates erectile dysfunction. A recent study found that low testosterone is also independently associated with reduced IVF success even where sperm itself is healthy.[20] Many IVF clinics will advise a cut-off of between ten and twelve units per week as this is the point many deem alcohol to have a negative impact. However, particularly for men with pre-existing sperm dysfunction, keeping alcohol to below five units per week is worth the investment. Men with oligospermia (low sperm count) should either reduce the amount they drink to below five units or stop altogether.

These changes may take at least three months to start to translate into demonstrable improvements in a semen analysis, and even then the change may be gradual. The sooner you make the changes, the better.

Smoking

Perhaps obviously, cigarette smoking impairs fertility. Both partners should stop smoking, particularly while trying to conceive. Smoking has been shown to cause an imbalance in key proteins in sperm, increase oxidative stress, damage sperm DNA and reduce sperm mitochondrial activity. Paternal smoking can also affect the health of the child and studies show that children whose fathers smoke have increased risks of adverse health outcomes including childhood cancers.[21] Some of the damage caused by smoking may not be reversible, therefore it is vital to stop smoking immediately if you are trying to conceive. Similarly, the use of e-cigarettes or vaping results in noxious chemicals entering the body and should also be avoided as research has found these substances are damaging to sperm.[22]

Cannabis

Another significant source of sperm damage is the use of recreational drugs, with cannabis smoking being particularly well researched. A recent study showed that men who smoke marijuana at least once a week have a 33 per cent lower sperm count than men who do not use the drug.[23] As well as impacting sperm health, paternal cannabis smoking has the potential to have a negative effect on the health of their children. Many clinics will not proceed with any treatments for a period of at least six months after the cessation of illicit drug use because of the potential effects on the unborn child.

Anabolic steroids

Some men use anabolic steroids to build muscle as part of their gym routine without realising they are literally shrinking their testicles. Steroids are a large group of compounds that includes the naturally occurring sex steroids (oestrogen, testosterone and other androgens, and progesterone) and corticosteroids (e.g. cortisol), which are important for dealing with stress. Androgens play a crucial role in the development of male reproductive organs such as the epididymis, vas deferens, seminal vesicles, prostate and penis.

They are necessary for puberty, male fertility and male sexual function, and they also increase muscle bulk and strength. High levels of testosterone are secreted by particular cells in the testes known as Leydig cells, where the hormone is needed for spermatogenesis.

In the same way that synthetic oestrogens act as a contraceptive in women, illicit steroids containing testosterone will switch off sperm production, ultimately causing the testes to shrink as a result. Steroid use commonly leads to temporary or persistent problems with male reproductive function and sperm quality. The damage may not be recoverable, so this is a very serious issue.

Eating disorders and body dysmorphia

An important and often overlooked factor for men is that certain conditions can sometimes fuel the desire to use these drugs for bodybuilding to the detriment of their health including body dysmorphia and eating disorders. A gym obsession can sometimes be a sign of this kind of underlying issue, as can a very intense focus on particular foods or your next meal to build up your body to the point it is constantly on your mind. Men who have mental health issues or who want to lose weight can also lapse into anorexia.

Whatever is going on at an individual level, men experience similar pressures to women to look a certain way and to be 'manly' and protect their partner when going through any kind of challenge. If you're a man going through fertility challenges, remember to take care of yourself too. Always seek support and don't feel you have to face things alone. You can speak to your GP or get help from either fertility or eating disorder support groups.

Heat

Temperature is another significant factor when it comes to male fertility. Testes descend from the warmth of the body cavity in order to keep sperm cool, thereby acting as mini-refrigerators and taking the heat out of spermatogenesis. Cycling, rowing, saunas, hot baths and electronic devices in pockets and on laps all have the potential to heat up your testes. We have seen a man with severely oligozoospermic semen recover completely when the cycling season ended, for example. His sperm count fell dramatically again a few weeks into the next season, when he resumed vigorous training. Interestingly, male athletes can also develop hypothalamic hypogonadism (impaired testicular function that affects the ability to produce sperm – see page 191) similar to the hypothalamic amenorrhea (the absence of periods caused by things like over-exercising and weight loss – see page 212) seen in sportswomen, so always be conscious of extreme levels of exercise.

Tight underwear has also been shown to negatively impact sperm. We advise boxer shorts and avoiding tight trousers, Lycra shorts and leggings. Sitting in very hot baths and saunas for long periods should be avoided. We do not, however, recommend cold showers; it's important to maintain the balance the body seeks.

Environmental toxins

As well as affecting female fertility, endocrine disrupting chemicals (EDCs) may contribute substantially to male reproductive disorders, with many studies finding that various different pesticides and toxins damage sperm.[24] As well as concerns about a global decline in sperm quality, cases of certain congenital anomalies such as hypospadias (when the urethra opens through the underside of the penis), cryptorchidism (undescended testes) and testicular cancer are rising. It is believed that environmental pollutants containing oestrogens and other toxins may be to blame. Strikingly, the impact on male fertility begins while a baby is still in his mother's womb and research has shown that EDCs such as bisphenol A (BPA) can impair development of the prostate of male embryos.[25]

Recent research into couples trying to conceive has also found that exposure to environmental toxins causes epigenetic changes in sperm that can reduce IVF success and increase the chance of miscarriage.[26] Parabens are a group of compounds that are now thought to be toxic to both male and female fertility. Parabens are preservatives that are widely used in foods, cosmetics, toiletries and medications, and have historically been viewed as non-toxic. However, they are known to have a weak estrogenic effect in the body and growing evidence contradicts the assumption that these compounds are safe, especially in terms of reproductive function. In particular, parabens are known to impact mitochondrial function in the testes.

Heavy metals are also toxic to sperm production, especially lead, cadmium and mercury, as are a number of chemicals (pesticides: dibromochloropropane, chlordecone, ethylene dibromide; glycol ethers – used in inks, paint and adhesives). It's important to be aware if you have to work in the presence of environmental toxins that can affect fertility and ensure that the area is well-ventilated and you are provided with appropriate protective clothing and respiratory protection.

There is also a growing body of evidence to suggest air pollution can also negatively impact male fertility.[27] If you live in a city or on a busy road, getting out into the countryside for exercise or avoiding exercising at rush hour can make a difference.

Here are some other steps you can take to reduce your toxic load, which can be beneficial for both male and female fertility:

- Avoid drinking water from plastic bottles and heating food in plastic containers as both of these things can be a source of BPA exposure.

- Eat organic food where possible, washing non-organic produce.

- Limit toiletries that contain phthalates and parabens and choose natural alternatives where possible.

- Ensure any heavy metal exposure is kept to a minimum, including making sure there are no lead water pipes feeding into your home water supply, and avoiding tin foil and aluminium-containing antiperspirants.

- Avoid excessive consumption of tinned foods where possible and affordable. Frozen foods are a better option than tinned (they actually retain some nutrients better than fresh food) and choose glass jars over tins where possible.

Psychological factors

Things are starting to change but, historically, men have been neglected when it comes to infertility and fertility treatment – emotionally as well as physically. We have conducted focus groups with our male patients and they tell us that it feels like 'it's all about the woman' and that there is 'nothing they can do'. This can all be incredibly disempowering for men, especially when their masculinity is literally under the microscope. This is exacerbated by the fact that society conditions men not to show their emotions and many are reluctant to make their feelings known, even to their loved ones. Men often feel they need to support their partner and that they have to be the strong one. For men reading this, please know that you are a vital part of the process and it's important that you are taken care of too. Your feelings matter and it is healthy to feel and express emotions.

The latest WHO guidance now recommends that men who are experiencing fertility problems are thoroughly assessed for general health, diet and lifestyle factors that may affect fertility and the health of their children. While it is extremely important to have the appropriate medical investigations, which are covered in the next part of the book, overall there are many things you can do yourself that have the potential to improve sperm health and fertility. Making these changes will also help improve your general health and well-being; healthier sperm not only means a healthier baby, but a healthier you, too.

PART 2

When You Need Medical Help

This next part takes you through all the steps that you need to take if you haven't been able to conceive naturally and need medical help on your fertility journey. If you think you may have a problem with your fertility then first seek the advice of a doctor who has a full understanding of reproductive health.

Chapter 11

How and When to Seek Help

A S A GENERAL rule, you should seek advice if you have been trying for a baby for more than a year. If you have irregular periods or a past history of a pelvic issue, then you might want to seek help earlier. Also if you are in your late thirties or forties it is worthwhile getting checked as soon as you decide to start trying. We believe that there is no harm in getting some simple tests done, which may be reassuring or, on the other hand, point to problems that may require help.

For most people the term 'subfertility' is more appropriate than 'infertility' as the vast majority of people attending fertility clinics have the ability to conceive naturally, it is just taking longer than it should and help may be required.

FIRST STEPS

Your GP should be the first person you contact to discuss your fertility. Most GP practices will have a website outlining their special interests; it is worthwhile speaking to a GP who has an interest in reproduction and women's health, even if this isn't your usual doctor. You may initially be seen by one of the nurses rather than the doctor – this doesn't matter as long as you see someone who understands what tests are required and when they should be done. For example, all too often we find that blood tests to measure hormones are taken at the wrong time in a woman's cycle and this makes all the difference when interpreting the results (see page

159). Most GPs can organise the basic tests for both you and your partner, so it is important that you attend together. You should also ask to be referred to the specialist infertility clinic at your local hospital.

Infertility clinics

Depending upon the size of your nearest hospital the clinic may be run by a gynaecologist with a 'special interest' in infertility or a team of reproductive medicine specialists. If your local hospital is relatively small then the clinic may be limited in what it can offer and you may be referred to a larger reproductive medicine service, which will usually be in a teaching hospital.

Infertility clinics are usually run by obstetricians and gynaecologists, who are specialists trained in all aspects of women's health and the care of women during pregnancy. Some gynaecologists have additional qualifications and accreditation in reproductive medicine, which requires several additional years of training in order to be able to manage more complex problems and provide treatments such as *in vitro* fertilisation (IVF). Specialists in reproductive medicine are also trained to know how to investigate and manage male fertility problems, even if their main qualification is as a gynaecologist, so don't worry if you see a specialist and there are problems on the male side. If the male partner requires surgery or more complex treatments then you may also be referred to an andrologist, who is usually a urologist (a consultant who deals predominantly with kidney and bladder problems) with a special interest and training in male fertility. All large reproductive medicine centres should have access to an andrologist.

The costs

In the UK you should be able to access initial investigations through the NHS. There are, however, eligibility criteria for NHS-funded fertility treatments and these vary around the UK and may depend upon factors such as your age, body mass index (BMI) and whether you or your partner have children already. Unfortunately, there is what's known as a 'postcode lottery', which we have been campaigning to abolish for many years. It's important to find out what your local eligibility criteria are so that you know where you stand.

If you are not eligible for NHS funding then you will have to self-fund. Most NHS reproductive medicine centres will also provide self-funded (or 'private') care and so you won't necessarily have to go to a private clinic. In the UK the Human Fertilisation & Embryology Authority (HFEA) licenses all IVF clinics and provides information on success rates in order to help you to make a choice. Of course, where you live will also make a difference as it is important to choose a clinic that is easily accessible as most fertility treatments require many visits to the clinic.

Facilities for fertility treatment and funding criteria vary around the world and so if you don't live in the UK it's important to check out your local situation.

The age factor

A recent study suggested that for couples who would like a 90 per cent chance of having a family of three, it's probably necessary to start trying by the age of 23.[1] For those who wish for two children, start around the age of 28, and if you wish for only one then you could wait until you are in your early thirties, say 32.

But what if you are older than this? It may take a year or so before you realise that you may have a problem, a few months to be investigated and referred to a fertility clinic, and then, if you need additional testing or treatment, time will have marched on. Unfortunately, the chance of any treatments working will decline with age as well.

As a general rule it is thought that a woman is extremely unlikely to have fertile eggs in the five years before she goes through the menopause, and in the five years before that her fertility will be significantly reduced. There are always exceptions of course. Furthermore, while IVF can be used to try to improve fertility it cannot enhance the fertility potential of the eggs. This is why the chance of conceiving with IVF drops rapidly from about the age of 37, is very low during a woman's early forties and simply doesn't work over the age of 45. Many high-profile cases of celebrities having babies in their late forties and even older will be as a result of using donated eggs (see page 205), although this isn't usually spelt out in the media articles that publicise these reports.

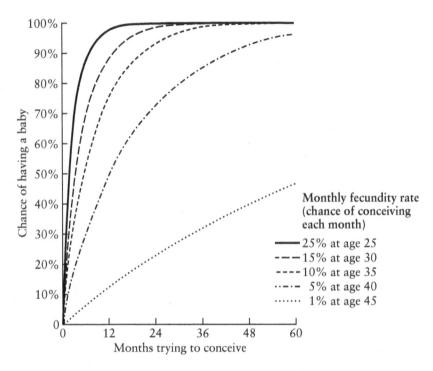

Average chance of conception over time

Weight and fertility treatments

We have already discussed how weight can impact general health and fertility for men and women (see Chapters 2 and 6). From a medical perspective, we also need to consider this in relation to how you may respond to fertility treatments. Women who are overweight respond less well to drugs that are used for ovarian stimulation for the treatment of both anovulation and assisted conception, although this does not always equate to a reduction in ongoing pregnancy rates. Also, being overweight may affect the safety of procedures, for example the ability to see ovaries on an ultrasound scan or the provision of safe anaesthesia and surgical procedures.

YOU MIGHT NEED HELP IF . . .

Guidelines for the investigation of subfertility suggest that a couple should have been trying to conceive for at least 12 months before any tests are performed. Issues that may suggest the need for earlier investigation for women include:

- having irregular cycles
- painful periods
- a history of sexually transmitted infection (STI) or pelvic infection
- previous major surgery in the abdomen or pelvis, or a history of pregnancy problems (such as miscarriage or ectopic pregnancy)

For men:

- a history of STIs
- a history of problems with development of the testes
- surgery on the testes
- surgery for an inguinal hernia
- a history of mumps after puberty

Your medical assessment will start with a series of basic investigations for both partners. These can include:

- a general health screening by your GP

- a sexual health screen

- assessments to check whether you are ovulating, including progesterone testing

- other hormone blood tests and an ultrasound scan

- a semen analysis (see page 186)

What happens next will depend on the results of your investigations. In the next two chapters we will look at what will happen medically once you seek assistance. Once the decision has been taken to commence investigations it should be possible to:

- perform basic screening tests within a month or two

- provide a management plan, which may involve reassurance, more detailed investigations or treatment

A SHARED PROCESS

We encourage you to attend the clinic together as a couple. It is our practice to send patients copies of correspondence so that they have a written record of what has been discussed. Not only does this help to avoid confusion, it also increases confidence that everyone is included in the communication 'loop'.

Chapter 12

Investigating Female Fertility

Your GP should provide general health screening and preconception counselling, including the appropriate use of preconception vitamin supplements for both you and your partner (see page 23). It is also important to ensure that you are up to date with screening for cervical cancer and that you are immune to rubella (German measles), which can cause serious developmental problems for the baby if you catch it while pregnant.

SEXUAL HEALTH SCREEN

A sexual health screen, with either blood tests or swabs looking for infections such as chlamydia, is usually performed on both partners. *Chlamydia trachomatis* infection is the commonest sexually transmitted infection (STI) in the UK and the commonest cause of damaged or blocked fallopian tubes. It often goes undiagnosed, which may cause inflammation of the cervix, tubes and endometrium in women (cervicitis, salpingitis and endometritis respectively) and in the urinary tract and parts of the testes in men. Symptoms can be mild and the majority of people with infection are asymptomatic, and therefore are not treated.

When getting tested for chlamydia, you will either have a swab of the cervix or a urine test. If chlamydia is found then there is up to a 90 per cent chance that you have damaged fallopian tubes.

The infection bacterial vaginosis (BV – see page 96) is also picked up on a swab and causes up to 50 per cent of vaginal infections, yet often goes unrecognised. BV is associated with complications following gynaecological surgery, first and second trimester miscarriage and premature labour. There is also an increased risk of miscarriage after *in vitro* fertilisation (IVF) in women found to have BV.

You may be tested for BV by your fertility clinic, though many doctors prescribe routine antibiotics during IVF treatment as a prophylaxis against infections, and this will also treat BV if present.

A blood test to assess hepatitis B and C and HIV status is also required before proceeding with assisted conception treatments.

ASSESSMENT OF OVULATION

If your menstrual cycle is regular (it doesn't vary by more than a couple of days either side of a cycle length of between 23 and 35 days), it is likely that you are ovulating. The first part or follicular phase of the cycle is when the egg-containing follicle grows in readiness for the release of a mature egg (oocyte). This phase of the cycle can vary in length from about 9 to 21 days, and is only 14 days in a 28-day cycle (see Chapter 1 for more on this).

Ways to check for ovulation at home

It is important to have an idea of your 'fertile window' – that is the time in your cycle when it is most likely that you can conceive (see page 60). There are also ways of testing whether you are ovulating at home:

- **Basal body temperature (BBT):** some women like to check their BBT every morning at home with a sensitive thermometer. The rationale behind the use of BBT measurements is that progesterone, released after ovulation, will raise the BBT by 0.2–0.4°C, although between 10 and 75 per cent of ovulatory cycles fail to show an adequate rise in BBT. A 'flat' chart therefore does not necessarily mean you haven't ovulated, and we therefore don't recommend their routine use. Furthermore, they can cause stress without telling you in advance when you are going to ovulate.

156

- **Cervical mucus:** you can monitor your cervical mucus to predict when it is receptive to sperm (the so-called 'Billings method'). This can be used to determine the best time to get pregnant.

- **Mid-cycle pain:** you may be also aware of pelvic discomfort (*mittelschmerz*) around the time of ovulation and this can also be used as a guide to when to have sex. The discomfort is usually felt on the side of ovulation and is nothing to worry about – it is probably caused by a combination of the ovary being swollen by the egg-containing follicle and the release of fluid from the follicle at the time of ovulation. It is interesting that ovaries ovulate on alternate sides more often in young women, while those over 40 years of age are more likely to have successive ovulations from the same ovary.

- **Home testing kits:** you can also buy ovulation detection kits to use at home. These kits test for hormones in the urine. The simplest way to test is by measuring luteinising hormone (LH) in the urine to identify the pre-ovulatory surge and help predict when to have sex, so that sperm is waiting for the egg when it is released. We recommend that you calculate your anticipated 'fertile window' (see page 61) and start testing your urine the day before. Some advocate testing urine morning and evening, but this is probably more than is required and so a morning check on its own is fine. The most advanced monitors measure both oestradiol and LH in the urine and can be expensive. Women with polycystic ovary syndrome (PCOS) may produce a high level of LH and so can have false positive results when using kits.

- **Menstrual cycle regularity:** if your menstrual cycle is regular (frequency of 23–35 days, with no more than 2–3 days' variation each month), there's a greater than 95 per cent chance that you are ovulating, so the use of BBT charts or urinary testing kits has limited value. Up to 75 per cent of women with an erratic cycle are also found to be ovulating. Therefore, for most women, the most important thing is to have regular sex during their cycle. This is good for your relationship and also for the health of sperm – long gaps between ejaculations may lead to poorer quality sperm, which is produced daily and declines in function the longer it is stored. For the best-quality sperm, it's best to have sex every two to three days in the follicular phase of the cycle and, if possible, daily for two to three days at the predicted time of ovulation. Try to avoid timed intercourse 'to order'.

- **Menstrual cycle length:** the luteal phase (second half) of the cycle can last for between 10 and 17 days. Sometimes it is shorter, but usually this happens at random and is not due to a repeated problem with the secretion of progesterone. Some specialists have described the concept of 'luteal phase deficiency' (LPD), but this is somewhat controversial medically as there is no evidence that giving hormone treatment for additional 'luteal support', with either progesterone or human chorionic gonadotrophin (hCG), improves pregnancy rates in natural cycles.

Testing for ovulation with your doctor

To check whether you are ovulating, your doctor will test the level of progesterone in your blood. If it's greater than 30nmol/L, this suggests you are ovulating, although the only real way to know for certain that an egg is released is if a pregnancy occurs. It is difficult to know when to take the blood if a woman has an erratic cycle – and impossible if she has no periods at all (amenorrhoeic). If the progesterone is 15–30nmol/L it is likely that ovulation has occurred, but the timing of the test may have been incorrect. It is then necessary to check the timing of the blood test in relation to the date of your next period and repeat the test in the following cycle (sometimes two progesterone measurements in the same cycle are helpful).

Your GP should be able to arrange the measurement of progesterone. Sometimes a fertility clinic may also arrange a combination of serial ultrasound scans and hormone measurements (follicle-stimulating hormone (FSH) and LH in the early follicular phase and progesterone in the luteal phase). The combination of a corpus luteum seen on ultrasound and an elevated serum progesterone concentration provides the best possible evidence of ovulation, although only a pregnancy will confirm that an egg was actually released from the follicle.

OTHER HORMONE BLOOD TESTS AND ULTRASOUND SCAN

In addition to progesterone, your initial investigations will usually include a series of hormone blood tests, known as a baseline hormone (endocrine) profile, and an ultrasound scan. The hormone profile is best done during the first three days of your cycle and includes tests for FSH, LH and oestradiol. The assessment of anti-Müllerian hormone (AMH) as a measure of ovarian reserve, however, is not cycle-dependent (see page 160). The normal reference range for a particular hormone may vary depending on the laboratory as the type of testing kit can differ between labs. This means the reference ranges may differ too, which makes it difficult to describe normal values.

If a woman is either not having periods (amenorrhea) or having infrequent periods (oligomenorrhea), a random blood sample has to be taken and is best repeated once or twice at intervals of at least a week in order to get an idea as to what's going on. Hormone blood tests together with a pelvic ultrasound scan, to assess how your ovaries are working and the thickness of your endometrium, will together usually be enough to make a diagnosis.

TESTING OVARIAN RESERVE

It's not possible to count the numbers of eggs within the ovaries without removing a whole ovary or taking a surgical biopsy – neither of which are practicable! We therefore have to estimate your 'ovarian reserve' by measuring hormones in the blood. For many years, FSH was measured to give an indication of how the ovary is working. An ovary that is functioning efficiently only needs a little FSH to keep it ticking over. An ageing or inefficient ovary, on the other hand, needs more FSH to stimulate the growth of follicles and so the level of FSH goes up as ovarian reserve goes down and age increases. In recent years we have had a more direct marker of ovarian reserve in the form of AMH, which declines with falling ovarian reserve. We therefore tend to measure AMH rather than FSH, when the test is available (see below).

Testing follicle-stimulating hormone (FSH)

FSH is often still measured, however, and high levels indicate lower ovarian reserve. Generally, if FSH is higher than 10IU/L on more than one occasion, the ovaries are unlikely to be ovulating eggs with a good fertility potential. A woman with an elevated FSH will not respond as well to ovarian stimulation as the drugs contain FSH as the active ingredient. When the serum concentration of FSH is above 15IU/L the chance of releasing a fertile egg is slim and levels greater than 25IU/L are suggestive of the menopause or premature ovarian insufficiency (POI – see chapter 24, page 329).

Even if ovulation is occurring when serum FSH is high, the fertility potential of the egg within the follicle is unfortunately significantly impaired. This means that even when fertilisation does happen, there is a higher chance of a chromosomally abnormal embryo developing, which in turn increases the risk of miscarriage and chromosomal abnormality in the fetus.

Antral follicle count (AFC) and anti-Müllerian hormone (AMH)

As well as FSH, you may have other tests in order to get a clearer picture of your ovarian reserve. This includes measuring the volume of your ovaries (which goes down with age and ovarian reserve), counting the number of small antral follicles on an ultrasound scan (the AFC) and testing AMH in the blood. It has even been suggested that these tests may help determine a woman's future fertility over forthcoming years – although the evidence for longer term predictions is still to be conclusively confirmed and there is debate about the widespread use of ovarian reserve testing outside of the context of planning infertility treatment (see page 260).

The main thing that affects ovarian reserve is age, although the rate of ovarian ageing can vary significantly from person to person. The transition from normal fertility to subfertility, sterility and then menopause is individually based on your genetic predisposition, combined with lifestyle and environmental factors. How your ovaries respond to stimulation during fertility treatment is the ultimate test of how they are functioning, but you only find this out after the event. Predicting how your ovaries might respond to stimulation based on measurements of ovarian reserve (see below) is one of the most important aspects of your fertility treatment. We use these measurements to decide how much of a particular drug is needed to get the best possible result. This is part of what is known as your stimulation protocol (see page 256). Women with a 'normal' ovarian reserve should ideally develop 8–15 follicles, with a corresponding number of oocytes, during routine stimulation for IVF.

Measuring AFC

When you have a pelvic ultrasound scan, the number of antral follicles in each ovary will be counted (see below). The total number of follicles in both ovaries visible on the scan is your AFC. AFC is a good predictor of poor ovarian response to stimulation for IVF and similar to a measurement of AMH because it is these visible follicles that produce AMH.

Testing AMH

AMH is produced by the ovarian follicles and appears to be a better indicator of how many follicles you have left (ovarian reserve) than FSH, partly because it does not fluctuate through the menstrual cycle. A higher AMH means you are more likely to get more mature eggs, embryos and clinical pregnancies during IVF treatment. Furthermore, women with polycystic ovaries have more follicles and higher AMH levels than those with normal ovaries, and so measuring AMH has been proposed as the best way to assess polycystic ovaries using a blood test.

Levels of AMH reduce slowly over time and so having repeat blood tests, say at 12-month intervals, may be useful as a long-term predictor of how your ovarian reserve is changing over time. This kind of repeat testing can be useful in assessing your reproductive health generally and possibly also to predict the age of menopause.

A hot debate in the fertility sector in recent years has been whether a measurement of AMH or AFC is best – we tend to measure both. They are actually very similar in being able to predict both the response of ovaries to stimulation during IVF treatment and the likely number of eggs that will be collected. The ovarian reserve and number of eggs also correlates with their fertility potential – in other words, the chance of an egg fertilising and developing into a healthy embryo. This isn't a hard and fast correlation as a woman's age also has a significant bearing on this – a young woman with a low AMH is still likely to have better quality or more fertile eggs than an older woman with the same measure of AMH.

Ultimately, the ovarian reserve tests give a guide rather than an exact prediction of fertility. It is only when a woman's ovaries are stimulated for IVF and the eggs collected that a more accurate assessment of egg quality can be made by then looking at the rate of fertilisation of the eggs and the subsequent embryo development. It is not possible to assess the genetic make-up of an egg without destroying the egg, but it is possible to assess the genetic make-up of an embryo by taking a biopsy of the cells (see page 303).

Unfortunately at the moment there are no proven treatments that can slow down, halt or reverse the ovarian ageing process, despite some claims that have been made about various drugs and other therapies, but you can eliminate habits that are known to be harmful, such as smoking (see page 22).

TESTING LUTEINISING HORMONE (LH)

Depending on your symptoms and results of other blood tests, LH is sometimes measured. LH is released from the same cells in the pituitary gland as FSH, under the influence of gonadotrophin-releasing hormone (GnRH), which is released in pulses from the hypothalamus at the base of the brain. LH secretion by the pituitary is very sensitive to the levels of oestrogen in the blood. When oestrogen levels are low, for example in a woman who is under-weight, LH levels in the circulation are lower than FSH, while the surge of LH (and FSH) that happens before ovulation is primed by rising oestradiol secretion from the ovary (see page 169).

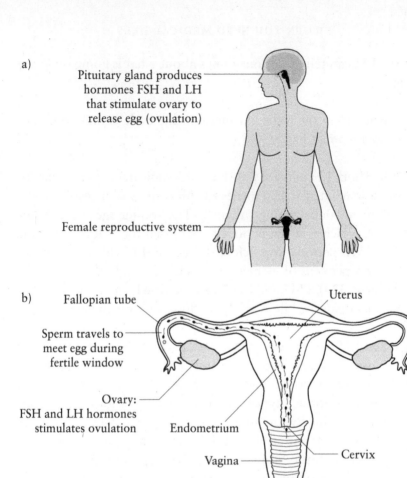

a)

Pituitary gland produces hormones FSH and LH that stimulate ovary to release egg (ovulation)

Female reproductive system

b)

Fallopian tube

Uterus

Sperm travels to meet egg during fertile window

Ovary: FSH and LH hormones stimulates ovulation

Endometrium

Vagina

Cervix

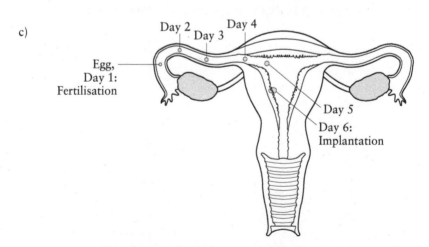

c)

Day 2

Day 3

Day 4

Egg, Day 1: Fertilisation

Day 5

Day 6: Implantation

Female reproductive system and the journey to conception;
a) Hormones stimulate ovulation; b) Sperm fertilises egg;
c) Egg travels to uterus and implants

Testing LH can tell us various things about what is going on in the body:

- When LH in the follicular phase of the cycle is high, this suggests a woman has PCOS.

- When both LH and FSH are high, this indicates either the menopause in women in their forties and fifties or ovarian insufficiency/failure in women younger than 40. The average age of the menopause, which is when periods have ceased for at least a year, is 51. When periods stop before the age of 40 (which happens in about 5 per cent of women), this is known as POI (see chapter 24, page 329). FSH and LH levels rise slowly in the years before the menopause while AMH goes down as women get older.

- When LH is very low (usually < 2IU/L or below the range of the assay) along with very low FSH, periods are usually absent (amenorrhea) and this combination of results suggests a non-functioning hypothalamus or pituitary gland, or hypogonadotrophic hypogonadism (see page 196). Gonadotrophin (that is FSH and LH) measurements are best interpreted together with the findings of a pelvic ultrasound scan as the combination of ovarian appearance, endometrial thickness (as a reflection of oestrogenisation) and serum oestradiol levels allows us to make a diagnosis in most cases.

HOW HORMONES CHANGE IN DIFFERENT CAUSES OF ANOVULATION

FOLLICLE-STIMULATING HORMONE	LUTEINISING HORMONE	OESTRADIOL (OESTROGEN)	DIAGNOSIS
Normal	Elevated or normal	Normal	PCOS
Normal or slightly low	Low	Low	Hypothalamic amenorrhea, due to being underweight or over-exercising
Low	Low	Low	Hypothalamic amenorrhea, due to hypogonadotrophic hypogonadism. Pituitary failure
Elevated	Elevated	Low	Ovarian insufficiency (failure)
Elevated	Elevated	High	Possible pre-ovulatory surge

TESTING ANDROGENS

Another test that you may have is for the androgen hormones – predominantly testosterone. Androgen hormones are secreted by both the testes and the ovaries. Androgens are steroid hormones and there are different ways in which one hormone is converted that can affect the normal balance of these vital substances in the blood. Oestrogen is made from testosterone, for instance, and so all women have some testosterone in their blood just as all men have some oestrogen. The blood test is looking for changes in the balance between the different hormones.

The normal female range for total serum testosterone (T) depends on how it is tested. Normal T is 0.5–3.5nmol/L when measured by traditional methods, but should be less than 1.8nmol/L when a newer way of testing (mass spectroscopy) is used. You need to know the normal range for your particular test so that you can understand your results.

Androgen blood tests that fall outside the normal range can give us further information about your reproductive health:

- The most usual cause of high testosterone is PCOS. Most women with PCOS, however, have a normal T level (about 70 per cent in our experience). If you also have your sex hormone binding globulin (SHBG) tested (normal range 16–119nmol/L), your doctor can calculate your 'free androgen index' (FAI) [(T x 100)/SHBG], which should be less than 5. Being overweight can often mean the FAI is high while the total testosterone is in the normal range.

- The level of testosterone in your blood fluctuates, with higher levels in the morning, in the luteal phase of the menstrual cycle and in summer compared with winter. Levels also decline gradually with age.

- A very high testosterone result means your doctor has to check you don't have other rare conditions that cause androgen excess. These include late-onset congenital adrenal hyperplasia (CAH), Cushing's syndrome and androgen-secreting tumours. We do this by measuring other types of androgen hormones. Late-onset CAH can be mistaken for PCOS and is rare in the UK, but more common in some Mediterranean populations and Ashkenazi Jews.

- Tests for other androgen hormones are not usually part of routine testing but include 17-hydroxyprogesterone, dehydroepiandrosterone sulfate (DHEA-S) and androstenedione. If levels are very high your doctor would then need to ensure you don't have a tumour of the ovaries or adrenal glands. This is checked by ultra-sound or computed tomography (CT) scans.

THYROID FUNCTION

As well as testing sex hormones, a fertility clinic will test your thyroid hormones as thyroid disease is common in women, and even mild disturbances of thyroid function may have a profound effect on fertility and the health of a pregnancy. Women often have no symptoms with thyroid disease; 'biochemical hypothyroidism' is when the hormone levels are outside of the normal range in the absence of any symptoms.

The thyroid gland, situated in the neck, secretes thyroxine, which is a hormone needed for the health of most bodily functions. It is especially important for the normal growth and development of the fetus, including, most significantly, the fetal brain. You need sufficient iodine in your diet to produce thyroxine and getting enough before you conceive is especially important (see page 53). The production of thyroxine is stimulated by thyroid-stimulating hormone (TSH), which is produced by the pituitary gland. If the thyroid becomes underactive, the pituitary secretes greater amounts of TSH to ensure that enough thyroxine is made.

When you have a thyroid screen, tests are conducted and interpreted as follows:

- As a starting point, your TSH (range 0.5–4.0U/L) will be tested to assess thyroid function.

- If TSH is elevated, this suggests an underactive thyroid (hypothyroidism). In this case, measuring free thyroxine (T_4) (9–22pmol/L) as well as TSH is helpful.

- If you have an overactive thyroid (hyperthyroidism), your TSH will be low and free T_4 will usually be elevated.

- If the free T_4 is normal, then free tri-iodothyronine (T_3) (4.3–8.6pmol/L) is measured.

While a TSH level of less than 4.0U/L is required for general health, many reproduction specialists have historically considered a level of less than 2.5U/L necessary for good reproductive health, with a higher level being associated with a reduced chance of having an ongoing pregnancy.

We therefore advise as follows:

- If the measurement of TSH is greater than 2.5 we suggest that it is repeated and thyroid autoantibodies measured.

- If TSH is still elevated after retesting, a low dose of thyroxine medication is recommended.

It is essential that thyroid disease is treated and thyroid function stabilised prior to conception. Hypothyroidism in particular is very bad for the developing baby.

TESTING PROLACTIN

You may have your levels of prolactin tested as part of your fertility investigations, particularly if you have irregular periods. The hormone prolactin causes the breasts to make milk and increases during pregnancy and breastfeeding. Mild elevations in prolactin levels may be associated with stress and may occur simply as a result of having blood taken. Prolactin levels vary day to day and, if elevated to more than 1,000mU/L, the test should be repeated. If levels are still high, you will need further investigations, including magnetic resonance imaging (MRI) of the pituitary gland. If you have slightly raised prolactin levels, this can indicate PCOS or hypothyroidism.

TESTING OESTROGEN

While oestrogen is an extremely important hormone for female health and for the normal development of the endometrium, measuring it isn't that helpful when investigating infertility. The main form of oestrogen is oestradiol and levels tend to be at their lowest during days 1–3 of the cycle (usually less than 100pmol/L). Levels then start to rise with follicular growth. At the time of ovulation, levels are usually 500–1,000pmol/L, but can vary quite widely.

If you have absent or irregular periods, it's often more helpful to have an ultrasound scan, both to look at the appearance of your ovaries and to assess the thickness of your endometrium. If you have low levels of oestrogen, your endometrium will be thin and it will only thicken in the presence of oestrogen. The number of follicles in the ovaries also gives more of a clue as to what is going on.

THE PELVIC ULTRASOUND SCAN

A pelvic ultrasound scan is an extremely important part of your initial investigations to look at both the uterus and ovaries. Most GPs can order this test at the start of investigations, although sometimes it isn't done until after the first hospital visit.

You may initially have a transabdominal scan, where the ultrasound probe is placed on the abdomen together with ultrasound jelly, which helps the person scanning to see the internal organs, including, if necessary, the kidneys and other structures in the abdomen. You will need to have a full bladder when you have a transabdominal scan. This helps to ensure the images are clear. This can be quite uncomfortable and so in the fertility clinic a transvaginal scan is usually performed, with a probe placed within the vagina to look at the pelvic organs. A transvaginal scan also provides clearer images of the pelvic structures.

Not all women will need further assessment after a pelvic ultrasound scan, but it's helpful to understand exactly what your specialist is looking for so that you have confidence that you're having everything you need in terms of investigations and are able to recognise the relevance of any symptoms.

Transabdominal ultrasound

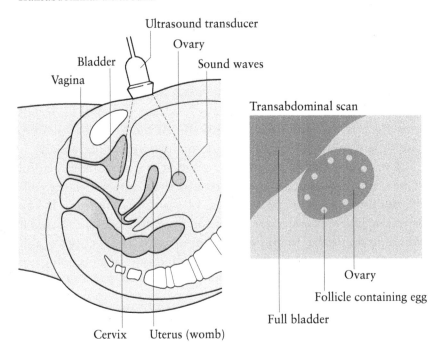

Ultrasound transducer

Ovary

Bladder

Sound waves

Vagina

Transabdominal scan

Ovary

Follicle containing egg

Full bladder

Cervix   Uterus (womb)

Transvaginal ultrasound

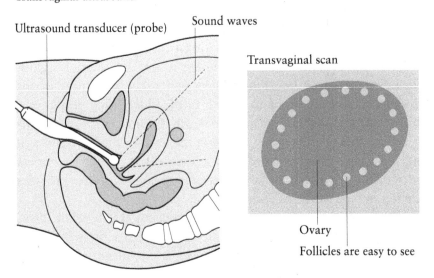

Ultrasound transducer (probe)   Sound waves

Transvaginal scan

Ovary

Follicles are easy to see

Differences between transabdominal and transvaginal ultrasounds

Ovarian appearance (morphology)

Your ovaries can vary considerably in appearance, depending upon your age and the stage in the menstrual cycle, and these factors are taken into consideration when you have a scan.

One of the most important things we look at in terms of your fertility is the number and size of your follicles (see page 161). We can see the small, antral follicles when they reach a certain size (around 2mm in diameter) and several of these are usually visible during a normal cycle. Only one usually grows to become the dominant follicle (about 10mm) and the others fade away. The dominant follicle continues to grow until it is about 20–25mm and, when it reaches this size, the egg is released during ovulation. Once it has released the egg, the follicle then changes to the 'corpus luteum', which produces progesterone.

The number of follicles that can be seen on your scan will depend on your age and how well your ovaries are working. The number of follicles also gives an indication of your ovarian reserve (see page 160). Sometimes more follicles are visible than expected:

- **Multicystic ovaries** can be seen in girls around the time of puberty and also in women recovering from amenorrhea caused by weight loss. These multicystic (or multifollicular) ovaries are normal in size or slightly bigger and usually have six or more medium-sized follicles (also – incorrectly – referred to in these conditions as 'cysts') that are 4–10mm in diameter. This happens when the normal growth pattern of follicles is disrupted because the woman isn't having a normal cycle with regular ovulation.

- **Polycystic ovaries** have at least 20 cysts (2–9mm in diameter) throughout the ovary. The volume of the ovary can be double that of a normal ovary (more than 10ml (cm^3) compared to about 5ml of a normal ovary). The follicles or 'cysts' of the polycystic ovary do have the potential to grow and ovulate when exposed to the right hormonal signals.

Ovarian cysts

As well as an AFC and a careful assessment of ovarian morphology, you will also be checked for potential problems such as ovarian cysts, fibroids and polyps during your baseline ultrasound scan (see also Chapter 16).

After an egg is released, the remaining part of the follicle – the corpus luteum – can get bigger and form a cyst that may remain in the ovary for a few weeks. This can cause pain and may affect the timing of the next cycle. Occasionally a follicle may continue to get bigger without releasing an egg. This is called a 'functional' follicular cyst and may also cause pelvic discomfort and disrupt the menstrual cycle. Corpus luteum cysts and functional follicular cysts often go away by themselves but they can sometimes linger and may need surgery. Large cysts may cause the ovary to twist (known as ovarian torsion). This may cut off its blood supply and urgent surgery is needed to untwist the ovary and fix it to prevent it from twisting again. Thankfully, most ovaries recover and so can be preserved. It's also rare for ovaries to twist with cysts that are less than 5cm in diameter, but bear in mind that you should be monitored with repeat scans for any cyst if it measures more than 3cm.

If there is any concern about a cyst then you should have a blood test to measure what are known as tumour markers (such as CA125) to make sure the cyst is not cancerous (malignant). Sometimes surgery is need to remove cysts, both to check for the type of cyst and test for cancer and also to help the ovaries work better.

Other types of cyst include:

- Endometriomas: cysts in the ovaries in women with endometriosis.

- Dermoid cysts ('mature cystic teratoma'): may contain a number of components including fat, hair, bone and even teeth.

While it is unusual for ovarian malignancy (cancer) to occur in young women, all complex ovarian cysts need to be evaluated carefully and removed surgically if there is any doubt.

Fluid in the fallopian tubes

Your fallopian tubes and other pelvic structures will also be looked at during your baseline ultrasound scan. If you have fluid in your fallopian tubes (hydrosalpinges), the tube(s) should be removed as it can't function (even if opened up surgically). The fluid may also get into the uterus (womb) cavity and prevent an embryo implanting. The fallopian tubes are removed during a laparoscopy operation (see below).

Endometrial assessment

Another important part of your initial scan is an assessment of your endometrium (the lining of the womb). In the early follicular phase, the endometrium appears as a thin line, which then thickens in response to the oestrogen produced by the growing follicle. The endometrium then takes on a characteristic 'triple line' appearance. The endometrial thickness in the early follicular phase is usually 2–5mm, by the time of ovulation it is ideally about 8–10mm and in the mid-luteal phase it may reach 14mm or more. The chances of pregnancy are lower if the triple line appearance isn't seen on the scan or if the thickness before ovulation is less than 6–7mm. We have occasionally seen pregnancies when the endometrium is as thin as 4mm, but during fertility treatments there are ways to try to get it to grow thicker, with a combination of hormones and other drugs.

OTHER INVESTIGATIONS

As well as these initial tests, you may have further investigations depending on symptoms, underlying medical conditions and family history. This may happen at the same time as your initial tests or after your doctor has seen your initial test results.

Testing glucose tolerance

If you are overweight, especially if you also have PCOS, a metabolic assessment is helpful to assess insulin resistance (see page

81). We have already learnt that metabolic health is important for fertility (see Chapter 6). Insulin resistance occurs when the insulin receptors in muscle cells and elsewhere become less efficient at allowing insulin to help glucose enter into cells, where it is a vital source of energy. Because glucose can't get into cells if you have insulin resistance, it builds up in the blood and eventually this can lead to the development of type 2 (late-onset) diabetes. This is what we test for in a glucose tolerance test (GTT). Blood levels of glucose are measured fasting and then again two hours later after consuming a sugary drink containing 75g of glucose.

Insulin levels in the blood also rise with insulin resistance, but insulin is not tested directly as it's difficult to do. The glycosylated haemoglobin (HbA1c) may be measured instead as this gives a longer term overview of how well your body controls blood sugar.

Chromosomal analysis

You may be offered investigations to look at chromosomes and certain genes if you have POI. This may identify both the cause and any risk of transmitting congenital genetic problems to your children.

Autoantibodies

Women with POI sometimes have ovarian autoantibodies or signs of other autoimmune disease (such as thyroid disease or pernicious anaemia). The presence of autoantibodies alerts your specialist to the risk that these conditions may arise in the future.

Thrombophilia and antiphospholipid syndrome

If you have suffered from recurrent miscarriage, you should be tested for lupus anticoagulant and anticardiolipin antibodies. You may also benefit from a full thrombophilia screen to assess how efficiently the blood clots, which can have a bearing on implantation (see Chapter 20 for more on this).

Assessment of the fallopian tubes and uterine cavity

The next part of your investigations is to check to see if the fallopian tubes are open and that the internal structure of the uterus (endometrial cavity) is normal in size and shape, as this is where a pregnancy needs to grow and develop. Tubal infertility is diagnosed in between 15 and 50 per cent of women with subfertility. Abnormalities of the uterus that are present from birth occur in about 4 per cent of women. They can sometimes affect fertility and may also increase the risk of miscarriage and premature delivery. For example, a unicornuate and bicornuate uterus may affect both fertility and miscarriage risk. On the other hand, an arcuate (heart-shaped) uterus appears to have little effect on either (see page 240).

There are certain circumstances in particular where you will need these investigations, for instance, if your initial test results, including a semen analysis (see page 186), don't show any problems that explain why you haven't conceived or if you need treatment to help you ovulate (see Chapter 14). Assessment of the fallopian tubes is done by ultrasound, X-ray or laparoscopy to see if they are open and look normal, although the fact that they are open doesn't necessarily mean that they are functioning normally.

The traditional screening test is the X-ray hysterosalpingogram (HSG), which provides an internal image of the shape of the uterine cavity and the fallopian tubes. An HSG is a simple test and has few complications. A plastic or metal cup is placed over the end of the cervix or a narrow tube is passed into the cervical canal. Fluid (contrast medium) is then slowly and gently injected while X-ray imaging of the pelvis enables a live view as the fluid travels through. A water-soluble contrast medium is usually used and will be absorbed after an hour. Alternatively, an oil-based medium is sometimes used. This may increase the chance of natural conception after the procedure, possibly because plugs of mucus are dislodged by the oil.

You should ideally have an HSG within ten days of your period when there should be no risk of a pregnancy, though you should always have a pregnancy test beforehand as a precaution. We also advise avoiding unprotected sex during the cycle in which the HSG is performed because X-rays can damage the early developing pregnancy if you were to conceive. If you have an erratic menstrual cycle then drugs (a progestogen) are used to stimulate an artificial bleed after first ensuring a pregnancy test is negative.

The HSG can be uncomfortable, especially if there is either tubal spasm or a tubal obstruction. It is sensible to take a painkilling tablet (such as mefenamic acid, ibuprofen or diclofenac) 30–45 minutes before the procedure. One small study also showed women who took 1,000mg of evening primrose oil capsules daily for two days before a HSG had less pain than women who took a placebo, so you could also try taking this in addition.[1] Preparation for the HSG takes about five minutes and the actual duration of the procedure is usually no more than five minutes.

During the procedure, various problems such as blockages can be detected. Fallopian tubes usually get blocked (occluded) at the ends: either near the uterus or the ovary. The latter results in a build-up of fluid called a hydrosalpinx. Adhesions around the tube where it sticks together in places can also be detected. These can be removed to open up the tubes during a subsequent operation (laparoscopy – see below).

Ultrasound contrast hysterosalpingography (or hysterosalpingo-contrast sonography, HyCoSy)

An alternative procedure is to have an ultrasound instead of an X-ray as part of your HSG. This allows your specialist to look at your ovaries and uterus, as well as checking your tubes, which means they can assess you for other problems such as fibroids or congenital (from birth) abnormalities of the uterus and cervix. Fibroids are not usually seen on an X-ray but, when they are, it's not possible to tell whether it's a fibroid or polyp and so an ultrasound will help to make the distinction. Fibroids can cause tubal obstruction and can sometimes disrupt implantation, though it's not clear whether removing them surgically helps unless you also have blocked tubes (see page 237).

Your clinic may have the facilities to perform HSG, HyCoSy or both, and your specialist will be able to discuss which is most suitable for your situation.

Laparoscopy and hysteroscopy

If problems are identified during your ultrasound scan or HSG, or if endometriosis is suspected, you will be referred for an operation known as a laparoscopy to examine the pelvis internally, which provides more information than an HSG but is a more invasive procedure that also requires an anaesthetic. If an HSG shows your fallopian tubes to be clear and functional, then a laparoscopy usually shows the same. If, however, the HSG suggests a blockage, this tends to be confirmed by a laparoscopy in about 40 per cent of cases (the fallopian tubes can often go into spasm during an HSG, which wrongly indicates that there may be a blockage).

You are more at risk of problems with your fallopian tubes if you have previously had a pelvic infection. In this case, it is sensible to proceed straight to laparoscopy, to allow you both to be fully assessed and also potentially treated surgically at the same time. The same applies if you have had previous abdominal surgery, for example for peritonitis (infection) following appendicitis or surgery for inflammatory bowel disease (IBD). A history of painful periods (dysmenorrhea), pain during intercourse (dyspareunia) or pelvic pain generally might suggest the presence of endometriosis, although this is a condition where symptoms often do not correlate with severity of the condition (see page 109). Women who have had a previous emergency caesarean section may also be at greater risk of tubal subfertility than those who have had an elective caesarean.

What happens during a laparoscopy?

Although a laparoscopy requires a general anaesthetic, it is usually performed as a day case, so you can go home the same day. One incision is made just below the belly button, through which the scope is inserted (a flexible tube attached to a camera so the surgeon can see what's going on). A further one or two incisions are made lower down the abdomen – usually to the left and right – through which the instruments used to operate can be inserted. Each incision is usually 5–10mm and so should heal with barely a scar. It can take a few days to get back to normal after a laparoscopy, depending upon the nature of the operation. We usually recommend one to two weeks off work and the avoidance of strenuous exercise or driving a car for four weeks.

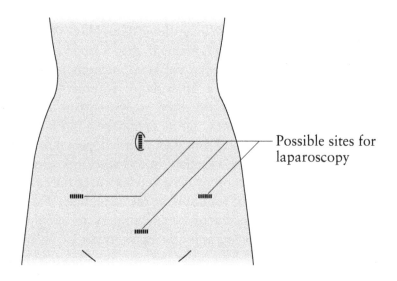

Possible sites for laparoscopy

Laparoscopy incision sites

A hysteroscopic evaluation of the uterus is often included when a laparoscopy is performed. This means having a thorough look using a hysteroscope (a tube attached to a camera). Although this doesn't usually detect significant abnormalities, the procedure is simple and safe and allows a detailed assessment of the shape and structure of the uterus (see page 240). It also allows the specialist to identify polyps, fibroids and adhesions.

The surface of your uterus, bladder and bowel will also be inspected during your laparoscopy. The ovaries are also examined for signs of follicular activity and ovulation, and for their general appearance and the presence of endometriosis. Endometriosis (see Chapter 17) tends to occur on the surface of the ovary, where it can develop into cysts (endometrioma) and elsewhere in the pelvis as small inflammatory nodules and scarring. There is evidence that even mild endometriosis may adversely affect fertility and so ablation, with diathermy (heat) or laser, may be performed during the initial laparoscopy. Endometriosis can take on a number of appearances and so the pelvis is inspected in a careful and systematic way.

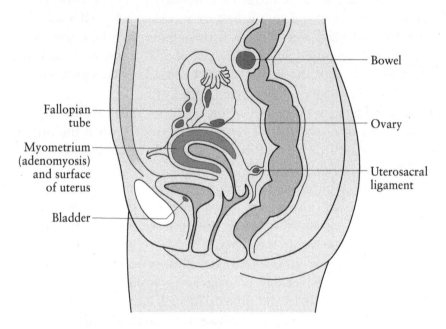

Bowel

Fallopian tube

Ovary

Myometrium (adenomyosis) and surface of uterus

Uterosacral ligament

Bladder

Common sites of endometriosis; endometriosis can affect fertility by creating an inflammatory environment and distorting reproductive organs

Methylene blue dye is injected through the cervix and the ends of the fallopian tubes to check they are clear. This doesn't confirm they can function well, however. This is because the fallopian tube is very delicate and has fine fronds at the 'fimbrial' (ovary) end to capture the egg as it is released during ovulation, and fine hair-like structures and muscle that help waft the egg and sperm together so that fertilisation can take place within the tube. The fertilised egg is then gently moved down to the uterus, where implantation should then occur.

Fine adhesions around the ovaries and fallopian tubes can often be cut through and treated at the time of the initial laparoscopy. The easiest way to envisage adhesions is to imagine a fine spider's web that covers the surface of the pelvic organs and causes them to stick to each other, thereby preventing them from functioning normally. Adhesions usually develop after infection or other inflammatory conditions such as endometriosis or TB.

Sometimes surgery on the tube can be helpful, although these days if the tube is very damaged it is unlikely to function normally even after surgery and so it is best to move on to IVF. If a tube is swollen and filled with fluid (a hydrosalpinx) it is best removed during the laparoscopy, as described above. It has been shown conclusively that the removal of hydrosalpinges significantly improves the chance of conception with IVF.

If a pregnancy occurs when one or both tubes are damaged there is an increased risk of ectopic pregnancy – when the pregnancy starts to develop outside the womb, usually within the fallopian tube (see page 285).

If the initial ultrasound scan showed you have a cyst that needs attention, this will also be removed during your laparoscopy. Cysts are removed carefully in order to preserve the valuable egg-containing tissue within the ovary.

While a laparoscopy is a fairly straightforward operation, there are small risks of bleeding or damage to structures such as the bowel, vessels, bladder and ureters. In such an eventuality it may be necessary to open up the abdomen through a larger incision (laparotomy) to deal with the problem. The risk of complications is about 1:1,000 and diagnostic laparoscopy carries a mortality of 1:12,000.

UNEXPLAINED INFERTILITY

If you haven't conceived after one year of trying and if all the investigations in both partners haven't identified a problem (see also Chapter 13), you have what we call unexplained infertility. This is when it is especially important to look at your general health, diet and lifestyle for both partners, as discussed in Part 1 (pages 22–58).

The natural pregnancy rate in couples with unexplained infertility has been reported as between 2 and 4 per cent per menstrual cycle. One study reported conception rates of 15 per cent of couples with unexplained infertility within one year and 35 per cent within two years.[2] And the cumulative chance of pregnancy over three years has even been reported as being 80 per cent. In other words, there's still a fair chance that you may get pregnant naturally in the absence of any identifiable problems. Therefore, it has been suggested that treatment should be deferred until the couple has been trying to conceive for two to three years, as before this time treatment may not improve their chances over natural conception. This will, of course, depend upon your age and how quickly you feel you may wish to progress with treatments (see Chapter 18).

Many fertility centres have their own specific areas of interest and research, which they then promote as the missing cause of unexplained infertility. Thus it is possible to come up with long lists of possible and subtle causes of infertility, many of which cannot be proven with certainty and few of which have treatments that have been shown to enhance fertility. Bear in mind that couples with normal fertility can also have abnormal test results, so teasing out why you haven't conceived can be complicated. Once the well-known and obvious causes of infertility have been excluded, if you end up with a diagnosis of unexplained infertility, your treatment should follow clear protocols (see page 249 and Chapter 18). It's always important to remember that subfertility is rarely absolute and many couples conceive naturally even after they have been trying for quite a long time – sometimes even after they have undergone various treatments.

MAIN CAUSES OF SUBFERTILITY

Studies of populations of patients with infertility indicate that approximately 10–25 per cent have unexplained infertility; 20–30 per cent ovulatory dysfunction; 20–35 per cent tubal damage; 10–50 per cent sperm dysfunction; 5–10 per cent endometriosis; and 5 per cent coital dysfunction (problems with sexual function).[3] A degree of subfertility is found in both partners in 30–50 per cent of couples, as usually a couple's subfertility is a relative rather than an absolute barrier to conception.

The most important factors that predict your chance of getting pregnant are how long you have been trying and your age. How quickly you want to progress to fertility treatment depends on many things, including how anxious you may feel about wanting to get pregnant, financial considerations and whether you would prefer to conceive naturally.

When the time comes to seek medical treatment, there are various options for managing unexplained infertility. We shall discuss some of the therapies that have been used and explain the medical journey that we use in practice in Chapter 18.

Chapter 13

Investigating Male Fertility

A T THE SAME time the woman is being investigated, it's vital the male partner is also assessed. The key test of male fertility is a semen analysis. Ideally this should be assessed on at least two occasions because of the natural variation that occurs in sperm counts and function. If the semen analysis is normal then further investigations are not usually necessary. On the other hand, if problems are identified, the man should be examined to ensure that there are no abnormalities of his genitalia and a general examination performed to assess general health, body weight and signs of hormone deficiency. A sexual health screen, looking for infections such as chlamydia, is also usually performed (see page 24). There are various issues that can be picked up during these initial checks.

HORMONE PROBLEMS

If a man has a deficiency of androgen hormones (the main one being testosterone) then the symptoms that he has will depend upon how long the deficiency has been there. General symptoms include lack of energy, reduced sex drive, weight gain and reduced beard growth. If the deficiency started before puberty he may have a high-pitched voice, small, soft testes and penis, lack of adult hair and decreased muscle mass. If testicular insufficiency (hypogonadism) develops after puberty the skin becomes fine and there may also be growth of the breasts (gynaecomastia).

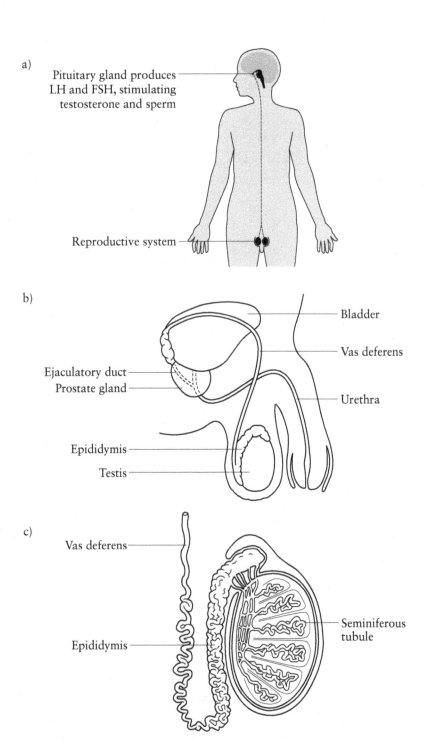

a)

Pituitary gland produces
LH and FSH, stimulating
testosterone and sperm

Reproductive system

b)

Bladder

Vas deferens

Ejaculatory duct
Prostate gland

Urethra

Epididymis
Testis

c)

Vas deferens

Seminiferous
tubule

Epididymis

Male reproductive system; a) Hormones stimulate sperm development;
b) The penis and testes; c) Testis and vas deferens

A history of undescended testes in childhood and subsequent surgery to bring the testes into the scrotum (orchidopexy) has important implications for future fertility and is often associated with a low or absent sperm count. Testicular size can be measured using a device called an orchidometer and is normal if over 15ml in volume. Small testes that are soft are usually associated with low gonadotrophin (follicle-stimulating hormone and luteinising hormone) levels in the blood and may respond to hormone treatment. Small testes that are firm typically have scar tissue (fibrosis), which is usually associated with severe and permanent destruction of the sperm-producing tissue, even though androgen hormone (testosterone) production may be normal. Testicular lumps or uneven testicles may need further investigation by ultrasound to look for cysts and tumours.

VARICOCELE

Another possible problem is a varicocele, which is a swelling of the testicular veins within the scrotum that is best felt when standing. It may cause discomfort and possibly reduced fertility. Varicoceles are more common on the left, because the veins drain differently on the left and right sides.

Approximately 10–20 per cent of men have a varicocele compared with 30–40 per cent of those attending infertility clinics. If you're found to have a varicocele, it can be graded and investigated by ultrasound scan and other imaging techniques. Varicoceles can affect semen parameters, which may worsen with time, but a bigger varicocele doesn't mean worse sperm dysfunction.

Surgery to treat varicoceles is usually performed via an incision in the groin, with the aim of ligating (tying off) the spermatic vein(s). Alternatively, embolisation of the vessels to block them can be performed by an experienced radiologist. The most recent studies do now suggest a benefit, although the evidence is still accumulating, it is contentious and there is still no clear consensus, other than to operate if there is pain associated with a varicocele.[1]

INFECTION

If you notice changes in seminal colour or smell, you may have an infection of the epididymis, prostate or seminal vesicles. You should therefore have a semen sample sent for assessment by a microbiology laboratory and further testing.

THE SEMEN ANALYSIS

In order to have a semen analysis, a man has to produce a sample by masturbation into a clean, dry container and deliver it to the laboratory within 30 minutes – most fertility clinics have private rooms on site, so samples can be assessed quickly. It's important to abstain from ejaculation for three days before the test: this fixed period of abstinence not only improves the standardisation of the test, but more than five days' abstinence is associated with a decrease in motility despite an increase in sperm number. A large study of over 9,000 semen samples found that men with normal sperm parameters had similar semen characteristics when the period of abstinence ranged from one to ten days, after which they declined, whereas men with a low sperm count (oligospermia) had better samples after shorter periods of abstinence (less than three days, and in many cases one day of abstinence was preferable).[2]

Sperm counts and motility in different samples from the same healthy, fertile man can vary significantly, so be cautious about relying on results from a single test. It's best repeated on two or more occasions, ideally three months apart. In most cases, two semen analyses will be enough. There may be regional differences in semen quality dependent both on the ambient temperature (with counts being higher in the cooler winter months) and environmental exposures or lifestyle differences. Sperm production by the testis takes ten to twelve weeks and so an abnormal semen specimen is a reflection of testicular function approximately three months previously. Equally, a good result can worsen if there are negative changes in diet and lifestyle.

The current World Health Organization (WHO) criteria for the semen analysis are shown in the table below. (At the time of writing the WHO is re-evaluating these criteria and the proposed new values have been included below.)

SEMEN PARAMETERS (WHO, 2010)		NEW VALUES PROPOSED BY WHO, 2021
Standard tests	*Lower reference limit*	
Volume	$\geq$ 1.5ml	$\geq$ 1.2ml
pH	7.2–8.0	
Sperm concentration	$\geq$ 15 x 10^6/ml	$\geq$ 16 x 10^6/ml
Total sperm count	$\geq$ 39 x 10^6/ejaculate	$\geq$ 39 x 10^6/ejaculate
Motility (within 60 minutes of ejaculation)	$\geq$ 25% with rapid progression (category 'a')	$\geq$ 30%
	$\geq$ 40% with forward progression (categories 'a' and 'b')	$\geq$ 42%
Vitality	$\geq$ 75% live (categories 'a', 'b' and 'c')	$\geq$ 54%
	< 25% dead (category 'd')	< 20%
Morphology	$\geq$ 4 % normal forms	$\geq$ 4%
White blood cells, a sign of infection	< 1 x 10^6/ml	
Antisperm antibodies	< 50%	

Although the link between male fertility and results from a semen analysis is not always clear (it only takes a single good sperm cell to reach the egg from an ejaculate of millions!), the chance of natural conception falls significantly when the motile sperm concentration is less than 5 x 10^6/ml. When the total count is low there is often a corresponding reduction in motility. The concentration of progressively motile sperm consistently appears to be the most predictive factor for fertility.

Impaired sperm morphology (teratozoospermia)

Sperm morphology (shape) provides a good reflection of sperm function. The acceptable percentage of normal sperm is 4 per cent as men appear to make millions of abnormal sperm (it only takes a single sperm remember!), so there is a built-in redundancy. It is now felt that teratozoospermia on its own has little influence on fertilisation, pregnancy or live births. A compilation of a number of good studies has also shown that the use of intracytoplasmic sperm injection (ICSI) does not improve the outcome when morphology is poor compared with *in vitro* fertilisation (IVF) alone.[3] Recent advances in the analysis of sperm morphology include the use of intracytoplasmic morphologically selected sperm injection (IMSI). With IMSI, the embryologist uses a high-powered microscope to

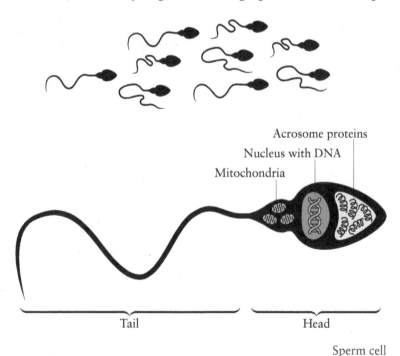

Sperm cell

closely examine the finer details of the structures within motile sperm. There is, however, still some debate about the benefit of this technology.

Reduced sperm motility (asthenozoospermia)

Reduced motility means the sperm doesn't swim so well and this can be caused by infection, antisperm antibodies (see page 190) or defects within the sperm tail. You can get misleading results if there is no facility to produce a sample near the laboratory and there is a delay between production and arrival at the laboratory. In other words, the sperm isn't sluggish – it's taken too long for sperm to be tested. It is also vital to ensure that the sample has been delivered directly into a pot and not into a condom as they often contain lubricating or spermicidal agents, which will kill off sperm. Lubricating jelly, soap or water can also cause sperm death, so avoid these, too. Good hygiene when producing the specimen also prevents contamination and so it is important to wash your hands and penis before producing the sample.

Some men have difficulties producing a specimen, in which case there are inert silicon condoms that can be used to collect sperm during vaginal intercourse. If producing a sample is a problem and fertility treatment is going to be required, it is sensible to consider freezing sperm as a back-up in case the pressure to produce a sample on the day of treatment is too much.

Infection

Sometimes bacteria are found in the semen analysis. Bacteria are most often thought to come from contamination at the time of sperm production as when the analysis is repeated there isn't usually an underlying infection. If a lower genital tract infection is suspected, a Stamey–Meares test should be performed. This involves collecting three small samples of urine in succession. The first indicates urethral infection, the second (a mid-stream specimen) urinary infection and the third, collected after prostatic massage (which requires a clinician inserting a finger up the man's anus and massaging the prostate gland), prostatic infection.

OTHER SEMEN PARAMETERS

Though not used in routine testing, there are other sperm tests available.

Testing for sperm DNA fragmentation

Sperm function can be damaged by what's known as oxidative stress caused by reactive oxygen species (ROS – see page 199). High levels of ROS are produced as a result of infection or inflammation. Seminal plasma (fluid) contains a rich concentration of antioxidants to try to protect sperm from these toxic effects, which may cause genetic (DNA) damage to the sperm and potentially also to a resultant embryo. Testing sperm for DNA damage (fragmentation) has therefore become more common and some believe it to be better at predicting chance of pregnancy than traditional semen parameters.

There are many different tests available but doctors don't agree as to whether they help or what can be done for men based on their results. There is some evidence for the use of diet and nutritional supplements (see Chapters 3 and 4), although this is still largely an area of ongoing research.[4] One well-conducted study showed that nut consumption can improve DNA fragmentation for instance (see page 137).[5]

Antisperm antibodies (ASABs)

Another factor that can affect male fertility is the presence of ASABs on the surface of sperm. ASABs are proteins produced in the testes that can cause sperm to stick together. ASABs may develop in men when the blood–testis barrier breaks down, for example after injury or surgery, such as vasectomy, and they may affect motility and fertilisation.

We don't have good treatment options for ASABs and, though there are different tests available to detect them, there is no medical consensus on which test is the best. If ASABs are high enough to cause a problem for fertility, other parameters will be affected (such as motility or agglutination) and so routine testing is not needed. The levels of ASABs are considered to be significant when more than 50 per cent of the motile sperm are affected.

Corticosteroid treatment was used in the past (more than 30 years ago), but the benefits were limited and serious side effects common, and so IVF with ICSI offers the best chance of a pregnancy.

HORMONE TESTING

If a man has severe oligospermia or any of the symptoms we described above that suggest hormone problems, he will need some blood tests to check levels.

Testosterone

One of the most important hormones to measure is testosterone. Levels vary across the day, with the highest levels in the morning. The time of the test is therefore important if the result is border-line. It's then best to compare with timing and measurements taken on other days. The normal range is 10–35nmol/L.

Follicle-stimulating hormone (FSH) and luteinising hormone (LH)

FSH and LH are two other hormones that are often tested. Nor-mal levels of both FSH and LH should be less than 10IU/L (although it is important to know the normal range for your local laboratory).

Problems that hormone testing can help identify include:

- The combination of azoospermia (no sperm in the ejaculate) with normal-sized testes and normal testosterone, FSH and LH suggests there is a physical blockage of sperm (see below).

- Low levels of all three hormones indicate problems in the hypothalamus or pituitary gland. Men who fall into this cat-egory can see improvements in sperm with hormone therapy.

- High FSH and LH with low testosterone level can indicate primary testicular failure, which means the testes aren't capable of producing sperm. Very occasionally a few live sperm have been found when a biopsy of the testes has been taken, which have then been used for IVF/ICSI. Unless the testes are really tiny (e.g. less than 2ml), it's therefore worth discussing the possibility of having a biopsy with your andrologist if you fall into this category to see if any sperm can be collected. Any sperm collected can then be frozen immediately after the procedure.

Testicular exploration and biopsy

If a physical blockage is suspected, surgery may be needed to open up the scrotum and examine the testis under anaesthetic. If an obstruction is found, it may be possible to fix it as part of the operation (see page 204). It's really important to make sure facilities are available to freeze sperm whenever surgery is performed on the testis. This doesn't always happen so it's useful to check this as a patient. Sperm can be stored in case the procedure is unsuccessful, and then used later for IVF. A biopsy of the testes will help diagnose severe oligospermia or azoospermia. How well sperm production (spermatogenesis) is working can also be assessed during the operation.

Chromosomal analysis

If from the above tests, primary testicular failure is suspected, a genetic profile (karyotype) test is needed to make a diagnosis as to the cause. You will be offered genetic counselling if a problem is found.

A karyotype test is usually recommended for men with azoospermia and for men with semen parameters that are severely impaired (severe oligospermia – a count of < 5 million/ml) as there is a higher risk of problems with the chromosomes, including the sex chromosomes. One such condition is Klinefelter syndrome (sometimes called Klinefelter's, KS or XXY), when there is an extra X chromosome. Genes for sperm production sit on the Y chromosome, so other problems with the Y chromosomes can affect sperm production, including where very short sections of the chromosome are deleted – these are called microdeletions and they may be passed on to the male children of men who need IVF/ICSI. These microdeletions may be found in 7 per cent of infertile men and in up to 2 per cent of normal men.

Another problem known as congenital bilateral absence of the vas deferens (CBAVD) means a vital part of the anatomy involved in sperm production is missing and is associated with mutations in the cystic fibrosis (CF) gene (see page 199).

OTHER CAUSES OF MALE INFERTILITY AND TREATMENT

We can't always find a reason for male factor infertility and only a small proportion of men will get a clear diagnosis as to the cause. Most will fall under the heading of 'idiopathic' male factor infertility (that is, 'no cause has been found') for which there are no specific medical therapies, although there is a lot of interest in lifestyle, diet and vitamin supplements (see page 135).

It may sound strange, but the semen analysis results do not guide us to a specific underlying problem in the man, so we rarely identify a specific dysfunction to treat. Instead, most therapies are based on enhancing sperm quality *in vitro* – that is, in the laboratory, with either intrauterine insemination (IUI) or, more usually, IVF with or without ICSI. While couples with severe male factor infertility are likely to benefit from IVF/ICSI, 'mild to moderate' male subfertility is poorly defined and treatment strategies vary.

Concern has been expressed that having the option of IVF and ICSI (see Chapter 18) has stopped us trying to understand the causes of male infertility. We believe that our goal should be to give couples the chance to conceive naturally rather than send them straight into assisted conception programmes, which are stressful, costly and not without risks – largely borne by the female partner.

As well as concerns about a deterioration of semen quality globally, the incidence of certain congenital anomalies, such as hypospadias (when the urethra opens through the underside of the penis), undescended testes and testicular cancer, is also rising. It has been suggested that environmental pollutants containing oestrogens and other toxins may be to blame, and we look at those in detail on page 120.

Undescended testes (cryptorchidism)

Boys who are born with undescended testes have a 40 per cent rate of abnormalities in the epididymis and vas deferens, compared with 0.5–1 per cent in the normal population. These abnormalities affect the ability of the immature sperm cells (gonadocytes) to develop into mature sperm cells (spermatogonia), which should have happened by the age of six months. Spermatogonia in turn start to develop further into primary spermatocytes by the age of three years. This process is delayed and doesn't happen in boys with testes that remain undescended after the age of one year.

Most men with a history of undescended testes are fertile but have a reduced sperm count. The undescended testis produces few, if any, sperm after surgery to fix the testis in the scrotum (orchido-pexy) as the shrunken testis is lacking in sperm-making cells. When both testes are undescended in adult men, they have a very poor prognosis for fertility. While it is thought that surgery should be performed at a very young age (preferably one to two years), if it is left much later than this it doesn't make much difference to future fertility whether boys have the operation early or late in the age range of four to fourteen years. Hormonal therapy, started at any age, does not appear to help.

Very early cancer (carcinoma *in situ*) has been found in undes-cended testes that have not been brought down before the age of ten years and, if left, this is likely to develop into testicular cancer. Men who have had surgery to fix undescended testes have an increased risk of developing testicular cancer in both testes – although it is much greater if the testes remain undescended. Early orchidopexy, before the age of five years, may decrease this risk.

Measles, mumps and rubella

Having a mumps infection after puberty can be serious for male fer-tility as it may significantly affect spermatogenesis. We advise having the MMR (measles, mumps and rubella) vaccination if you haven't already had it. This prevents infection and therefore the development of inflammation of the testes (orchitis) that happens with mumps.

Chickenpox

Chickenpox can also cause severe orchitis. If this happens, it is essential to try to minimise damage to the testes, which occurs as pressure increases inside the testes during infection. Steroid treatment may help and occasionally an operation is needed.

Sexually transmitted infections

Chlamydia trachomatis is now the most common sexually transmitted infection (STI) in developed countries, causing both male and female infertility. Gonorrhoea may cause irreversible obstruction of the spermatic ducts, but infection can be prevented with the use of barrier methods of contraception.

Injuries

Severe trauma to the testes can cause permanent damage and also increase the risk of the subsequent production of ASABs (see page 190). You should therefore wear appropriate protection when participating in contact sports, such as rugby, cricket and football.

Occupational factors

If you are exposed to environmental toxins in your workplace, be aware that this can affect fertility (see page 145). Do what you can to limit exposure including minimising time spent in toxic environments where possible, wearing a mask and ensuring the space is well-ventilated.

Drugs

While the effects of many medicines on spermatogenesis are reversible, some can have a permanent effect – for example some of the treatments for inflammatory bowel disease (IBDs). Sometimes the side effects of drug therapy have to be weighed up against the benefits of treatment, but there are often alternative medications.

Chemotherapy/radiotherapy

If you need to have chemotherapy or radiotherapy for the treatment of certain cancers, always ensure that you're able to freeze sperm before treatment starts (see Chapter 23). If you are very ill, it may be difficult to produce a sperm sample so ask to do this as soon as possible. Although the quality of the sample may be poor, it is usually sufficient for future use in IVF with ICSI, so it's definitely worth doing.

Age

Fertility declines with age in men as well as women, though to a lesser degree (see pages 12 and 17). So, while men have fathered children into their nineties, there is an increase in the rate of fresh genetic mutations in sperm with increasing paternal age that lead to some inherited congenital defects (such as Marfan syndrome, Apert syndrome, Duchenne muscular dystrophy, haemophilia, bilateral retinoblastoma and achondroplasia) and an increased risk of autism developing in children. Sperm numbers and function do tend to decline with age, although there is no predictable pattern. While the decline is most noticeable after the age of 55, even men older than 35 have been shown to have half the chance of achieving a pregnancy compared with men younger than 25.

Hormone problems: Hypogonadism

Hormonal (endocrinological) dysfunction as a cause of male infertility is uncommon but responds well to treatment. There are a few congenital causes of male hypogonadotrophic hypogonadism – a syndrome where the testes fail because of low levels of gonadotrophin hormones from the pituitary gland. One is Kallmann syndrome (see page 213 for the female equivalent), which causes delayed puberty, as may pituitary tumours and other rare pituitary problems.

Hypogonadotrophic hypogonadism is treated by injecting gonadotrophins either in the form of human chorionic gonadotrophin (hCG) 1,500–2,500IU twice weekly or human menopausal gonadotrophin (hMG) 150IU two to three times a week.

Testosterone is used as a hormone replacement treatment for men whose testes are not producing sufficient levels for health and well-being, but should not be given when trying to father a child as it will suppress sperm production, in a similar way to oestrogen in the contraceptive pill that suppresses ovulation in women.

If fertility is not required, or after a pregnancy has been achieved, it is important to be given maintenance testosterone if you are a hypogonadal man. It may also be sensible to consider freezing some sperm before starting testosterone just in case it is needed in future (see page 323).

General health factors

We looked at the effects of alcohol, body weight, diet, smoking, exercise, testicular warming, drug use, anabolic steroids and other factors that can affect male fertility in Chapter 10. Remember that sperm takes about twelve weeks to be made, so if you are found to have a sperm problem then any change in lifestyle may take at least three months to take effect. There are also seasonal variations in semen quality, with a decline during summer months, which may be enough to render some men subfertile.

As well as being overweight, any chronic debilitating illness may lead to infertility in men. There are also a few notable conditions that particularly affect male fertility, including diabetes, chronic renal failure and thyroid disease. An acute illness can also result in a temporary loss of sperm production. It is therefore important that your specialist notes any illnesses in the past three months when reviewing the results of semen analyses.

Oligoasthenozoospermia

The majority of men with subfertility have oligoasthenozoospermia (reduced sperm numbers of low motility and morphology) of unknown cause. At present, little can be done for this in the way of direct medical treatment, although assisted conception procedures such as IUI or IVF (with or without ICSI) may be of benefit.

Azoospermia

If you have azoospermia (absence of sperm), it may be due to a hormonal deficiency, genetic abnormality or absence or obstruction of the vas deferens and spermatic ducts. There are some chromosomal causes of azoospermia, such as Klinefelter syndrome (see page 192), occurring in 1:500 males. There are other genetic abnormalities that may result in either azoospermia or severe impairment of fertility including microdeletions of the Y chromosome (see page 192).

Even if you do have azoospermia, it's possible that you have a small area of normal sperm production within the testes. As many as 50 per cent of men with supposed untreatable infertility may produce sperm. It's possible to recover sperm either from the ejaculate using special sperm preparation techniques (such as MERC – multiple ejaculation, resuspension and centrifugation) or from the testes themselves, using a surgical technique that targets different areas of the testes (TESE – testicular sperm extraction, see page 201). This increases the chance of finding an area that is producing sperm. Although numbers of sperm found may be low, if mature sperm are present, they can be frozen as there will usually be sufficient for ICSI. There is, however, a high rate of chromosomal abnormalities in the sperm if levels of FSH are high and these may possibly be transmitted to children conceived by ICSI.

Usually, in a man with normal fertility, the concentration of motile sperm in the ejaculate decreases with each successive ejaculation, but it's different if you have oligozoospermia or asthenozoospermia. In these cases, it actually seems to be good for sperm concentration to have multiple sequential ejaculations. The best timing is intervals of either 1–4 hours or 24 hours where either similar or more motile sperm is found in the second ejaculate when compared with the first (hence MERC preparation for assisted conception – see above).

If you are a man with subfertility, we therefore advise having sex or masturbating at least daily, if not twice daily, around the time of ovulation instead of following the usual advice given to men with normal fertility (alternate day intercourse). If you need fertility treatment, there's a possibility that the sperm sample you produce on the day of the IVF egg collection may be suboptimal and so it is sensible to have sperm frozen as a back-up before you start treatment (see page 323).

Oxidative stress and reactive oxygen species (ROS)

We discussed the potential for sperm to be damaged by ROS and the lifestyle factors that make it worse on page 199. This damage may affect the membrane and thereby motility of the sperm and prevent it fertilising an oocyte. Furthermore, ROS may also directly damage sperm DNA and this affects the father's genetic contribution to the embryo. A number of supplements have been used to combat the effects of ROS, which we discuss in detail on pages 33 and 55.

Obstructive azoospermia

No underlying cause can be found in over half of patients with obstruction of the epididymis. However, infection is often the cause, particularly in developing countries, and include gonorrhoea, chlamydia, filariasis, tuberculosis and bilharzia.

Congenital bilateral absence of the vasa deferens (CBAVD)

Two-thirds of men with CBAVD also have genes that cause cystic fibrosis (CF), without having symptoms of this serious condition. It is possible to use sperm extracted from the epididymis by percutaneous epididymal sperm aspiration (PESA – see page 201) to achieve a pregnancy, but the fertilisation rates are lower. Furthermore, half of the children born by these techniques will have CF mutations and the male children may have the same problems as their fathers. Both partners should have genetic screening before treatment to assess the risk of a child being affected by full-blown CF. Testing can then be performed in either the pre-implantation embryo or during pregnancy, if both parents are found to be carriers of the gene. Mutations in the CF gene are sometimes also found when there is severe oligospermia.

Surgical trauma and vasectomy

Surgical obstruction of the vas deferens may happen by accident during childhood surgery for a hernia in the groin area or during the repair of a hydrocele (build-up of fluid) of the testis. A vasectomy is the deliberate blockage of the vas deferens to make a man infertile.

Microsurgical reconstruction of the vasa to reverse a vasectomy

It is possible to reverse a vasectomy by surgically reconstructing the vasa, but the original surgery is associated with high levels of ASABs and the success of reversal declines with increasing time after five years since the initial vasectomy operation. Reversal probably shouldn't be attempted after ten years. Furthermore, sperm should be extracted during surgery and frozen at the time of the attempt at reversal in case the procedure is unsuccessful.

You should only consider a vasectomy reversal (surgical reconstruction of the vasa) by a skilled urologist with good success rates. This should mean up to 97 per cent for successful surgery and a pregnancy rate of 76 per cent if you are within three years of having a vasectomy. If you had a vasectomy more than 15 years ago, these success rates should be 76 per cent and 30 per cent respectively.

Karen and Peter: Treatment following a vasectomy

Peter (45) had two teenage children from a previous relationship and had been with Karen (38) for three years. He had a vasectomy ten years ago. He was healthy with normal hormone levels. Karen had also been checked and was healthy too, but with a reduced anti-Müllerian hormone (AMH) level for her age. We discussed the possibility of a vasectomy reversal. However, given the length of time since the vasectomy and Karen's age and low AMH, we agreed that IVF would give them the best chance of having a baby. We performed a PESA and were able to freeze enough sperm potentially for six attempts at IVF combined with ICSI. We stimulated Karen in a short protocol with the maximum dose of medication, but were only able to obtain six eggs, of which four were mature and injected with sperm. Three eggs fertilised and a beautiful blastocyst embryo was transferred. Karen conceived and the baby is due this coming summer.

Surgical collection of sperm

If vasectomy reversal fails or if the operation isn't feasible, it may be possible to collect sperm surgically from either the epididymis or the testis. The different techniques are:

- PESA (percutaneous epididymal sperm aspiration) works well for simple cases and can be done under local anaesthetic. A fine needle is passed into the epidermis, which is the reservoir of the sperm.

- MESA (microsurgical epididymal sperm aspiration) may be performed under general anaesthetic, with an incision made into the testis to extract the sperm.

- If this fails, a TESE (testicular sperm extraction) can be attempted. This requires a bigger operation and incision into the testis to search for sperm.

With all these techniques sperm is frozen for use in IVF combined with ICSI as there isn't usually enough good-quality sperm for either insemination or conventional IVF (see Chapter 23).

IDIOPATHIC MALE FACTOR INFERTILITY: WHEN NO CAUSE HAS BEEN FOUND

If there is no obvious reason for problems with sperm, as is the case in around half of men, the only options are assisted conception: IUI or IVF with or without ICSI (see Chapter 18). In the past, a number of drugs have been tried but without any effect and so they should no longer be offered.

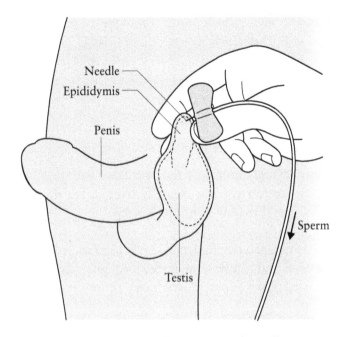

PESA operation to collect sperm

Sexual dysfunction and psychosexual problems

Problems with sex are more common than you may think and trying to conceive can put you under even more pressure (see page 60). Counselling can help and your clinic should be able to refer you for specialist support.

Erectile dysfunction

Good nerve function, adequate hormone levels and a healthy blood supply to the penis are all needed to have an erection, but things can go wrong. Impotence and erectile dysfunction may be caused by various issues, ranging from psychological (anxiety, depression), to hormonal problems, diabetes, certain drugs (e.g. blood pressure medication), multiple sclerosis, major abdominal surgery, prostate surgery and spinal cord injury. Around 80 per cent of cases of erectile dysfunction have a cause, usually due to reduced blood supply, with 20 per cent due to psychological or emotional factors (psychogenic). Regardless of the cause, you and your partner may benefit from counselling (see page 275).

You will usually be given tablets (sildenafil, tadalafil or vardenefil) initially to treat the problem. If this doesn't help, the next step is either an injection into the penis or a pellet of prostaglandin El (alprostadil) or papaverine inserted into the opening at the end of the penis (urethra). This needs to be done very carefully and with the help of your doctor at first. Inflatable penile prostheses have also been used with varying degrees of success.

If you aren't able to ejaculate, you can try massage using a vibrator at the base of the penis either yourself or with the help of your partner. If it works, you can then collect the semen and try self-insemination at home. If it doesn't, the next step is to try electroejaculation using a rectal probe, which needs to be done by a properly trained professional because of the risk of developing very high blood pressure (autonomic dysreflexia). Electroejaculation has also been used successfully for men with spinal cord injuries. Semen quality tends to decline with time after the injury and so the collected sperm often has to be used for IVF/ICSI rather than intravaginal insemination or IUI.

Retrograde ejaculation

Retrograde ejaculation is another fairly common problem where sperm is ejaculated backwards into the bladder rather than through the penis and may occur after prostate surgery, with diabetes or multiple sclerosis. The diagnosis is confirmed by finding sperm in a urine specimen collected after ejaculation. Drugs such as ephedrine hydrochloride can be tried initially. If these don't work, sperm can be collected by inserting a catheter into the penis after ejaculation and washed immediately in the laboratory before insemination. It is important to first alkalinise the urine by taking oral sodium bicarbonate.

Testicular failure

Sometimes we find that the testicles themselves have failed, which can happen for various reasons, including high levels of FSH and

LH, congenital defects, viral orchitis (e.g. mumps), trauma, testicular torsion, cancer or toxins. Hormone therapy doesn't help but, in recent years, there has been progress in treating men with azoospermia and high levels of FSH, where previously the only option was donor insemination. If the testes are not completely shrunken and at least one is of a normal size, a biopsy of the testes can be attempted as sperm can sometimes be found, which can be used later for IVF with ICSI. It may even be worthwhile considering biopsy of small testes as a few sperm can sometimes, albeit rarely, be collected.

INTRAUTERINE INSEMINATION (IUI)

Intrauterine insemination (IUI) is a form of fertility treatment where a prepared sperm sample is inserted directly into the womb. IUI can be used if you need to use donor sperm or sometimes for the treatment of 'mild' male infertility, the rationale being that using a prepared sample of sperm may confer some benefit. IUI may be performed in a natural cycle or with mild stimulation of the ovaries, using letrozole or gonadotrophin injections (which carry the risk of multiple pregnancy). Unfortunately, neither stimulated nor unstimulated IUI for male infertility has shown any real benefit and so they are no longer recommended.[6] The management of male factor infertility was revolutionised by the advent of ICSI, by which a single sperm is injected into an oocyte (egg) to achieve a viable embryo and pregnancy. (See Chapter 18 for more on IUI, IVF and ICSI.)

Historically, IUI has also been used to treat unexplained infertility, but IVF is more commonly used as it is much more successful (see Chapter 18). There has been quite a bit of controversy surrounding the use of IUI in the management of unexplained infertility, either with or without ovarian stimulation. Overall, IUI with ovarian stimulation appears to have a potential, albeit relatively limited, role. In the UK, however, the National Institute for Health and Care Excellence (NICE) guidelines do not currently recommend the use of IUI with ovarian stimulation because of the risk of multiple pregnancy, hence it is not funded by the National

Health Service and this has caused a lot of debate and some unhappiness.

DONOR INSEMINATION

If the various treatment options that we've covered so far don't work or aren't suitable for you, you may wish to consider donor insemination (DI). This is usually needed if you have no sperm production at all and no possibility of either stimulating sperm with drugs or collecting sperm surgically, or if there is a genetic disease that will be carried and transmitted in the sperm. Donor sperm is also used to help lesbian women and single women to conceive (see pages 313 and 311). It is essential, indeed mandatory, to have careful counselling from a qualified counsellor about the implications of using donor sperm so that you have an opportunity to fully explore your feelings on the matter (see page 275).

Selecting donors

While you can buy sperm online by private arrangement, either with individuals or certain 'services', we strongly advise against this because it is essential to receive properly conducted treatment with full support from trained medical and counselling staff in a licensed clinic.

If you select sperm through a properly licensed clinic, you can be confident that the selection and screening of sperm donors will be scrupulous. This is not only to ensure that the frozen sperm has a good chance of achieving a pregnancy, but also to prevent the transmission of disease to the woman receiving it during treatment. While the ideal would be to use donors with proven fertility, in reality many donors are students or young men who may not have fathered any children. Donation in the UK is considered to be altruistic and so donors are not paid; however they do receive a small reimbursement for 'expenses'. This is tightly regulated by the Human Fertilisation & Embryology Authority (HFEA).

In the UK, the HFEA stipulates that donated sperm is frozen for at least six months so that the donor can be retested for infections such as HIV and hepatitis B and C after this period of time – just in case they weren't evident at the start of the donation process. For these reasons fresh sperm is no longer used for DI treatment and highlights the risk of finding sperm donors online. Screening of donors also includes a thorough medical history, including family history of genetic disease, clinical examination to exclude infections (herpes, human papillomavirus, chlamydia), semen culture and blood screening for hepatitis B and C, HIV, syphilis and cytomegalovirus. The donor's blood group (rhesus status) and chromosomal analysis are also assessed. Additional screening for CF is also performed.

Matching the donor with the recipient

If you decide to go down the route of donor sperm, you will usually be matched with a donor based on the characteristics of the male partner of the recipient. This typically means physical appearance (race, hair and eye colour, height and build) and sometimes blood group (both ABO and rhesus factor), although the latter more for family rather than medical reasons, as these days with genetic testing it is easy to find out whether or not two individuals are related. If you are part of a same-sex female couple or a single woman, the characteristics will be discussed and agreed so that a suitable match can be made.

In some countries, most notably the USA, it is possible to choose donors (of both sperm and eggs) from a database that includes photos and much more in the way of physical characteristics and personal details. While some people like this concept, it does tend to over-commercialise the whole process.

The female partner should always have routine fertility investigations to ensure there aren't any problems (see Chapter 12). Investigations can be kept to a minimum if she is young and healthy, with regular periods and no history of gynaecological disease. At the very least she should be immune to rubella and be ovulating. Unless tubal damage is suspected from the medical history, she would normally have between three and six cycles of DI before a test of tubal patency (see page 233), though a pre-treatment ultrasound scan of the pelvis is a good idea to ensure that there are no abnormalities of the uterus or ovaries.

Timing of insemination

Initially, the woman will usually have a series of ultrasound scans to make sure she is ovulating. The number of clinic appointments can then be minimised by testing for ovulation at home. This also helps choose the right timing for treatment and is done with kits that test for LH in the urine (morning and evening) at the time of the mid-cycle surge. As soon as there is a positive result for LH, this means ovulation is about to happen, so the female partner should contact the clinic and go in for the insemination. Most insemination treatments are done in a natural cycle, although sometimes a human chorionic gonadotrophin (hCG) injection is needed to trigger ovulation and time insemination accurately. This will usually involve prior monitoring of the growing follicle with ultrasound scans.

Sperm is usually passed through the cervix into the uterus via a fine plastic straw – intrauterine insemination (IUI). This simple process has been shown to be more effective than simply leaving

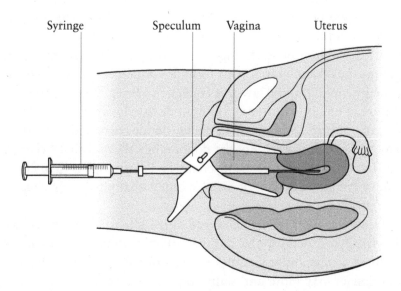

Syringe   Speculum   Vagina   Uterus

Transferring sperm (insemination) or embryo into uterus

the sperm in the top of the vagina or cervix (intracervical insemination). One insemination is sufficient; some clinics try double insemination on consecutive days, but there is no evidence that this improves the chance of pregnancy.

The chance of conceiving using frozen sperm in a single month is around 10–15 per cent, and if you try each month, you have a 40–50 per cent chance of conceiving after six months and a 70–80 per cent chance if you keep trying for a year if the woman is under the age of 35 years. If you haven't been able to achieve a pregnancy after 6–9 cycles of treatment, the next step is to consider IVF, with donor sperm.

Genetic origins

If you're considering fertility treatment and need donor eggs or sperm, it's important to think through the implications and agree how you will manage telling your children about their genetic origins as they grow up. Gamete donation used to be anonymous in the UK, except when it was intentionally undertaken between people who know each other. There was considerable pressure from some of the people born as a result of donated gametes to learn more about their genetic origins. They pointed out the anomaly that adopted children have the right of information about their birth parents, but that children born from donor gametes were denied it. Therefore in 2005, the law was changed to bring the right to information of children born as a result of donated gametes in line with that of adopted children. As a result, donor-conceived individuals may find out the identity of the donor when they reach 18 years of age. Interestingly, despite being counselled to do so, less than 20 per cent of couples who use donated sperm actually tell their children how they were conceived.

However, since the law changed in the UK to allow the release of identifying details, the number of men donating sperm has declined significantly. Couples in need of treatment now have to wait longer, pay more and sadly sometimes give up. There is also big business nowadays in the import of donated sperm from overseas, which is permissible provided that the sperm originates from a clinic that is regulated to the same standards as UK clinics.

Sperm from a single donor cannot legally be used after ten families have been achieved, because of the theoretical risk of 'paternal siblings' meeting in years to come and wishing to have children without knowing their own origins. The HFEA keeps a central record of all donors and resultant pregnancies, but the genetic origins of the child are not recorded on the birth certificate. Many people who use donor sperm keep additional samples from the same donor for future use after conceiving their first child so that their siblings are genetically related and also likely to have similar features.

Chapter 14

Ovulation Matters

B EING AWARE OF what your body is telling you about your
reproductive health can really help when it comes to need-
ing medical treatment. One of the most significant factors is
understanding whether or not you are ovulating. If you have very
irregular periods, long gaps between periods or, sometimes, no
periods at all, this may mean you are not ovulating. These situations can be grouped together with the term 'anovulatory infertility'
or anovulation.

The steps that can be taken to manage this are first to correct
any underlying disorder (such as nutritional deficiency in those
who are underweight) and optimise health (by losing weight in
those who have polycystic ovary syndrome (PCOS) and are overweight) before starting treatment to stimulate regular unifollicular
ovulation – that is with the release of a single egg. We have already
looked at the first two (see Chapters 3 and 6), so in this chapter we
will focus on ovulation.

CHECKING YOUR TUBES

There are a few things that need to be checked before starting ovulation induction therapy, including an assessment of your tubes to
ensure they are clear and functioning (see Chapter 16). There are
some specialists who believe that, if there is no firm suggestion of
a problem (e.g. past history of pelvic infection or pelvic pain), you
can have treatment to help you ovulate for three to six months

before you need to have your tubes checked. In order to minimise the risks and also to ensure a cost-effective approach to treatment, we feel that an assessment of tubal patency is appropriate in every woman before starting.

ASSESSING YOUR CYCLE

If you suffer from anovulatory infertility, you may either have a complete absence of any cycles (amenorrhea) or infrequent, irregular periods (oligomenorrhea), particularly if you have PCOS. Amenorrhea is sometimes termed primary – where periods never started – or secondary, that is, the periods have stopped. All causes of secondary amenorrhea can also cause primary amenorrhea, although there are some rare causes of primary amenorrhoea that will come to light when an adolescent hasn't yet started her periods because important structures haven't developed normally: for example, the hypothalamus or pituitary may be abnormal, the womb may not have developed at all or it may be there but there is a blockage preventing the flow of menstrual blood.

There are four main causes of absent or irregular periods: hypogonadotrophic hypogonadism, high levels of prolactin, ovarian insufficiency and PCOS (which is the most common and accounts for about 90 per cent of cases). We have covered ovarian insufficiency, which either causes periods to stop altogether or irregular periods in its early stages due to low anti-Müllerian hormone (AMH), in Chapter 12 and we will cover PCOS in detail in the next chapter.

Hypogonadotrophic hypogonadism

One common reason for problems with periods and ovulation is something called hypogonadotrophic hypogonadism. This means low levels of the gonadotrophin hormones – follicle-stimulating hormone (FSH) and luteinising hormone (LH) – that cause the gonads (ovaries or testes) to stop working – 'hypogonadism' – and can be caused by problems either with the pituitary or hypothalamus.

The most common causes of hypogonadotrophic hypogonadism that lead to problems with periods and ovulation include:

- **Being underweight:** In women who are underweight, LH levels are often lower than FSH levels.

- **Eating disorders:** Anorexia nervosa can impact FSH and LH levels and lead to amenorrhoea. Bulimia is another eating disorder that can affect fertility, and both conditions tend to cause problems with periods and ovulation. While fertility doctors can treat the physical aspects of these conditions, it's important to seek psychological help to address the underlying causes and also support you during pregnancy (see also Chapters 6 and 9).

- **Exercise:** Over-exercising can disrupt the menstrual cycle, and period problems are common in athletes undergoing intensive training. Between 10 and 20 per cent have oligomenorrhea or amenorrhea, compared with 5 per cent in the general population. Amenorrhea is particularly common in endurance athletes (e.g. with long-distance running). Up to half of competitive runners training 80 miles per week may have no periods. The main factors are low weight and percentage body fat, which is why gymnasts, runners and ballerinas tend to have greater problems than swimmers. The physiological changes are similar to those seen with starvation and chronic illness. You don't have to be a professional athlete for exercise to cause problems, however, so always discuss your exercise levels with your doctor if you are having problems with your periods.

- **Unknown cause:** Sometimes the cause simply isn't known ('idiopathic hypogonadotrophic hypogonadism') and we recommend following the dietary and lifestyle guidance we covered in Part 1 (chapters 3 and 4) alongside medical treatment. Sometimes eating more can help, even if you are not underweight, but we recommend seeking professional advice first.

Rare causes of hypogonadotrophic hypogonadism include a tumour of the pituitary and/or hypothalamus, diseases such as tuberculosis and sarcoid, being overweight and Kallmann syndrome, a rare condition where the nerve cells that secrete gonadotrophin-releasing hormone (GnRH) from the hypothalamus to the pituitary fail to develop (see page 196). Kallmann syndrome is diagnosed if periods have never started and FSH and LH levels are unrecordable; there is often also a deficiency of the sense of smell (anosmia) and/or colour blindness.

Treating hypogonadotrophic hypogonadism

If you are found to have hypogonadotrophic hypogonadism (sometimes abbreviated as hypog hypog or simply HH), then you will first need hormone replacement therapy (HRT) to give you an artificial menstrual cycle and healthy levels of oestrogen until the time is right for you to start trying for a pregnancy, and then ovulation induction. Ovulation is best stimulated with GnRH, delivered by a mini pump that delivers the hormone in pulses under the skin every 90 minutes, which provides the most natural treatment to address the underlying hormone imbalance with little risk of multiple pregnancy. However, the GnRH medication is no longer manufactured for this use and the drugs are no longer available in the UK. The alternative is human menopausal gonadotrophin (hMG) injections that contain both FSH and LH rather than alternatives containing FSH alone.

Weight and hypogonadotrophic hypogonadism

You may gain weight and reach a normal BMI but still not resume regular periods. This is because sometimes the body resets itself and simply won't start ovulating naturally, so you will need medication to help. In some cases, high levels of exercise continue to suppress the hypothalamus, in which case your LH levels will still be low. Furthermore, approximately 20 per cent of women have PCOS, which only comes to light when they put on weight, and PCOS is also associated with an increased rate of eating disorders.

If you are underweight, you could be treated with gonadotrophin injections to help restore ovulation, but it is not in the baby's best interests to be pregnant when severely underweight as there is significant risk of intrauterine growth retardation (IUGR), prematurity, still birth and neonatal problems. Therefore, it is vital to first gain weight and correct any nutrient deficiencies before treatment and conception to prevent the avoidable risks to the unborn child.

Nila and Bodhi: Periods stopped due to being underweight

Nila (33) and Bodhi (35) had been together for eight years and had been trying to conceive for two years. Nila was a keen gymnast as a child and very slim. She went through puberty later than her friends and didn't start her periods until she was 16, when she weighed 50kg with a BMI of 20. She then became very anxious about her eating habits and restricted her diet. Her weight fell to 45kg and her periods stopped for a couple of years. She was prescribed the contraceptive pill, which gave her a regular cycle. When she stopped, her weight was 47kg and once more she did not have any periods. When we met Nila, her ovaries had a multicystic appearance and her hormone profile indicated hypogonadotrophic hypogonadism. We provided her with a full nutritional assessment and a diet plan. After six months she had gained her target weight of 50kg, but was still not having periods. She responded well to ovulation induction treatment with gonadotrophin injections and conceived during the third cycle.

Hyperprolactinemia: Overproduction of prolactin

Prolactin is a hormone secreted from the pituitary gland to trigger milk production from the breasts during breastfeeding (lactation). This acts as a natural contraceptive by (usually) switching off the menstrual cycle to allow time for a mother to breastfeed one baby before conceiving another. Aside from the very high levels produced during pregnancy and breastfeeding, there are many causes of a mildly elevated prolactin level, some of which can also cause problems with the menstrual cycle. These include stress, hypothyroidism and various medications. A recent physical or breast examination can also temporarily raise prolactin. If prolactin levels are more than 1,000mU/L, this suggests a problem and the test should be repeated. If the second result is still high, it is likely that there is a benign pituitary tumour that is producing the excess prolactin hormone. Sometimes the levels can reach the tens of thousands.

Treating hyperprolactinemia

If the level of prolactin is only slightly elevated and you're having regular periods, then there is no evidence that treatment to reduce prolactin levels will improve fertility. On the other hand, if your periods have stopped because of high prolactin, then you will need treatment. The main symptoms are usually caused by low oestrogen (vaginal dryness, dyspareunia – pain during intercourse) and reduced libido (sex drive). Prolonged oestrogen deficiency can also lead to osteoporosis. You may also get some milk production from the breasts (galactorrhea), which happens in up to a third of women with high prolactin. In about 5 per cent the tumour can affect the optic nerve, which sits at the base of the brain on top of the pituitary gland, and cause eyesight problems (loss of peripheral vision).

Tumours can be seen on computed tomography (CT) and magnetic resonance imaging (MRI) scans and usually shrink quickly with medical treatments, such as bromocriptine or cabergoline, which are taken as a weekly, twice-weekly or daily tablet. Surgery to remove a tumour is complex and reserved for cases when drugs don't work and fail to shrink the tumour, or if there are intolerable side effects from the drugs.

Chapter 15

Polycystic Ovary Syndrome (PCOS)

POLYCYSTIC OVARY SYNDROME (PCOS) is the commonest hormonal disturbance in women and is the main cause of problems with periods and ovulation, accounting for 85–90 per cent of cases of anovulatory infertility. Aside from menstrual cycle disturbances (irregular or absent periods), the most significant problems that women with PCOS experience are difficulty in controlling body weight and skin problems (acne and unwanted hair growth on the face or body). Not all women with PCOS experience all of the symptoms and many women have relatively mild symptoms. Furthermore, a woman's problems may change over time. In particular, gaining weight can make PCOS symptoms worse.

If you have some of these problems and haven't had a diagnosis, it's important to be investigated for PCOS. This will involve an ultrasound scan and blood tests. It's possible to have polycystic ovaries, as seen on ultrasound scan, without the full-blown syndrome. This happens in around 20–30 per cent of women whereas a smaller proportion will have symptoms of PCOS – perhaps 10–15 per cent. This does depend on where you come from, as there are worldwide and ethnic variations in the prevalence of the syndrome.

WHAT ARE POLYCYSTIC OVARIES?

Polycystic ovaries contain many small follicles (incorrectly termed 'cysts') that each contain an egg and have started to grow, but do not reach a mature size and instead remain at a size of about

216

2–5mm in diameter. The diagnosis is best made by an ultrasound scan, which visualises the ovaries and the small cysts within them (see page 159). A polycystic ovary usually contains at least 20 of these small follicles or cysts and with modern ultrasound machines many more may be visible (these days we expect to see at least 20 per ovary, while a few years ago the diagnosis was made when 12 were seen). Sometimes blood tests show characteristic changes in hormone levels, although these changes are not universal and can vary considerably from person to person.

The ultrasound picture is not always clear and some women with PCOS may have an ultrasound scan that does not clearly demonstrate polycystic ovaries. This isn't a problem as the syndrome is defined by the presence of at least two out of the following three characteristics:

1. Signs or symptoms of high androgen hormones – predominantly testosterone – namely, unwanted facial or bodily hair, loss of hair from the head, acne or an elevated blood level of testosterone itself. If the testosterone is much higher than expected additional tests may be performed to look for other causes of androgen excess, for example tumours of the ovaries or adrenal glands and other rare hormonal conditions (such as late-onset congenital adrenal hyperplasia or Cushing's syndrome).

2. Irregular or absent menstrual periods, after other causes for these have been excluded by simple blood tests to measure the other hormones – follicle-stimulating hormone (FSH), luteinising hormone (LH), oestradiol, prolactin and thyroid function.

3. Polycystic ovaries on an ultrasound scan.

Women with polycystic ovary *syndrome* may have elevated levels of:

- Testosterone: an ovarian androgen hormone that influences hair growth and is also converted to oestrogen.

- LH: a pituitary hormone that influences hormone production by the ovaries and is important for normal ovulation.

- Oestrogen (oestradiol): an ovarian hormone that stimulates growth of the womb lining (endometrium).

- Insulin: a hormone that is principally involved in the utilisation of energy from food, which when elevated may stimulate the ovary to overproduce testosterone and prevent the follicles from growing normally to release eggs and hence cause the ovary to become polycystic. Indeed, it is high levels of insulin that is thought to be one of the main problems for women with PCOS. Insulin becomes more elevated in women who are overweight. Insulin in the blood is not routinely measured, but often other signs of problems of insulin action are (see below).

- Anti-Müllerian hormone (AMH): a measure of the ovarian reserve (or how fertile the ovaries are) and correlates with the number of small follicles seen on the scan.

There are also many other subtle hormonal abnormalities that may affect ovarian function and influence the menstrual cycle, fertility, bodily hair growth, body weight and general health.

INVESTIGATIONS

Standard blood tests include measurements of the following hormones: testosterone, LH, FSH, thyroid hormones and prolactin. Sex hormone binding globulin (SHBG) – the protein that carries testosterone around the blood – is also sometimes, but not always, measured. AMH is a more recent test that may also sometimes be suggested.

Glucose tolerance test – a sugary drink – is given first thing in the morning on an empty stomach and blood taken at the time of the drink and then again after two hours. This helps to see how well the body handles sugar in food and is a screening test for diabetes.

In essence it helps to assess the action of insulin. A measure of gly-cosylated haemoglobin (HbA1c) is another way of assessing the long-term effects of blood sugar levels and is also used to screen for diabetes and monitor the long-term control of diabetes.

Cholesterol levels (best done first thing in the morning before anything is eaten or drunk) are also a useful indicator of long-term health, especially for women with PCOS who are overweight.

An ultrasound scan of the pelvis allows visualisation of the ovaries and also the womb – it is important also to measure the thickness of the womb lining (endometrium), for reasons explained below.

CAUSES

It is now thought that having polycystic ovaries may run in families and so there is some evidence of a genetic cause, although there are probably a number of genes involved, and for a condition that is so common there are likely to be a number of genetic and environmental influences for the development of PCOS. Some women may have polycystic ovaries and never have symptoms – or, for that matter, never know that they have polycystic ovaries. Ovaries do not suddenly become polycystic, but women who have polycystic ovaries may develop symptoms at any time, for reasons that are not always clear. A gain in body weight is often the precipitating cause for the development of symptoms. The appearance of polycystic ovaries does not tend to disappear, although symptoms may improve, either naturally or as a result of therapy.

It appears that one of the fundamental problems is with over-production of insulin due to inefficient handling of energy from food. While the extra insulin is working hard, it is ineffective in turning carbohydrates from food into energy and instead they are turned into fat. The high level of insulin has other effects in the body, including stimulating the ovaries to overproduce androgens (mainly testosterone), which then inhibits normal ovulation and also leads to longer term effects, such as the development of type 2 diabetes, high cholesterol levels and an increased risk of cardiovascular disease (heart attack and stroke).

The balance of hormones is affected by body weight and being overweight can greatly upset this balance and make the symptoms of PCOS worse. Being overweight is commonly associated with PCOS and this increases the risk of heart disease and high blood pressure in later life. Many clinics now measure cholesterol levels and if they are abnormal dietary advice is given. A high-fibre, low-fat and low-sugar diet at a young age, together with regular exercise, may help to reduce problems such as high blood pressure and heart attacks when older. Smoking cigarettes seriously worsens the risk of developing these problems. Another problem sometimes seen over time is the development of 'late-onset' or type 2 diabetes, in which blood sugar levels stay abnormally elevated. If this occurs it is then necessary to modify the dietary intake of carbohydrates and sometimes to take medication. The risk of both cardiovascular disease and diabetes can be reduced by keeping to the correct weight for your height.

The small cysts in the ovaries do not get larger, in fact they eventually disappear and are replaced by new cysts. The cysts (follicles) are on average 2–5mm and no greater than 9mm. If a follicle starts to grow and develops into a mature follicle it should then ovulate when it is about 20–25mm in diameter. Ovulation may occur regularly, for example once a month in women with PCOS who have regular periods, or less frequently in those with long gaps between their periods. The cysts are not the type of ovarian cyst that require surgical removal – such cysts are usually 50mm or larger and often have a different appearance. Furthermore, the cysts of the polycystic ovary do not lead to ovarian cancer.

Women with PCOS and infrequent or absent periods are at risk of excessive growth of the endometrium as a result of constant stimulation by oestrogen in the absence of progesterone, which is only produced by the ovaries after ovulation. It is important that the endometrium is shed on a regular basis to prevent this from happening as, if the endometrium becomes too thick, it may sometimes develop into cancer of the womb (endometrial carcinoma). The endometrium can be seen on an ultrasound scan and if it appears too thick or irregular, a hysteroscopy and endometrial biopsy procedure is advised in order to examine the endometrium under a microscope.

TREATMENT

Menstrual irregularities

While this book is all about fertility, if you have PCOS you may experience different symptoms at different stages in your life and may require treatments when you are not trying for a baby. Irregular and unpredictable periods can be unpleasant and a nuisance as well as suggesting irregular ovulation and the risk of endometrial thickening. The longer the intervals between periods, the more likely they are to be heavy due to the increasing build-up of the endometrium. If you're not trying to conceive, the easiest approach is the use of a low-dose combined oral contraceptive (a contraceptive pill). This will result in an artificial cycle and regular shedding of the endometrium. Some women cannot take the pill and require alternative hormonal therapy to induce regular periods, such as a progestogen/progesterone for ten days every one to three months, depending on an individual's requirements.

We believe that it is important to have a period at least once every three to four months to prevent abnormal thickening of the womb lining. An alternative is to use a progesterone secreting coil (for example, a Mirena intrauterine system) that releases the hormone progesterone into the womb, thereby protecting it and usually resulting in reduced or absent menstrual bleeding.

Skin problems

If you have high androgen (testosterone) levels, the skin may be affected. Acne may appear on your face, chest or back. Sometimes there is also unwanted hair growth on the face, chest, abdomen, arms and legs. These problems may be more prominent in women with darker hair or skin, simply because the unwanted hair is more noticeable than in fairer people. There are also ethnic differences in the way the hair follicles respond to the hormones. A less common problem is thinning of hair on the head, although if this occurs it is rarely serious. Being overweight probably causes the worst problems for women with PCOS by aggravating imbalances of the hormones that control ovulation and affect skin and hair growth.

Physical treatments to remove unwanted hair, such as electrolysis, laser therapy and waxing, may be helpful while waiting for medical treatments to work, and are the only real options for women who wish to conceive as drugs are either contraceptive or dangerous for the developing baby. Electrolysis and waxing may be expensive and should only be performed by properly trained therapists as scarring can result from unskilled treatment. Shaving can help some women and, contrary to popular belief, does not make hair grow back faster.

Any combined oral contraceptive pill is likely to improve acne and unwanted hair growth by suppressing the production of testosterone from the ovaries and also raising SHBG levels, which mops up testosterone already in circulation. Some contraceptive preparations contain specific anti-androgen hormones, such as cyproterone acetate and drospirenone, although they don't appear to be much better in controlling the symptoms of PCOS. Spironolactone is an effective preparation, particularly for women who are overweight or who have high blood pressure (for whom the contraceptive pill may not be allowable). There are also other hormone treatments and drugs, such as isotretinoin, that can be effective, but also bring with them more potentially serious side effects and must not be taken when trying to get pregnant. Topical preparations such as eflornithine may be helpful, but also cannot be used while trying to conceive.

Weight, nutrition and modifiable factors

Being overweight worsens the symptoms of PCOS, yet it can be very hard to lose weight and there isn't a simple solution. Having PCOS does not in itself make you gain weight, but women with PCOS find it easy to put on weight as their metabolism works inefficiently to deal with food. Regular physical exercise (at least 20–30 minutes of hard exercise, 5–7 days per week) will increase the body's metabolism and significantly improve the ability to lose weight and improve long-term health.

Diet and lifestyle

The recommended first-line treatment for women with PCOS is a dietary and lifestyle approach, but in practice this usually means your doctor will encourage you to lose weight. In reality, there is much more that you can do in order to optimise the different parameters associated with PCOS, including menstrual cycle irregularity, insulin resistance and hormonal disturbances. The principles that we covered in Part 1 are especially important for women with PCOS in terms of following a healthy, balanced diet and optimising all nutrient levels and the gut microbiota. Indeed, it has been suggested that the changes in the gut microbiota following bariatric surgery may be the underlying factor that improves fertility and PCOS parameters in the women treated, so always pay attention to digestive symptoms.

Women with PCOS are disproportionately affected by low vitamin D when it comes to *in vitro* fertilisation (IVF) outcomes, so your nutrient status takes on an added significance if you suffer from this condition. One study showed that vitamin D and calcium supplementation together may improve menstrual regularity, hyperandrogenism, weight loss and fertility in women with PCOS.[1] Other studies have found that micronutrient supplementation for a period of three months improves PCOS parameters including the ratio of LH to FSH and serum testosterone levels.[2] This particular supplementation protocol included folic acid, vitamin E, omega-3, co-enzyme Q10, catechin (a flavonoid) and glycyrrhizin (liquorice extract). In our patients, we find that additional zinc, magnesium and vitamin B_6 are usually needed. Interestingly, various animal and laboratory studies show that zinc inhibits the enzyme (5-a reductase) that converts testosterone into dihydrotestosterone and that vitamin B_6 increases this effect.[3] Dihydrotestosterone is the more potent androgen that leads to typical symptoms in PCOS of acne, hirsutism and sometimes alopecia. However, the effects of zinc in terms of 5-a reductase and related symptoms in women with PCOS have not been well studied in humans and the underlying processes are complex. Likewise, data is mixed in terms of the effects of fatty acids on 5-a reductase, and vitamin D was found not to have an effect in one study, contrary to what you may read online.[4] Again, we urge caution in terms of sourcing information online that often presents early or suggestive evidence from animal and laboratory studies as established scientific fact for humans.

As a starting point, we recommend testing and ensuring adjusting supplementation according to individual results before considering any kind of standardised supplementation protocols from studies.

Other significant factors include exercise and food choices, with exercise improving menstrual cycle regularity in women with PCOS. As we've seen, the data is still mixed in terms of the effects of dairy on PCOS, though it is possible that cow's milk may worsen symptoms (see page 40). Soy is likely to be beneficial for women with PCOS, as is reduced carbohydrate and slightly higher levels of protein. Including some protein with each meal, as outlined in Chapter 3, is therefore particularly important, but ensure you eat a balanced diet. A very high-protein or ketogenic diet is not recommended and ensuring sufficient intake of whole grains and dietary fibre will feed the bacteria in your gut and fuel exercise adequately.

Avoiding refined carbohydrate is especially important for women with PCOS. Having only one meal a day that is 'carb-heavy' (for example, one that includes a small or medium-sized jacket potato or a portion of brown rice) is a good rule of thumb. This may look like poached eggs, grilled tomatoes and spinach or scrambled eggs and home-made guacamole for breakfast, a chicken salad for lunch and a fish or tofu Thai curry with vegetables and a medium portion of brown rice for your evening meal. Including five portions of beans and legumes per week will help to ensure good intake of fibre. Don't forget to include two or three portions of fruit daily and a snack of nuts and seeds to ensure a good spread of nutrients. As always, adjust portion size so that you feel satisfied after each meal and properly hungry by the next. The proportion of macronutrients that is optimal for each of us varies, and some people find they need more carbohydrate than this. We recommend monitoring your response carefully when changing your diet and seeking professional advice where needed.

Once all the different dietary and lifestyle factors have been optimised, we routinely see improvements in symptoms including regularisation of the menstrual cycle, weight loss and return of ovulation. Some patients who have struggled with symptoms and subfertility for years are able to conceive naturally purely through natural interventions. At the very least, taking these steps will help put you in the best possible place prior to any medical treatment that may be needed.

Therapeutic supplements

After making the necessary changes to diet and lifestyle and addressing the underlying factors that are individual to you, including nutrient levels, there are certain additional steps that may be helpful in improving symptoms. It is beyond the scope of this book to cover them all in detail, but there are various supplements that have been tested in women with PCOS. One that has seen a growing evidence base to demonstrate benefit, especially when it comes to fertility, is myo-inositol.[5] Inositol is a naturally occurring substance in the B vitamin family found in foods including nuts, seeds, oranges, grapefruit and melon, to name a few. Numerous studies have shown improvements to hormonal parameters of PCOS, including significantly decreased levels of testosterone and dehydroepiandrosterone sulfate (DHEA-S) and increased levels of SHBG following inositol supplementation.[6] Research has also shown improvements in metabolic factors in terms of fasting insulin and fasting glucose.[7] When it comes to fertility, studies have demonstrated that frequency of the menstrual cycle and ovulation rates both increased following supplementation with inositol and no serious adverse events.[8] In other words, inositol seems to be safe to take.

Evidence to suggest the number of women having a healthy baby increases following inositol supplementation is also starting to emerge. A recent small study concluded that the combination of two different forms of inositol (myo-inositol and D-chiro-inositol) at high doses of D-chiro-inositol improved the pregnancy rates and live birth rates and also reduced the risk of ovarian hyperstimulation syndrome (OHSS) in women with PCOS undergoing IVF treatment with intracytoplasmic sperm injection (ICSI).[9] Over half – 55.2 per cent – of women in the group treated with the combined inositol supplement went on to have a baby compared with 14.8 per cent in the control group, so this is significant indeed (perhaps implausibly so and may be due to the small number of patients), and the effects need to be demonstrated in larger trials. Overall, however, evidence supports a 40:1 ratio between myo-inositol and D-chiro-inositol for the treatment of PCOS.[10] Myo-inositol has also shown to be beneficial in preventing gestational diabetes and early studies indicate it is safe to supplement during pregnancy, though it is especially important to seek the advice of your treating doctor before taking any supplements while pregnant.[11]

Finally, supplementation with the protein alpha-lactalbumin may improve absorption of myo-inositol, which is impaired in some patients. Taken together, alpha-lactalbumin and inositol may increase the chance of experiencing benefit but, importantly, alpha-lactalbumin is a protein derived from milk and should not be taken by those with milk allergies or intolerances.

One caveat with this type of supplement or nutraceutical is that it is important to start any additional supplements that may offer therapeutic potential *after* you have optimised your individual nutrient levels. Sometimes these products can lead to sufficient improvements to help you conceive, but there may still be underlying deficiencies that lead to poorer outcomes.

Other supplements that have shown benefit in women with PCOS include cinnamon (improved antioxidant status, insulin resistance and serum lipid profile) and evening primrose oil together with vitamin D (significantly improved various parameters including triglycerides and cholesterol). These supplements have not been suitably tested in terms of fertility, and care should always be taken in the weeks leading up to fertility treatment and in the second half of your cycle when you may become pregnant.

TREATING INFERTILITY

Various factors influence how well the ovaries function and fertility is adversely affected by being overweight. The first-line approach is therefore lifestyle changes and weight loss. Once these have been addressed, there are other treatments that can be used to induce ovulation.

Medication

The first drug to try is usually either letrozole or clomiphene citrate (both come as tablets) and if these don't work the alternatives include daily hormone injections of a drug that contains FSH or alternatively an operation performed by laparoscopic ('keyhole') surgery in which the ovaries are cauterised (where a small hole is made using heat – called ovarian diathermy or 'drilling').

These treatments must be monitored by ultrasound observation of the developing follicle in the ovary. This means you have to attend the fertility clinic on a regular basis in order to prevent the main side effect, which is multiple pregnancy. The aim of the treatment is to induce the release of only one egg. Another risk of treatment is OHSS, when the ovaries respond oversensitively and can make the individual very unwell.

Both letrozole and clomiphene are taken for 5 days starting on day 2 of your period. Sometimes a bleed has to be brought on artificially with a short course of an oral progestogen (such as medroxyprogesterone acetate). The monthly chance of conception is about 20 per cent and will depend upon other factors too, such as your age and body weight. If you don't ovulate initially then the dose may be increased.

Gonadotrophin therapy

If you still don't ovulate, the next stage is gonadotrophin therapy, which involves daily injections of a preparation that contains predominantly FSH but also often LH too. The injections are subcutaneous – just under the skin – and so are quite easy to self-administer. Gonadotrophins are available in the form of urinary-derived human menopausal gonadotrophin (hMG) and human chorionic gonadotrophin (hCG), which contains FSH and LH or genetically engineered (recombinantly-derived) FSH, LH and hCG. There is no difference in results irrespective of which drug is used. The main risks of gonadotrophin therapy are overstimulation and multiple pregnancy, and so a low-dose protocol should be used and monitored very carefully.

It can be extremely difficult to predict the response to stimulation of a woman with polycystic ovaries – indeed this is our biggest challenge as doctors when giving treatment to kick-start ovulation. The polycystic ovary often looks quite inactive, at least on the ultrasound scan, and then it suddenly responds to stimulation as lots of follicles start to get bigger at once. Therefore, it can be very challenging to stimulate the development of a single dominant follicle – remembering also that there are two ovaries.

Ovulation should occur in 70–80 per cent of cycles of which the majority should result in the release of only one egg, thereby reducing your chance of having a multiple pregnancy. You should be closely monitored and treatment suspended if two or more follicles develop, as the risk of multiple pregnancy obviously increases.

Ovulation does not need to be triggered if you're taking letrozole or clomiphene, whereas if you're having gonadotrophin therapy, you will need a single injection of hCG when there is at least one follicle of at least 17mm in its largest diameter and no more than a total of two follicles larger than 14mm in diameter. If too many follicles develop, hCG is withheld, and you will be advised to refrain from sexual intercourse (as the eggs can still sometimes be ovulated even if hCG hasn't been given).

Because gonadotrophin therapy is usually only given if you are resistant to letrozole or clomiphene, you will still have a good chance of conception over time as it has been shown that the use of gonadotrophin ovulation induction is even better used as first-line therapy. However, this has to be balanced by the convenience of tablets and the high costs of the gonadotrophin injections.

Lily and James: PCOS

Lily was 28 and had never had a regular cycle. She and James had been trying for a baby for three years before they came to see us. At that time, Lily was having a period once every six months or so. Our initial investigations identified that she had PCOS. She was also very overweight with a BMI of 38 and was going to need to lose 12kg to get her BMI down to under 30, which would enable her to be eligible for NHS-funded treatment. We explained that the reason for losing weight was more than just enabling access to NHS funding as it would also increase her general health, improve the prospects of responding to treatment and also the likelihood of having a normal pregnancy with a healthy baby.

They did conceive naturally but unfortunately experienced an early miscarriage, which very probably was due to Lily being so overweight. She attended our preconception course and was highly motivated. James was also a little overweight and so together they supported each other to lose weight by joining a gym, cooking meals together from scratch and avoiding snacking between meals. Once Lily's weight had reduced, her periods became more frequent but were still very irregular, occurring every 35–48 days or so. We started letrozole treatment, initially at a dose of 2.5mg, which did not stimulate ovulation, and so we increased it to 5mg, but this was still unsuccessful. We then embarked upon treatment with daily hMG injections, which we monitored very closely with ultrasound scans. Lily continued to lose weight during these treatments and they conceived with the second cycle and now have a healthy baby boy.

Metformin

One treatment that has been popular in recent years is metformin. Because it lowers insulin, which causes some of the problems associated with PCOS, it was expected to improve symptoms. Initial studies appeared to be promising, suggesting that metformin could improve fertility in women with PCOS. However, more recent large trials have observed limited beneficial effects of metformin.[12]

The role of metformin in the management of PCOS is therefore limited and you should only take it if you have impaired glucose tolerance (usually assessed by a glucose tolerance test – see page 218 – or the measurement of HbA1c in the blood) or type 2 diabetes.

Surgical ovulation induction

If you have PCOS and you don't respond to clomiphene, an alternative to gonadotrophin therapy is laparoscopic ovarian surgery.

This takes away the risks of multiple pregnancy and OHSS and you won't need intensive ultrasound monitoring. Furthermore, this surgery (ovarian diathermy) will be just as effective as routine gonadotrophin treatment if clomiphene doesn't work for you. This surgery may be especially beneficial for you if you have PCOS and you're not ovulating, you fail to respond to clomiphene and also have consistently high levels of LH, need a laparoscopic assessment of the pelvis or live too far away from the clinic to be able to attend for the many monitoring scans needed when having gonadotrophin treatment. You are more likely to respond better to laparoscopic ovarian diathermy (LOD) if you are slim with high LH levels.

Surgery does, of course, carry its own risks (see page 180) and must be performed only by fully trained laparoscopic surgeons. A concern is the possibility of ovarian destruction leading to ovarian failure, an obvious disaster in a woman wishing to conceive, although this should not occur with careful treatment and minimal diathermy to the ovary.

Although ovarian diathermy appears to be as effective as gonadotrophin therapy in the treatment of women with PCOS who do not respond to first-line therapy, it does take longer to get pregnant. Around half of those treated still need drugs to stimulate ovulation (either clomiphene or gonadotrophin injections). The greatest advantage for LOD is the need for less monitoring and that multiple pregnancy rates are considerably reduced.

IVF in women with polycystic ovaries

If you haven't conceived after between six and nine monthly treatment cycles then there are likely to be other things preventing you getting pregnant aside from not ovulating. The next step in your treatment is therefore IVF. IVF should be the end-of-the-line treatment for PCOS, but many patients with the syndrome may be referred for IVF, either because there is another reason for their infertility or because they fail to conceive despite ovulating (whether spontaneously or with assistance) – i.e. their infertility remains unexplained. Furthermore, as approximately 20 per cent of women have polycystic ovaries as detected by ultrasound scan, and many will have little in the way of symptoms, they may be referred for treatment for other reasons (for example, tubal factor or male factor). These women with asymptomatic polycystic ovaries are likely to respond sensitively to stimulation during IVF and are at increased risk of developing OHSS.

As with ovulation induction, if you have polycystic ovaries, the response to stimulation will be very different from that of normal ovaries. IVF depends on inducing many follicles to grow, and the polycystic ovary tends to have a more 'explosive' response with the development of lots of follicles in response to stimulation, which is associated with very high levels of circulating oestrogen. In some cases, this may result in OHSS, which is more common in women with polycystic ovaries.

Your risk of OHSS will be lower if your stimulation protocol includes gonadotrophin-releasing hormone (GnRH) antagonists rather than GnRH agonist protocols (see page 248). Furthermore, if you are at risk of OHSS, it is preferable to freeze all your embryos rather than do a fresh transfer as this has been shown to both reduce the risk of OHSS in women with PCOS and possibly also increase the chance of having a baby in the subsequent frozen embryo replacement cycle (see page 271).

IN VITRO MATURATION OF OOCYTES

In recent years, *in vitro* maturation (IVM) has attracted a lot of interest as a new assisted reproductive technique. The immature eggs (oocytes) are retrieved from the follicles of unstimulated (or minimally stimulated) ovaries. The oocytes are subsequently matured in an incubator (*in vitro*) for 24–48 hours. The mature oocytes are fertilised, usually by ICSI, and the selected embryos are transferred to the uterus two to three days later. Although IVM is labour-intensive compared with conventional IVF treatment, there are clinical advantages as you avoid large doses of gonadotrophins and, most importantly, avoid the risk of OHSS. Pregnancy rates are lower than with IVF and so IVM has not become a popular option.

Complications of treatment

If you have PCOS, you have increased risk of developing OHSS during ovulation induction and IVF. This happens when too many follicles are stimulated, leading to fluid building up in the abdominal cavity, chest and, sometimes, around the heart, with the symptoms of abdominal bloating, discomfort, nausea, vomiting and difficulty in breathing. Hospitalisation is sometimes necessary in order for intravenous fluids to be given to prevent dehydration, and blood thinning injections of heparin to prevent thromboembolism (blood clots in the legs and lungs). Although this condition is rare, it is a potentially fatal complication and should be avoidable with appropriate monitoring of treatment.

Multiple pregnancy is something else we want to avoid during fertility treatment, firstly because of the increased risk of problems in the babies and secondly because of the devastating effects on the family of caring for a large number of babies (see page 274). High-order multiple pregnancies (triplets or more) result almost exclusively from ovulation induction therapies. Careful monitoring is therefore required to prevent this from occurring.

The underlying principle of all methods of ovulation induction for women with PCOS must always be to use the lowest possible dose (of drug or surgery) to achieve the ovulation of only one egg and thereby avoid the significant risks of multiple pregnancy and OHSS.

Chapter 16

Pelvic Problems: Fallopian Tubes, Fibroids, Polyps and More

I N THIS CHAPTER we look at pelvic problems that might be linked with infertility, in particular problems with the fallopian tubes and uterus.

DAMAGED OR BLOCKED FALLOPIAN TUBES

For the egg to get to the uterus, at least one of your fallopian tubes needs to be functioning well. Tubal damage is usually caused by pelvic infection, with the commonest being *chlamydia trachomatis*. Infection may sometimes be asymptomatic or can cause severe pelvic pain, fever and the need for hospital admission. The degree of tubal damage can be graded. Mild forms distort the appearance of the tube and cause the fine hair-like cilia within the tube to be damaged. The cilia help to move the sperm to meet the egg for fertilisation to take place and then the fertilised egg back into the womb. This explains why tubes don't have to be blocked for them to stop working properly. Sometimes the fimbrial end of the tube near the ovary may be damaged, which affects its ability to receive the egg as it is released during ovulation. Adhesions around the end of the tube can also stop it functioning normally and, in severe cases, can encase the pelvic organs (uterus, tubes and ovaries) and cause a complete loss of fertility. Severe damage may block the tube either at its junction with the uterus (corneal end) or at the distal, fimbrial end, which can lead to the tube filling with fluid and forming a hydrosalpinx. Such a tube cannot ever function to achieve a pregnancy and the fluid within can get into the uterine cavity and prevent an embryo from implanting. A hydrosalpinx should therefore be removed (see page 176).

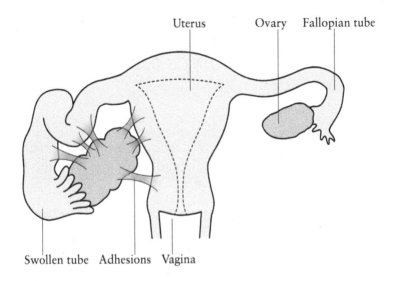

Uterus   Ovary   Fallopian tube

Swollen tube   Adhesions   Vagina

Damage to the ovaries or fallopian tubes can cause swelling and adhesions (where tissues and/or organs stick together)

What can we do about tubal damage?

In vitro fertilisation (IVF) has revolutionised many forms of fertility therapy, yet the question of IVF versus tubal surgery for mild to moderate tubal disease is sometimes still debated. IVF is a stressful and time-consuming treatment and each attempt offers only a single chance for pregnancy, unless embryos can be frozen for future use. Successful tubal surgery, on the other hand, can provide a permanent cure, with the possibility of more than one pregnancy. Furthermore, tubal surgery can be performed laparoscopically (often referred to as 'keyhole surgery', see page 286) rather than by open surgery, which requires a large incision into the abdomen and a longer recovery time, for the same results.

By the time the decision is made to perform tubal surgery you will have been thoroughly investigated. If there are coexisting fertility problems, for example sperm dysfunction, IVF is the way forward. Your age is another important consideration, as the success rates of IVF decline with age and in women over the age of 38 it is prudent to move on to IVF quickly rather than wait for tubal surgery to have a chance to work. Surgery is least likely to be of benefit when there is severe tubal damage with only a short length of normal tube or when there are extensive pelvic adhesions or an active disease such as endometriosis.

Selective salpingography and fallopian tube cannulation is a procedure to help check for blockages and identify where a blockage is. It can sometimes be used to open up the tubes without resort to surgery – a bit like unblocking a drainpipe. This is performed by a radiologist inserting a catheter into the tube at the time of a hysterosalpingogram (HSG, see page 175). You would usually have this done as an outpatient, though sometimes a general anaesthetic is needed.

Adhesions around the tubes interfere with pick-up of the egg and its transport along the tubes, while adhesions around the ovaries can prevent the release of an egg at the time of ovulation. When the tubes are patent and the ovaries freely mobile, adhesiolysis (a surgical procedure that cuts through the adhesions during a laparoscopy) will result in good cumulative conception rates (60 per cent in 24 months). Dense adhesions carry a worse prognosis than fine, filmy adhesions.

If you have a history of damaged fallopian tubes then you are at increased risk of an ectopic pregnancy (see page 285) and so you should always have a scan early in any future pregnancy to check that it is developing in the womb rather than the tube.

Reversing sterilisation

Surgery to reverse tubal sterilisation is often successful not only because there is a proven history of fertility, but also because damage from the original operation is usually to a very small portion of the tube. Pregnancy rates are between 60 and 80 per cent, with ectopic pregnancy rates usually less than 5 per cent. Your chance of having a baby in the 72 months after reversal of sterilisation is around 72 per cent if you are under the age of 37 years. Success rates over time are better with IVF and so the pros and cons need careful discussion. When taking cost-effectiveness into consideration, older women may be better proceeding straight to IVF (see Chapter 18).

In vitro fertilisation

Most women with tubal infertility are treated with IVF (see Chapter 18). If you have a history of repeated ectopic pregnancy there is a case for being sterilised prior to IVF, as developing a further ectopic pregnancy after the stresses of an IVF treatment cycle is very traumatic. The overall rate of ectopic pregnancy after IVF is 5 per cent (higher than normal) because transfer of the embryo into the womb does not ensure that it stays there. If you want to conceive, sterilisation is a big step, but if you have experienced ectopic pregnancies and have severe tubal damage, it can be easier to accept. If you have an ectopic after IVF and you have pre-existing tubal damage, it's best to discuss the option of sterilisation or salpingectomy (removal of the tube) before surgery for the ectopic pregnancy.

There is good evidence to suggest that having hydrosalpinges (fluid-filled damaged fallopian tubes) affects the outcome of IVF through their impact on the endometrium (womb lining), possibly due to toxic fluid getting into the uterus. This in turn can affect implantation. If the tubes are completely blocked and there are large hydrosalpinges there is a case for them to be removed before IVF as the chance of a live birth is doubled. The differences are more significant if you have hydrosalpinges in both tubes, and particularly so when they can be seen on an ultrasound scan.

FIBROIDS

Fibroids are areas of thickening of the muscle of the womb. They are common and increase in incidence with age. While they may be associated with heavier and painful periods, you may not be aware that they are there. The prevalence of fibroids is as low as 3 per cent in Caucasian women aged 25–32 years and 8 per cent in those aged 33–40, while rates have been reported as high as 80 per cent in those of Afro-Caribbean origin. You will usually have an initial ultrasound scan to assess whether you have fibroids, but magnetic resonance imaging (MRI) can be extremely helpful in giving more information about the position of multiple fibroids.

The exact location of fibroids is significant because it is thought that they are most likely to affect fertility if they either distort the endometrial cavity or they are partly embedded into the wall of the uterus (where at least 4cm is embedded). The main types of fibroids are:

- Serosal fibroids have the least impact on fertility and sit on external surfaces of the womb.

- Subserosal fibroids (in which at least 50 per cent projects out of the external surface) have a slightly bigger impact on fertility.

- Intramural fibroids that are partly embedded into the wall of the uterus but do not usually deform the cavity of the uterus have the next most significant impact.

- Submucous fibroids develop in the inner layer of the uterus and may protrude into the cavity of the uterus and so tend to have the most significant impact on fertility.

As with many aspects of the epidemiology of infertility, studies that have looked at the effect of fibroids on fertility are very mixed and can be difficult to interpret when it comes to thinking about the pros and cons of surgery.[1] There are many factors that need to be taken into consideration: the woman's age, the size, number and position of the fibroids, and other fertility factors.

Removal of fibroids

Until recently it was thought that fibroids should only be removed if they are causing a significant distortion of the uterine cavity or if they are blocking the first part of the fallopian tube. It is probably

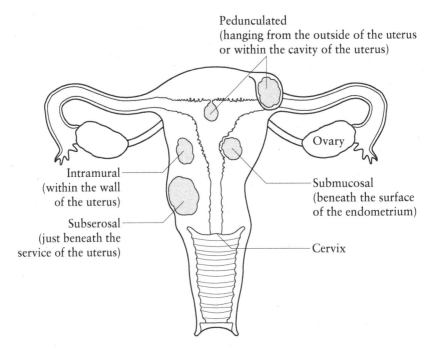

Pedunculated
(hanging from the outside of the uterus
or within the cavity of the uterus)

Ovary

Intramural
(within the wall
of the uterus)

Submucosal
(beneath the surface
of the endometrium)

Subserosal
(just beneath the
service of the uterus)

Cervix

Common locations of fibroids

not the presence of fibroids that affects implantation rates but rather the distortion of the uterine cavity that they cause – perhaps by affecting growth of the endometrium and altering the blood flow through the uterus. Fibroids may have adverse effects on pregnancy, with growth causing pain, miscarriage and preterm delivery; they may also cause the baby to lie in an abnormal position and so there is an increased need for caesarean delivery.

Surgery to remove fibroids is known as a myomectomy. It is a major procedure with potential risks to the uterus and may also cause extensive pelvic adhesions. Treatment with a gonadotrophin-releasing hormone (GnRH) agonist for six to eight weeks before your operation will cause significant shrinkage of the fibroids and their blood supply, which reduces bleeding during surgery. In recent years, a new drug – ulipristal acetate – has also been used for this purpose, although it is not a drug that we use because of concerns about side effects. Small submucosal fibroids can be removed hysteroscopically. There has yet to be a randomised controlled study of myomectomy before fertility treatment or, for that matter, looking at natural fertility.

Less invasive procedures than operative myomectomy are being evaluated for the management of fibroids, including uterine artery embolisation and MRI-guided laser coagulative necrosis or high-intensity focused ultrasound for the destruction of fibroids. The place of these techniques in the management of infertility is yet to be established. Furthermore, while uterine artery embolisation has become popular in the management of fibroids, it is not recommended for those who wish to preserve fertility because of the potential adverse effect on both uterine and ovarian blood supply – this is because the arteries that supply blood to the uterus are blocked off, as it isn't possible to selectively block off the blood supply to only the fibroids themselves. There is also an increase in adverse events during pregnancy, including miscarriage, an abnormally adherent placenta (placenta accreta), the need for caesarean delivery and heavy bleeding after delivery (postpartum haemorrhage), so we do not recommend embolisation in women wishing to conceive.

POLYPS

Polyps within the uterus are often found during initial investigations of the uterine cavity, during an HSG or at the time of hysteroscopy. If the polyp appears to be blocking the cornual opening of the tube, or if you also have abnormal bleeding, it should be removed. This can be easily done during a hysteroscopy. If, however, the polyp is an incidental finding during imaging of the pelvis, in the absence of symptoms, there is still debate as to whether surgery is beneficial – or, for that matter, the size at which a polyp may affect conception – as there is no clear evidence for an association between the presence of a polyp and infertility. It is our current practice to remove polyps > 1cm in diameter and if the patient is experiencing irregular bleeding or discharge, the polyp should be removed to exclude cancerous changes.

ASHERMAN'S SYNDROME

Asherman's syndrome may be picked up during either an HSG or hysterosalpingo-contrast sonography (HyCoSy) and is a relatively uncommon condition in which adhesions in the uterus prevent normal growth of the endometrium. This usually occurs after surgery to empty out the uterus (womb) after a miscarriage or termination of pregnancy. Other causes are infection or retained pieces of placenta (afterbirth) after a pregnancy. Intrauterine adhesions may be seen on an HSG and then inspection of the inside of the uterine cavity with a hysteroscope will confirm the diagnosis and enable treatment by cutting through the adhesions (adhesiolysis). If you have these adhesions, you may be amenorrheic because they obliterate the endometrial cavity and may have destroyed the ability of the endometrium to develop. Following surgery, a three-month course of a high dose of oestrogen with progesterone should be given to stimulate the regrowth and development of the endometrium. You will also have an intrauterine contraceptive device for two to three months, which may also help to prevent adhesions returning by keeping the walls of the cavity separated as your womb regenerates.

VARIATIONS IN THE SHAPE OF THE UTERUS (WOMB)

Approximately 5.5 per cent of women have differences in how the uterus has developed; so-called congenital uterine anomalies. Some may be associated with infertility and an increased risk for miscarriage, although many women conceive and might only be found to have a uterine anomaly during routine pregnancy scans.

The commonest anomaly is an arcuate, or heart-shaped, uterus, although this doesn't reduce fertility, so you do not need to worry if this is mentioned while you are being scanned. In women with infertility and miscarriage the septate uterus is the most common anomaly, but less common anomalies such as bicornuate, unicornuate and didelphic uterus are also associated with reduced reproductive performance, although there is little surgically that can be done in these cases.

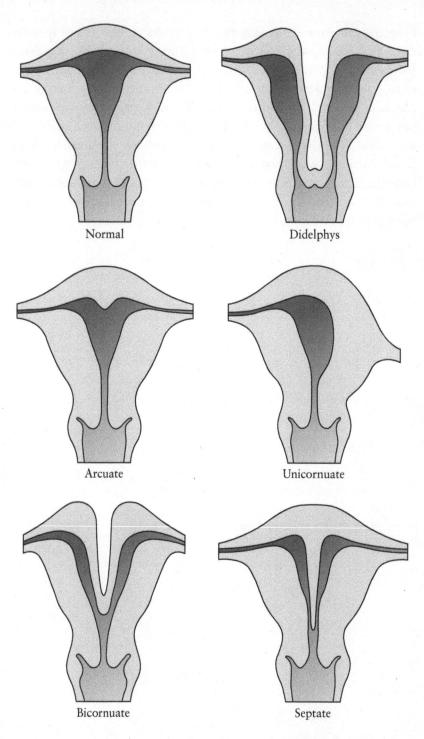

Normal

Didelphys

Arcuate

Unicornuate

Bicornuate

Septate

Different uterine shapes

Large intrauterine septa may result in an increased risk of miscarriage and, if a septate uterus is found during routine investigations for infertility, you should discuss the need for surgery with your doctor. It will depend on whether the abnormality is having an effect on fertility. The other consideration is risk of miscarriage if you go on to conceive. As a miscarriage is by no means a certainty, we would urge caution before major surgery on the uterus, which could further distort the uterus or lead to damaging adhesions forming. There have been no prospective studies that have answered this question, and so the current consensus in the UK is not to perform septum resection.

Chapter 17

Endometriosis

ENDOMETRIOSIS IS A common condition that can cause pelvic pain and infertility. The normal lining of the uterus (womb) is called the endometrium and endometriosis is where endometrial tissue develops outside the womb. Endometriosis therefore responds to the hormonal changes of the natural cycle in a similar way to the endometrium, leading to inflammation, particularly during your period. Endometriosis is a disease that affects the whole body and multiple organs including the brain. As well as causing inflammation, it can also impact behaviour, and increase the risk of depression, anxiety and sensitivity to pain. Endometriosis can be seen during a laparoscopy to investigate the pelvis as small dark red or blue/black spots that can occur anywhere on the outer surface of the uterus, ovaries and fallopian tubes, and can be scattered across the surface of the peritoneum (the surface lining of the abdominal cavity). (See figure on page 179.)

Endometriosis can cause scarring and adhesions, which may then result in internal structures sticking together and prevent normal functioning. Often cysts develop on the surface of the ovaries, which may grow to a significant size (several centimetres in diameter). Sometimes the bowel can stick to the uterus and ovaries, which may lead to pain when passing stools and bleeding from the rectum during menstruation. Nodules can also develop at the top of the vagina and in the bladder. In fact, endometriosis has been found in virtually every organ of the body. Endometriosis can also be associated with adenomyosis, which is when pockets of endometrium develop within the muscle (myometrium) of the uterus.

SYMPTOMS

The usual symptoms of endometriosis are:

- Pelvic pain, particularly during menstruation (dysmenorrhea) and also during sexual intercourse (dyspareunia). Severe endometriosis that causes dense adhesions in the pelvis and ovarian cysts may result in constant pain throughout the month. Fertility can also therefore be impaired.

- Erratic or unpredictable periods.

- Altered immune function. Interestingly, there is research ongoing looking at the impact of diet on endometriosis, so again we advise following the guidance in Part 1 and noting the impact of nutrition on immune function.

DIAGNOSIS

Endometriosis is usually diagnosed during a laparoscopy, which should be performed by an experienced gynaecologist who can both diagnose and treat the problem during the same procedure. The lesions are usually too small to be seen during an ultrasound scan of the pelvis, as they are usually just a millimetre or so across. If endometriosis has caused ovarian cysts, these will usually be visible by ultrasound as they tend to have a characteristic appearance. Magnetic resonance imaging (MRI) of the pelvis is better at detecting small lesions and is good at indicating whether other organs, such as the bowel, are affected.

When fertile women have a careful laparoscopic assessment of the pelvis, endometriosis is found in about 20 per cent of cases. There's a big variation when it comes to infertile women, however, with between 20 and 70 per cent of women having the same surgery showing signs of endometriosis. This is probably due to different levels of detail gynaecologists use to make the assessment, as well as variations in different groups of women. Further, not all endometriotic lesions have the classic blue/black pigmented appearance. Lesions that are less common appear as flame-like blisters, clear nodules, white plaques and scarring in the peritoneum. In addition, endometriotic lesions change both in position and with time. Some describe endometriosis as being like a field of mushrooms, with lesions appearing and disappearing at different times and in different places.

Blood tests

A number of markers for endometriosis that we can test for in the blood have been investigated, although none have been found to accurately predict the severity of the condition or whether it's likely to get worse. The most commonly used marker is CA-125. This is a protein that rises with endometriosis, acute pelvic inflammatory disease and ovarian cancer. While the levels tend to be higher in the latter two conditions than with endometriosis, there is considerable overlap. The cut-off concentration sometimes used for CA-125 is 35U/ml, below which endometriosis is unlikely to be present, but this isn't a reliable indicator. One area of research that may change this is the investigation of the role of micro-RNAs in endometriosis. Micro-RNAs are molecules involved in regulating how genes work that become faulty in endometriosis. Evidence suggests a number of different micro-RNAs could be tested in the blood to help diagnose the condition. Drugs targeting micro-RNAs may also offer potential for future treatment.

CAUSES

Various theories have been suggested for how endometriosis develops, but retrograde menstruation – when menstrual blood passes back through the fallopian tubes and out into the pelvis – is the most popular and plausible. Retrograde menstruation is common. It's seen in 75–90 per cent of women who have a laparoscopy while on their period. Menstrual blood does not always contain cells from the endometrium, however, and the factors that cause these cells to implant in the wrong places to cause endometriosis are uncertain. This is shown by the fact that only 1–20 per cent of women have endometriosis, compared to the 75–90 per cent who have retrograde menstruation.

If you have endometriosis along with some of the symptoms, you may have a genetic predisposition to developing problems and it can often run in families. The degree of endometriosis does not correlate with the symptoms of pelvic pain, dyspareunia and dysmenorrhea. It is also not possible to predict who will develop progressive disease that goes on to cause pelvic adhesions and ovarian cysts.

IMPACT ON FERTILITY

Severe endometriosis can affect fertility by distorting organs in the pelvis, with adhesions that smother the ovaries and tubes, and with ovarian cysts. However, while endometriosis is often found on the surface of the fallopian tubes, it does not tend to affect the inner part of the tubes and usually the tubes themselves are open.

There is still debate about how much endometriosis affects fertility unless there is pelvic deformity. Endometriosis changes the environment within the peritoneal (abdominal) cavity, including cells that deal with infection and inflammation and more inflammatory chemicals. These things have the potential to affect sperm motility, destroy sperm and also interfere with the pick-up of the egg by the fallopian tube, fertilisation and implantation.

TREATMENT

The management of endometriosis depends on your wishes, specifically whether your main concern is pain or infertility. If you want to conceive but pain is also a problem then you will usually have analgesics (painkillers), either alone or with surgery. Appropriate analgesics include the non-steroidal anti-inflammatory drugs (NSAIDs) – naproxen (250mg three or four times a day) and mefenamic acid (500mg three times a day) are particularly effective. There is some evidence that NSAIDs may prevent ovulation, but endometriotic pain is usually worse during menstruation rather than mid-cycle and so these drugs should be safe if you want to conceive. There is ongoing research into the impact of diet on endometriosis but no clear consensus as to the best approach, though there is some evidence to recommend the Mediterranean diet.[1] Antioxidant supplements including co-enzyme Q10, vitamin E (1,200IU) and vitamin C (1,000mg), NAC, alpha lipoic acid, bromelain and resveratrol may also be of benefit.

Medical therapy

Endometriosis changes during the menstrual cycle, with age and during hormonal therapy. Endometriosis responds to the fluctuating hormones across the cycle and reduces during pregnancy, when oestrogen and progesterone are high. Endometriosis may be suppressed with hormonal treatments. They are very successful in controlling symptoms but also suppress ovulation and so are contraceptive. With treatment, endometriosis eventually dies away but it takes several months for things to settle.

Other treatment options include the combined oral contraceptive pill (COCP) taken continuously without any breaks, the use of daily progestogen tablets (e.g. oral medroxyprogesterone acetate) or the use of long-acting injectable gonadotrophin-releasing hormone (GnRH) agonists. Side effects of the latter are those of oestrogen deficiency – hot flushes, reduced libido, acne and oily skin – and so if used for more than six months, a low dose of an oestrogen add-back preparation (such as tibolone) is important. This combats the symptoms of oestrogen deficiency and also minimises the risk of osteoporosis (thinning of the bones). However, these medications are more relevant to the chronic treatment of endometriosis in women who experience pain rather than for the treatment of infertility.

Drug treatment of endometriosis helps with the symptoms, but has not been shown to be beneficial for fertility as it does not increase pregnancy rates and, if anything, may actually reduce them. They are also contraceptive, so we don't recommend drug treatments if you want to conceive. Furthermore, they simply suppress endometriosis for the duration of the therapy and do not prevent progression of the disease.

Surgical therapy

Surgical treatment of endometriosis should ideally be performed during the diagnostic laparoscopy. Before surgery, you should be given appropriate information about what might be found and provide consent to treat any factors that might affect fertility during the one procedure. We routinely request consent from women having a diagnostic laparoscopy for the possibility of ablation of minor endometriosis or adhesiolysis (cutting through the adhesions). This doesn't add more than 10–15 minutes to the procedure. Severe disease is sometimes apparent without pre-existing signs or symptoms and, in these cases, a detailed discussion is needed before proceeding to more major surgery.

If you don't conceive within 6–12 months after surgery, the next step is *in vitro* fertilisation (IVF, see Chapter 18). If the aim of surgery was to remove active disease before IVF, then it is advisable to start GnRH agonist therapy after surgery to reduce the risk of the endometriosis coming back, particularly if there have been ovarian cysts. You should then start IVF after six to eight weeks as clinical pregnancy rates are significantly higher in women receiving the GnRH agonist in this way.

Laparoscopic surgery should only be carried out by appropriately trained and skilled surgeons as endometriosis taxes the skill of the surgeon more than any other disease in the pelvis. Though rare, the surgeon sometimes needs to separate affected bowel or bladder and the help of a colorectal surgeon or a urologist may be needed. If you have ovarian endometriotic cysts (endometriomata), they need to be removed very carefully to avoid destroying the valuable egg-containing tissue of the ovary. Removing them prevents the risk of problems during IVF.

Nina and Pau: Endometriosis

Nina (36) had always had painful periods. She was given the contraceptive pill when she was 15 to help and took the packets continuously without any breaks so that she didn't have any periods and so her symptoms were controlled. She and Pau

248

(also 36) had been trying to start a family for five years. When Nina stopped the pill her periods returned and were very painful, sometimes so bad that she had to take a day off work. She also found sexual intercourse very painful and so she and Pau didn't have sex often. It took them a while to pluck up the courage to see their doctor. When they did he performed the baseline tests, which didn't show up any problems, and so he reassured them and they continued to try for another year before seeing their doctor again, who referred them on to our fertility clinic.

I arranged for Nina to have a laparoscopy and found severe endometriosis in her pelvis, with lots of inflammation, adhesions around her ovaries and a large cyst on her left ovary. This was removed, as well as cauterisation of the endometriosis and cutting away the adhesions. Nina's fallopian tubes also appeared to be quite scarred, even though dye passed through them to confirm that they were open. After the surgery I felt that her fertility was improved but nonetheless, given her age and the degree of scarring from endometriosis, I advised that she take medication to suppress the endometriosis (a long-acting GnRH agonist) and proceed to IVF treatment. She responded well to the IVF and a very good-quality embryo was transferred, but a pregnancy didn't occur. We were able to freeze three embryos and she conceived with the first frozen embryo replacement cycle and now has a healthy daughter. Furthermore, there are two embryos left over for the future.

ENDOMETRIOSIS AND IVF

There is ongoing debate about the impact of severe endometriosis on the success of IVF with research suggesting that rates of fertilisation and implantation are impaired.[2] It is reasonable to suppress active endometriosis with a GnRH agonist for two to three months before IVF, particularly if it will form part of your IVF treatment protocol. If you have had previous surgery to the ovaries or you have reduced ovarian reserve, caution is needed as taking a GnRH agonist for too long might impact your response to stimulation with gonadotrophins later.

If you have endometriotic cysts, these can cause problems during IVF, as they can be accidentally pierced during the egg collection and this can then cause severe infection. Indeed, the only severe pelvic infections we have seen after transvaginal ultrasound-guided egg collection have been when an endometriotic cyst has pierced accidentally. Therefore, ideally, endometriotic cysts should be removed surgically before IVF, or if not they should be avoided during the egg collection procedure. If a cyst is entered accidentally during egg retrieval then you should have antibiotic treatment for seven days.

Chapter 18

IVF and Associated Treatments

I F YOU HAVE been diagnosed with blocked tubes, unexplained fertility, male factor infertility or polycystic ovary syndrome (PCOS) that hasn't responded to ovulation induction, the next step in your medical journey is assisted conception. For most people, this usually means *in vitro* fertilisation (IVF), though there are other options that are less commonly used, mainly for unexplained infertility, and these are explained on page 204. However, couples sometimes start IVF before all other treatments have been exhausted. While we do not encourage unnecessary delay, particularly in older patients, the notion that IVF is the high-tech modern answer to every couple's subfertility is incorrect. The stresses of IVF (and other assisted conception procedures) can be huge, and the treatment has risks and complications (for example, ovarian hyperstimulation syndrome (OHSS) and multiple pregnancy – see page 273).

For unexplained infertility, the aim of treatment is to boost your chance of a pregnancy above what you could achieve naturally – that is a 2–4 per cent chance of natural conception per month for couples who have been trying for over a year. This is definitely true for IVF; therefore unexplained infertility is one diagnosis where it's sensible to progress straight to IVF. Some like to proceed to fertility treatments quickly and others prefer to avoid high-tech treatments for as long as possible, but in women over 35 years, we believe that IVF should be offered as first-line therapy for unexplained infertility.

WHAT IS IVF?

'*In vitro* fertilisation' literally means fertilisation in glass. In practice, this means we collect eggs and sperm, prepare them in the laboratory and mix them in a Petri dish to ensure they are brought close together to give maximum opportunity for fertilisation before transferring the embryos that are created back into the womb, usually one at a time. Modern-day reproductive medicine is in reality still a young speciality, with Louise Brown, the first IVF baby, having been born less than 45 years ago, in 1978. Since that time, IVF has revolutionised the treatment of infertility and given people who once would never have been able to conceive the chance to have their own children. Reproductive medicine is still a rapidly evolving branch of healthcare that is subject to intense scrutiny and regulation. It involves cutting-edge science that allows us to create new life, which really is incredible. We understand, however, that if you have got to this point, you will also have been on a long journey, which can be challenging emotionally. We hope that by helping you understand your medical treatment in this ever-changing field, it will make the journey a little easier.

GONADOTROPHINS EXPLAINED

Gonadotrophin is the collective term for the two hormones produced by the pituitary: follicle-stimulating hormone (FSH) and luteinising hormone (LH). Together they help coordinate the growth of the follicle, the maturation of the egg within it and the production of the ovarian hormones (testosterone, oestrogen and progesterone) that prepare the uterus (womb) for a pregnancy.

These hormones therefore all work together in beautiful harmony to synchronise your menstrual cycle and the development of follicles in the ovary. First, LH stimulates the production of testosterone. Testosterone then gets converted to oestrogen within the follicle. This conversion needs an enzyme called aromatase, which in turn needs FSH to work.

Why gonadotrophins are important in ovulation and fertility treatment

LH also stimulates the corpus luteum (the 'shell' left behind after the egg is released) to produce progesterone after ovulation. Progesterone stays high during the first few weeks of pregnancy as the pregnancy hormone human chorionic gonadotrophin (hCG) from the placenta continues to stimulate the production of progesterone. Progesterone helps maintain the endometrium to prevent it shedding as a period and allows a pregnancy to continue. hCG is the hormone that is detected when you do a pregnancy test.

hCG is also very similar to LH, which is why it is used as an injection during IVF. It mimics the mid-cycle LH surge that happens just before ovulation and, when you're given it as part of your treatment, it triggers the maturation of the egg. Both the LH surge that happens in your natural cycle and an hCG injection during fertility treatment take about 40 hours to work and cause the release of an egg (ovulation). As well as causing the release of the egg, its action to start the maturation of the egg before ovulation so that it is ready to be fertilised by a sperm is a crucial part of your treatment. When hCG is used as the trigger during ovulation induction treatments, including intrauterine insemination (IUI – see page 204), the aim is to help you ovulate, whereas during IVF cycles the aim is solely to mature the eggs within the developing follicles. The egg collection is performed 35–36 hours after the hCG has been given in order to allow the eggs to mature, but also to collect them before they are released from the follicles by ovulation.

Gonadotrophins for fertility treatment

When women go through the menopause, the ovaries stop working and the levels of FSH and LH rise as the pituitary gland tries hard to stimulate the ovaries. It recognises that they are not working and so responds by producing even more FSH and LH. The FSH and LH are removed from circulation by the kidneys and so end up in the urine. Post-menopausal women therefore have high levels of FSH and LH in their urine. Historically, this has been purified to extract these hormones to produce what is known as human menopausal gonadotrophins (hMG). The pharmaceutical companies that manufacture hMG collect urine from thousands of post-menopausal women and purify it to remove impurities and any infectious material so that the products are safe. In a similar way, hCG is purified from the urine of pregnant women.

The hMG preparations contain FSH and LH in differing proportions depending on the formulation, and some have virtually all of the LH removed and contain FSH alone. Also there are some preparations that contain hCG as well as FSH. In the early days, the preparations were initially for intramuscular (into the muscle) use, but with purification and extraction of impurities they are now able to be given subcutaneously (just under the skin with a small needle).

Newer drugs for IVF

The problems of supply, collection, transport, storage and processing of an ever-increasing need for urine means that genetic engineering is now used to produce synthetic versions of the same hormones. This allows production of FSH, LH and hCG without the need for purifying human urine. These new drugs are known as recombinantly-derived gonadotrophins. The technology is very expensive but does mean 'pure' FSH, LH and hCG can be produced. They can also be modified to increase the length of time they are active. For example, there is a long-acting FSH preparation that continues to stimulate the ovaries for seven days, which means you need fewer injections during treatment.

While there are various advantages of recombinantly-derived gonadotrophins over earlier versions that were extracted from urine, there is no evidence for a clinical benefit. Aside from the improved logistics of the pharmaceutical process, controlled manufacture has led to a more consistent and pure product with less variability between batches. This used to be an issue when purifying enormous quantities of urine that varies from person to person. The supply is potentially unlimited and shortages should no longer be a threat to clinical practice.

Which drugs are most effective?

Quite a lot of research has been done to compare the different gonadotrophin preparations.[1] The studies are varied and include a mix of protocols and various comparisons of hMG, purified urinary FSH and recombinant FSH (rFSH). A number of analyses comparing the various types of gonadotrophin have been performed over the years, with varying conclusions. The current consensus is that the live birth rate is very slightly less with rFSH compared with hMG. Furthermore, hMG appears more cost-effective. There are no significant differences between hMG and rFSH with respect to the amount used, risk of miscarriage, cancellation of the cycle because of either under- or over-response or risk of OHSS. Therefore, in reality, it appears that there is no practical difference between the various gonadotrophin drugs with respect to how well they will work for you; that is, their ability to stimulate follicle development, the production of mature eggs, appropriate hormone production for endometrial development and pregnancy rates.

HOW IVF WORKS

IVF involves five main stages:

1. stimulation of the ovaries

2. ultrasound monitoring

3. egg collection

4. embryo transfer

5. luteal support

Sperm preparation is also needed, whether preparing a fresh sample provided on the day of egg collection or thawing of a frozen sample.

Stimulation of the ovaries

The first stage of your IVF treatment is to stimulate the ovaries to capture all the follicles that are growing at the start of the cycle (so-called 'superovulation') rather than with a natural cycle, where normal levels of the main hormone FSH generally only enables a single follicle to grow and ovulate. To stimulate the ovaries to allow more eggs to be collected as part of your IVF, higher doses of FSH are given than in a natural cycle. The aim is to stimulate 10–15 follicles, and collect mature eggs from the majority of them.

You also need to be given a second hormone (either a gonadotrophin-releasing hormone (GnRH) agonist or antagonist) to prevent ovulation, so that the eggs cannot be released and lost before they are physically collected from the ovaries during your egg collection.

IVF stimulation protocols have become increasingly simplified in recent years and there are different drug options for your clinic to choose for your treatment using either GnRH agonists or antagonists.

Agonist or long stimulation protocol

The 'long' protocol uses a GnRH agonist to switch off the natural menstrual cycle – known as pituitary desensitisation or down-regulation. This usually takes 10–14 days. GnRH agonists can be delivered by a nasal spray or as a short-acting daily or long-acting monthly subcutaneous (just under the skin) injection. You will be assessed by an ultrasound scan that will show that the endometrium is thin (< 5mm) and the ovaries are inactive. Some clinics measure hormones in the blood and start the next treatment when LH is < 5IU/L and oestradiol is < 150pmol/L (progesterone, if measured, should be < 3nmol/L). Most clinics, however, go by the scan alone.

Treatment with hormone injections containing FSH to stimulate your ovaries then starts at the beginning of your period (either day 1 or 2). Daily injections of the GnRH antagonist then follow on day 5 or 6 of stimulation or once the largest follicle(s) has reached a diameter of 14mm. Success rates seem to be better if you start on day 6 rather than using a flexible protocol. The GnRH antagonist acts immediately to stop you ovulating by inhibiting natural production of FSH and LH. Follicles will grow at different rates and we usually like to see at least three that are larger than 17mm in diameter. Any follicle bigger than 14mm is likely to contain mature eggs. Once the follicles have grown appropriately, the egg collection can be timed precisely 35–36 hours after an hCG injection. If the egg collection doesn't take place, the ovaries would be expected to release the eggs about 40–44 hours after the hCG injection.

Disadvantages of the long protocol: A disadvantage of the long protocol using GnRH agonists is the 10–14 days lead-in to treatment before stimulation can start. Not only does this extend the treatment cycle, but pituitary down-regulation (switching off the natural menstrual cycle) causes menopausal symptoms due to oestrogen deficiency (including hot sweats, mood changes and vaginal dryness). Some clinics prefer to start GnRH agonist therapy on day 21 of your cycle. They believe that desensitisation happens more rapidly than if it is commenced on day 2 of menstruation in the following cycle. A day 21 start, however, carries the risk of 'rescuing' a corpus luteum (the remnant of the follicle after ovulation) from the last natural ovulation. This can cause an ovarian cyst that can then disrupt treatment. Also a day 2 start virtually guarantees you are not pregnant (although GnRH agonists are not harmful to take if you are).

Antagonist or short stimulation protocol

Antagonist cycles are shorter and more popular than longer protocols as they are newer forms of treatment that are kinder on the body. Treatment can also be scheduled more easily as the combined oral contraceptive pill (COCP) or progesterone can be given for a short time to delay your period and therefore the start of stimulation. You may therefore be given one of these drugs before you start stimulation, which simply allows your egg collection to be scheduled more accurately – often to suit your clinic's timetable. The use of COCP or progesterone is usually stopped three to five days before stimulation commences.

The next stage is stimulation of the ovaries, and this part of the treatment is the same as for the long protocol above, including using the same criteria when monitoring the maturation of the eggs. Egg collection is then performed 35–36 hours later.

A single shot of a GnRH agonist can be used as an alternative to hCG in a short GnRH antagonist cycle. This strategy reduces the risk of OHSS because of the shorter time ('half-life') the agonist stays active in the body compared with hCG. If this approach is taken, luteal support (described below) has to be modified with either the combined use of progesterone and oestrogen supplementation or additional hCG in the luteal phase (at a low dose in order to minimise the risk of OHSS).

Advantages of the short protocol: GnRH antagonists in a 'short protocol' are a more recent development that have enabled us to skip the 10–14 days of down-regulation of the long protocol. Women usually prefer these protocols as they are shorter and have fewer side effects (for example, avoidance of symptoms of oestrogen deficiency during pituitary desensitisation). Furthermore, there is a similar probability of a live birth when either GnRH agonists or antagonists are used.

EGG DONATION, EMBRYO DONATION AND SURROGACY

IVF technology with donated eggs (see page 205) is necessary to assist women who have premature ovarian insufficiency (POI) – an early menopause – or an extremely low ovarian reserve (see page 159). If there are significant egg and sperm problems then embryos may be donated by couples who have completed their desired family through IVF and still have surplus embryos frozen. Surrogacy may be considered for women born without a uterus but with functioning ovaries or for those for whom carrying a pregnancy would be medically dangerous (for example, if there is severe heart disease) – see page 315.

Long IVF protocol

Embryo transfer

Oocyte (egg) collection

Trigger injection with hCG

Day one of period

| 1 | 2 | 3 | 4 | 5 | 6 | 7 | 8 | 9 | 10 | 11 | 12 | 13 | 14 | 15 | 16 | 17 | 18 | 19 | 20 | 21 | 22 | 23 | 24 | 25 | 26 | 27 | 28 | 29 | 30 | 31 | 32 | 33 | 34 | 35 | 36 | 37 | 38 | 39 | 40 | 41 | 42 | 43 | 44 | 45 | 46 | 47 | 48 | 49 | 50 | 51 | 52 | 53 | 54 | 55 | 56 | 57 | 58 | 59 | 60 | 61 | 62 | 63 |

Take GnRH agonist drug

Daily Gonadotrophin injections

Take progesterone

Short IVF protocol

Embryo transfer

Oocyte (egg) collection

Trigger injection with hCG or GnRH

Day one of period

| 1 | 2 | 3 | 4 | 5 | 6 | 7 | 8 | 9 | 10 | 11 | 12 | 13 | 14 | 15 | 16 | 17 | 18 | 19 | 20 | 21 | 22 | 23 | 24 | 25 | 26 | 27 | 28 |

Daily Gonadotrophin injections

Take GnRH antagonist drug

Take progesterone + oestradiol if had GnRH trigger

Protocols for long and short IVF cycles

Ovarian reserve and predicting response to stimulation

Predicting an individual woman's response to stimulation is the hardest part of fertility treatment: young women and those with polycystic ovaries tend to respond well (and may over-respond), while older patients and those with reduced ovarian reserve respond less well (see below). How you may respond to stimulation is based on your ovarian reserve and this is done by assessing your antral follicle count (AFC) and measuring your anti-Müllerian hormone (AMH) – see pages 160–2. Your specialist will plan the starting dose of the stimulation based on these results.

As ovarian reserve declines, so too does the chromosomal integrity of the eggs that are ovulated, so that there is a fall in the development of healthy embryos and a rise in the rates of miscarriage and fetal chromosomal abnormalities.

The response of the ovary to stimulation by gonadotrophins is the ultimate test of ovarian function and would help to decide the starting dose or stimulation protocol that best suits you. However, specialists only have this information after treatment rather than beforehand, so they can only use this information if you have had IVF before.

Having polycystic ovaries, whether or not there is overt PCOS (see Chapter 15), means your ovaries are likely to respond sensitively to stimulation and produce lots of follicles. This does not necessarily mean you will get the same number of good-quality eggs, however. Patients with polycystic ovaries are also at the greatest risk of developing OHSS during treatment.

Our recommended starting dose for stimulation for IVF is:

- 150 units of FSH or hMG if you are under the age of 38 years with normal ovarian reserve.

- 200–250 units if you are over the age of 38, depending on your baseline ovarian reserve tests.

- Maximum dose of 300–450 units if you have poor ovarian reserve or have responded poorly in a previous cycle (i.e. fewer than five oocytes collected).

There doesn't seem to be benefit in increasing the dose after you have started stimulation and follicles have started to grow (also known as being 'recruited').

If you have polycystic ovaries (whether or not there are signs of PCOS), we recommend reducing the starting dose, depending upon age and previous response to stimulation, and starting ultrasound monitoring earlier (day 6 or 7 of stimulation). Your specialist may also reduce the dose of FSH as soon as follicles greater than 10mm in diameter have been recruited. Your response should be reviewed after each cycle of treatment and the dose of stimulation adjusted according to this response.

Ultrasound monitoring

After stimulation has started, your ovarian response will be monitored by ultrasound scans. The dimensions of the growing follicles are recorded either daily or every other day, from around day 8 of stimulation, together with a measurement of endometrial thickness. The daily measurement of oestrogen in the blood is of little help in predicting either success or the development of OHSS and adds to the cost of treatment. The hCG 'trigger' is usually given when the leading follicle is at least 17–18mm in diameter and there are at least three follicles greater than 17mm.

There is current interest in the measurement of progesterone on the day of hCG, as there is some evidence that if it is high at that point, the outcome of treatment is less good.[2] In this case, there would be a case for freezing any embryos and using them in the future (see page 324). This approach hasn't been universally accepted and is an area of ongoing research.

Egg (oocyte) collection

The next stage of your IVF treatment is egg collection. You will usually have your ultrasound-guided oocyte retrieval (the 'egg collection') under light sedation with pain relief (combinations of benzodiazepines, midazolam, opiates and sometimes propofol are given intravenously). You may also be given a local anaesthetic into the top of the vagina. The procedure should be pain-free and you will be monitored during and after the egg collection. As you will be only lightly sedated, you may be shown the eggs on a closed-circuit video monitor attached to the embryologist's microscope. Most clinics do not allow your partner to be present for the egg collection because of the overall stress of the situation, in an unfamiliar environment, seeing a partner sedated and having an invasive procedure. Both partners can, however, be present at the embryo transfer (see below).

During the egg collection the ultrasound probe is inserted into the vagina. A long needle is passed through a needle guide; the needle is attached to plastic tubing, which in turn has a pump attached to the end to suck the fluid from the follicles and obtain the eggs. It isn't possible to see the eggs on the scan or with the naked eye and so the test tube with the fluid from the follicle is passed to an embryologist, who can identify the eggs by looking down a microscope. Sometimes it is necessary to inject some fluid through the needle to flush the egg out of the follicle.

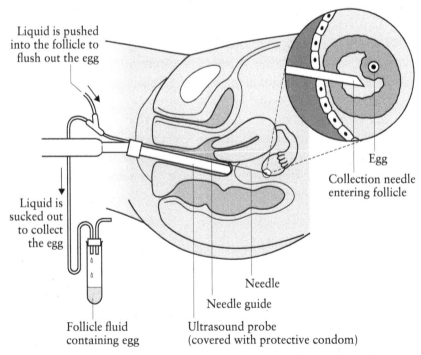

Liquid is pushed into the follicle to flush out the egg

Liquid is sucked out to collect the egg

Egg

Collection needle entering follicle

Needle

Needle guide

Follicle fluid containing egg

Ultrasound probe (covered with protective condom)

How oocytes (eggs) are collected from the ovary

The egg retrieval procedure should take about 15–20 minutes and is relatively free of risks. Occasionally there may be bleeding from the point at which the needle passes through the vagina and you may need a stitch. Less commonly, the ovary may bleed after the procedure and this may very occasionally require an operation to stop the bleeding. Infection is also an uncommon occurrence and many clinics provide prophylactic antibiotics to minimise any risk.

During the egg retrieval every follicle greater than 14mm in diameter is expected to have a mature egg and eggs are usually obtained from at least 90 per cent of follicles of this size. After the egg retrieval, the semen is washed and prepared. Sperm is usually added 1–6 hours later with 50–200,000 motile sperm being placed with each oocyte; 16–18 hours later the oocytes are examined to ensure that normal fertilisation has happened. If intracytoplasmic sperm injection (ICSI – see page 269) is needed, a single sperm is injected into each of the mature eggs.

Approximately 80–85 per cent of the eggs collected are expected to fertilise. They are then observed as they develop into embryos over the next five days. Traditionally, the dish containing the embryos was removed from the incubator on a daily basis to inspect their development. Nowadays we use a sophisticated incubator (known as an Embryoscope™) which has a time-lapse camera within to take a photo of each embryo every ten minutes so that the precise timing of each cell division can be observed in order both to identify which embryos are developing normally and to avoid having to remove them from the incubator and disturb the environment in which they are growing. We have published data showing that the use of the Embryoscope™ has significantly improved the success rates in our clinic.[3]

Embryo transfer

You will usually have an embryo transfer five days after the egg collection when the embryos have reached the blastocyst stage of development. A few years ago, the transfer was done on day 2 of development and then this was extended to day 3 and now to day 5. By this stage, we can better tell which are the highest quality embryos and so can choose the best for either transfer or freezing. Those embryos that do not develop normally are then discarded. Blastocyst transfer is thought to better mimic natural conception by synchronising the embryo development with the readiness of the endometrium for implantation. It also means that you have your embryo transfer when any uterine contractions following the egg collection have reduced.

The embryo transfer procedure usually takes five to ten minutes. A fine plastic catheter is inserted through the cervix into the uterus under ultrasound guidance (see diagram on page 207). A narrower catheter is then inserted inside this that carries your precious embryo into your womb. This means the specialist can see it clearly as it enters the middle of the uterine cavity. After the embryo transfer it is fine to go about your normal daily activities. Indeed, it's best to keep busy as the two weeks up to the pregnancy test are hard to cope with as you don't have to attend the clinic for regular scans and monitoring.

Single versus double embryo transfers

The aim, whenever possible, is to transfer a single embryo, as there is good evidence that the transfer of more than one good-quality embryo does not increase the chance of a pregnancy developing, but instead significantly increases the risk of a twin pregnancy to as high as 50 per cent. In the UK, a maximum transfer of two embryos is permitted in women under the age of 40 and three in those older (although if frozen embryos or donated eggs are being used it is the age of the woman at the time the eggs were collected that is considered).

Thus, the UK and many other countries nowadays have a policy of elective single embryo transfer (eSET) for all women with good prospects of success (young patients under 37 in their first or second cycle). Evidence suggests that by only transferring one embryo and freezing the spares for later transfer if the initial cycle doesn't work gives a similar live birth rate to that for double embryo transfers.[4] Plus, multiple pregnancy rates can be reduced to under 5 per cent. Furthermore, there is a significant benefit in terms of your pregnancy and child's health, because

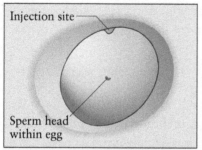

Egg after injection with sperm for ICSI

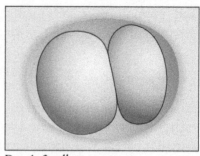

Day 1: 2 cells

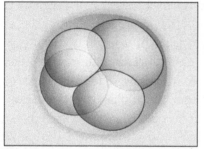

Day 2: 4 cells

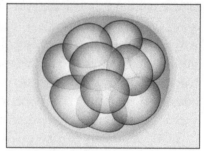

Day 4: morula

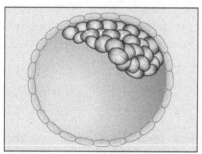

Day 5: blastocyst

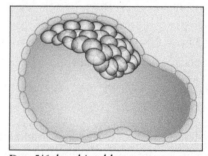

Day 5/6: hatching blastocyst

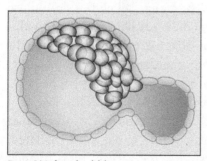

Day 5/6: hatched blastocyst

How the embryo develops

twin pregnancies have an increased risk of problems, most notably premature delivery of babies who need specialist intensive care and are at high risk of long-term disability.

Luteal support

Progesterone treatment to support the second part of the cycle and early pregnancy if treatment is successful (known as luteal support) is started on the day of egg collection. It is usually given as pessaries or injections and continued until the day of the pregnancy test. Some clinics continue luteal support for up to 12 weeks of pregnancy, although this is unnecessary particularly if progesterone pessaries have been used. No one protocol or means of delivery of luteal support has been shown to be superior to another, though most women tend to prefer vaginal progesterone to injections. While a number of additional medications have been proposed to enhance implantation, such as aspirin and intralipid, there is no evidence for any benefit.

hCG injections can be given, but most clinics these days give progesterone. hCG should be avoided if there is any risk of OHSS as it will continue to stimulate the ovaries, while progesterone instead replaces the production of progesterone from the ovaries. Many clinics, including our own, have now stopped giving hCG because OHSS is not always easy to predict.

'Mild IVF'

There has been much publicity about 'mild stimulation' and this has become very much a buzz word in some circles and used as a marketing strategy by some clinics. In reality, all clinics should use the lowest effective dose and tailor the treatment to the individual's needs, carefully assess the factors that can predict an individual's response and be prepared to modify the dose if there is an unexpected response. This indeed has always been our approach.

There are some clinics that offer 'natural cycle' IVF – IVF in a cycle that has not been stimulated by medication. This then relies on the ability to collect a single egg before it has been ovulated, which can be challenging. Furthermore, the success rates of such cycles are very low as it is common either to have no egg or for the egg not to fertilise and thereby have no embryo for transfer. Furthermore, contrary to what some clinics suggest, there is no evidence that this approach is beneficial for older women or those with low ovarian reserve.

WOMEN WITH LOW OVARIAN RESERVE

Women with low ovarian reserve who respond poorly to stimulation not only have fewer eggs but also their eggs will have reduced potential to fertilise and develop into healthy embryos. While much research has been carried out to try to improve the situation, in reality there is very little that can be done to enhance the quality/fertility of the eggs. There is often much publicity when a so-called 'breakthrough' has been made – for example, the infusion of platelet-rich plasma (PRP) – but, to date, there have been no large scientifically validated studies that have confirmed benefit.

Various adjunctive therapies that have been used in poor responders include dehydroepiandrosterone (DHEA), about which there has been much commercial publicity and consequent demand. Similarly, the addition of growth hormone has been proposed and a number of small studies have been performed, which when combined together have suggested there may possibly be some benefit.[5] There is, however, no good evidence from appropriately sized clinical trials that any adjuvants or particular protocols benefit women with reduced ovarian reserve by increasing their chance of having a healthy baby, which at the end of the day is what it's all about.

Pregnancy rates after IVF

Improvements in fertility treatment protocols and scientific advances in the laboratory mean that your chances of having a baby from IVF have increased steadily over the last few decades. Approximately 60,000 assisted conception treatments are performed annually in the UK and around 2 per cent of all births are IVF babies. Your chance of success with each cycle of treatment in the UK is more than 30 per cent per cycle and in larger units, like ours, it is 40–45 per cent for women under the age of 38. Many couples will still, however, need more than one treatment cycle. Often surplus embryos can be frozen if they are of good enough quality and they can then be used without you having to go through the full fresh cycle (see page 271). In our clinic, the cumulative live birth rate after three full cycles, including the use of frozen embryos, is about 85 per cent for those under the age of 38.

There are huge variations in both provision and outcomes of assisted conception treatments around Europe (and the globe). We have been campaigning for years for equality of access in the UK, where there still remains a 'postcode lottery' (see page 343) with funding dependent upon where you live, with most areas being under-resourced and not complying with the guidance that everyone should be entitled to three funded cycles of fresh IVF, including the use of all frozen embryos too. If this were the case, the majority would have a good chance of having a baby and not require the full three cycles in any case.

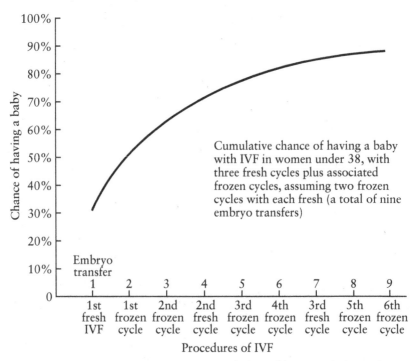

Cumulative chance of having a baby with IVF in women under 38, with three fresh cycles plus associated frozen cycles, assuming two frozen cycles with each fresh (a total of nine embryo transfers)

Chance of having a baby with IVF

Add-ons

There has been a lot of discussion in recent times about the use of 'add-ons' during IVF treatments. We believe, however, that the term 'add-on' is confusing and unhelpful. While the fundamentals of the IVF treatment cycle will be similar in different clinics, there will be some variations in what is provided and also what might be included in the costs of the package of care for those who have to self-fund. Some use the term add-on to refer to extras in the package that have to be paid for, while others refer to add-ons as additional therapies that may not yet be of proven benefit.

It is important to appreciate that reproductive medicine is a relatively new field and has pushed the boundaries of science in many exciting ways. It is also extremely highly scrutinised and regulated, especially within the UK. Any new treatment or adjunctive therapy needs to be properly studied and only introduced into routine clinical practice after it has been shown to be of proven benefit and safe – and certainly not charged separately for until this is the case. There are, however, different grades of evidence and sometimes new therapies are introduced when the evidence is still evolving. It is the responsibility of every clinic to explain fully every component of the treatment that you are going through and also the evidence behind any new components that are introduced.

INTRACYTOPLASMIC SPERM INJECTION (ICSI)

For you to have standard IVF, you need to have a semen sample with a good sperm count for a reasonable chance of success. This means there needs to be more than 500,000 motile sperm in the total ejaculate. In cases where the sperm count is lower, lab techniques can be used to help things along. ICSI involves the injection of a single sperm cell (spermatozoon) directly into the cytoplasm (ooplasm) of the egg. ICSI revolutionised the management of male infertility. It now allows men whose partners previously would have needed donor insemination to be the biological fathers of their own children. ICSI is used not only for men with very low sperm counts but also for those with obstructive azoospermia, after microsurgical or direct aspiration of sperm from either the epididymis or the testis.

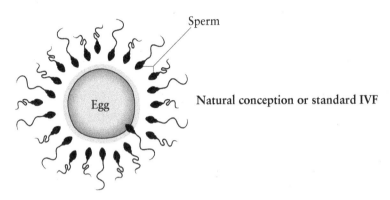

Natural conception or standard IVF

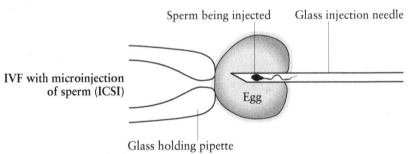

IVF with microinjection of sperm (ICSI)

Sperm being injected   Glass injection needle

Glass holding pipette

Natural or IVF fertilisation compared to ICSI fertilisation

Fertilisation rates with ICSI are in the region of 60–70 per cent, irrespective of the origin of the sperm, providing 90 per cent of couples with an embryo transfer and chance of a pregnancy. Pregnancy rates after ICSI are the same as after IVF and so there is no advantage in using ICSI if there isn't a problem with the sperm. ICSI is, however, sometimes offered to couples in whom fertilisation has failed during IVF in the absence of an apparent sperm problem.

Micromanipulation of the embryo can also be performed in the form of 'assisted hatching', which some believe improves implantation rates for patients with previous IVF failures. There is no good evidence, however, for its use and so we do not perform this procedure in our clinic.

We still have limited knowledge about how sperm mature in the body and the ways in which sperm are naturally selected for fertilisation. Most fertility therapies retain an element of natural selection, whether it be ovulation induction or IVF; that is, only 'good eggs' are likely to become fertilised or result in good-quality embryos that are suitable for transfer. We are not able to distinguish between 'good-' and 'poor-' quality sperm other than by a crude assessment of their appearance. There is some evidence for an increased rate of breakages in the DNA ('fragmentation') of sperm from men with subfertility.[6] The data on children born to date as a result of ICSI is largely reassuring with respect to major congenital abnormalities, but there is an increased rate of sex chromosome anomalies and a suggestion that male children may have increased rates of infertility themselves.

FROZEN EMBRYO REPLACEMENT CYCLES

Many IVF cycles result in the creation of surplus good-quality embryos that can be frozen for future use. If you're having a frozen embryo cycle, your embryo will be removed from storage in liquid nitrogen to thaw on the day of your transfer. Embryo survival is in the region of 80 per cent after freezing and thawing. You will usually have a thawed embryo transferred five days after ovulation in carefully monitored natural cycles. Most clinics, however, use a hormone-supported cycle as this is more predictable and also better for planning. If you're having treatment in an artificial cycle, you will first have a GnRH agonist to switch off your cycle and then oestrogen (tablets) to develop the endometrium for at least 12 days. A scan is performed to ensure the endometrium has thickened, usually to at least 8mm, and then progesterone is commenced (as either pessaries or injections, or a combination of both). The embryo transfer is planned after five days of progesterone if the embryos have been frozen at the blastocyst stage. The oestrogen and progesterone are continued until the pregnancy test two weeks later and then to twelve weeks' gestation if the treatment is successful. Alternatively, in a shorter cycle you may be given a GnRH antagonist, instead of the GnRH agonist, during the first seven days of the treatment cycle.

Freeze-all IVF cycles

There has been a lot of interest in the elective freezing (cryopreservation) of all embryos and later transfer of embryos in a subsequent frozen embryo cycle – so-called 'segmentation of IVF'. This is thought to help with healthy implantation when compared to the high hormone levels of a fresh cycle, especially when there has been a high response to stimulation. This approach has also been shown to improve live birth rates in the subsequent frozen embryo cycles, particularly for those women with polycystic ovaries, who are more prone to ovarian hyperstimulation.

PREGNANCY AFTER IVF

If your treatment is successful, the first stage of pregnancy when you get a positive result on a pregnancy test is known as a biochemical pregnancy. It's so called as you are testing for the presence of hCG (a biological chemical) in the serum that also shows up in urine – in the absence of hCG from any luteal support treatment. If you start bleeding before a gestational sac is seen on your first scan, the outcome of your treatment will be recorded as a biochemical pregnancy. Biochemical pregnancies shouldn't be used when advertising success rates and care must be taken when comparing the results of different clinics or studies to ensure that the same definitions of pregnancy have been used.

A clinical pregnancy is when you can see a pregnancy (gestational) sac inside your uterus on an ultrasound scan. The pregnancy is considered viable when your fetus can be seen with a beating heartbeat (at the earliest three to four weeks after the embryo has been transferred, when the pregnancy is by convention five to six weeks – as pregnancy traditionally is dated from your last period, which is two weeks before ovulation and so equivalent to two weeks prior to egg collection).

A baby born as a result of IVF treatment is recorded as a live birth, and this is the definition of successful treatment that clinics should use when publishing their results.

The major factors that determine the chance of an ongoing pregnancy from IVF treatment are the age of the woman, duration of infertility and number of previous pregnancies. Not surprisingly, couples who have achieved a pregnancy are more likely to do so if they try again. Indeed, many couples have now achieved their desired family size either through repeated attempts at IVF or by the transfer of frozen embryos obtained in a previously successful or unsuccessful cycle of treatment.

The miscarriage rate from IVF treatment is about 20 per cent and the chance of an ectopic pregnancy is approximately 5 per cent.

Multiple pregnancy

Twin pregnancies occur naturally in about 1 per cent (1:80) of all pregnancies. Most often two eggs are released at the same time and are fertilised separately to result in non-identical (dizygotic) twins – these account for about 80 per cent of twin pregnancies. When one egg is fertilised and the resulting embryo splits, identical (monozygotic) twins occur (about 1:250 pregnancies) – this can actually happen at a number of the stages of early development leading to identical twins developing in one pregnancy sac, two pregnancy sacs or even not dividing completely and becoming conjoined twins.

Triplet pregnancies are even less common, with a frequency of about 1:1,000 pregnancies. They are very rarely identical, but sometimes identical twins together with a third embryo can comprise a triplet pregnancy and this occurs more frequently after IVF, when multiple embryos are sometimes transferred (see below).

Multiple pregnancies carry increased risks. Approximately 25–30 per cent of twin pregnancies spontaneously reduce to singleton in the first trimester. Premature delivery, prior to 38 weeks, is three times as common with twins as with singleton pregnancies and usually occurs at around 34–36 weeks, and the risk of all other obstetric complications is increased (e.g. pre-eclampsia, abnormal bleeding, etc.). Triplet and quadruplet pregnancies further magnify the risks, with mean gestation at delivery of 33 and 31 weeks, respectively, and neonatal morbidity increased at least twenty-fold. Cerebral palsy rates have been reported as 2.3 per 1,000 singletons,

12.6 per 1,000 surviving twins and 44.8 per 1,000 triplets. In addition to the increase in long-term disability in survivors of multiple pregnancy, there are significant effects on family dynamics and the ability of parents to cope, as well as the potential detriment to any existing children.

The rate of multiple pregnancy has increased in recent years because of the development of assisted conception treatments, which initially resulted in the transfer of several embryos during IVF in the mistaken belief that this would increase the chance of getting pregnant. We now know that in young women, especially those under the age of 38, if a good-quality embryo is transferred into the uterus the chance of conception is not increased by the transfer of a second. So, with greater awareness and responsible practice, the trend is reversing. A few years ago, the multiple pregnancy rate after IVF was about 25–30 per cent; now it has dropped to less than 10 per cent – and even lower in the best clinics.

In the UK the legal regulations only allow the transfer of a maximum of two embryos in women under the age of 40 and a maximum of three in those over 40 undergoing IVF. In addition to IVF treatments, strict guidelines should be in place during ovulation induction protocols to ensure that no more than two eggs are released. Poorly monitored ovulation induction treatment (see page 227), whether by clomiphene citrate or gonadotrophin therapy, is still the cause of many multiple births.

Therapeutic fetal reduction (see page 348) may be offered at the end of the first trimester for high-order multiple pregnancies, but brings with it risks of infection and a 15–25 per cent chance for the whole pregnancy to miscarry. Fetal reduction is naturally very traumatic and is therefore best avoided by reducing the multiple pregnancy rate in the first instance.

SURROGACY

IVF surrogacy is an option for women with ovaries but without a uterus or for women for whom a pregnancy would be a medical risk (e.g. severe heart or lung disease). See page 315 for a detailed explanation of how surrogacy works.

COUNSELLING

All fertility clinics are obliged to have counsellors who are trained in all aspects of fertility therapy, so that they understand fully the social and legal implications of complex issues such as donation, fertility preservation and surrogacy. It is mandatory for you to have counselling when having these treatments and for donors and surrogates too, without any charge, whether through NHS or private clinics. In addition to implications counselling, you may benefit from support counselling, for support during treatment, after unsuccessful treatment or at other times, for example if you have experienced miscarriage or other complications. You may also need counselling to discuss options for moving from one treatment to another, such as using donor eggs rather than your own eggs, or the difficult discussion as to when to discontinue treatment altogether (see page 353).

Genetic counselling is also essential if you carry the risk of genetic problems or need treatments such as pre-implantation genetic testing (PGT – see page 300). These issues may be very complex and you may need several sessions in order to ensure you make the right decisions for you about which treatment to have and when.

Many people find it helpful to seek the support of other therapists, such as those who practise meditation, acupuncture, reflexology, yoga, etc. (see Chapter 25). These options may provide enormous comfort, support and therapeutic benefit. There is no substitute, however, for the detailed advice that can be provided by a properly trained fertility counsellor.

Chapter 19

Miscarriage, Ectopic and Other Pregnancies

ABOUT A QUARTER of all women will experience a miscarriage at some time in their lives and the risk remains similar if you have already had children. Miscarriage occurs in 15–30 per cent of all naturally-conceived pregnancies. This big range is a reflection of how early pregnancy has been detected as many women miscarry before they even know they are pregnant, sometimes having a period that is a little later or heavier than usual, or sometimes simply having what they perceive to be a normal period. We know this happens as there have been studies of large groups of women who have been asked to provide a daily urine sample to see if they have conceived and the frequency of very early miscarriage was found to be much higher than anticipated. Experiencing a miscarriage can be very distressing, so it's important to know that it doesn't mean you have a particular problem or that you are likely to miscarry again. Although we don't always find the cause of a miscarriage, understanding what has happened and the possible reasons can be helpful (we discuss recurrent miscarriage in Chapter 20).

UNDERSTANDING AND DETECTING EARLY PREGNANCY

Sometimes a very early miscarriage is termed a 'biochemical pregnancy' (see page 279). We don't think that this is a very helpful term, as it simply describes a measurable level of human chorionic gonadotrophin (hCG) in either the urine or blood, before any sign of pregnancy has become visible on an ultrasound scan. The hormone hCG is produced by the placenta (also known as trophoblast in early pregnancy) and is produced in order to stimulate the continued production of progesterone from the corpus luteum (the remnant of the follicle that released the egg – see page 11). Progesterone is important both for implantation and for supporting the early pregnancy, which is why it is used for luteal support in IVF treatments (see page 266). It used to be thought that the treatment with progesterone or hCG might prevent miscarriage, although this hasn't turned out to be the case, because the majority of miscarriages are as a result of the pregnancy not forming normally and having a genetic, or chromosomal, imbalance which occurred very early in the development of the embryo. This is not correctable by hormone treatment.

The hormone hCG can be detected in a urine pregnancy test when the levels are very low (25IU/L, sometimes also written as mIU/ml) – at about ten days after ovulation or a few days before your period is due. Some tests can detect an even lower level (6.25IU/L) – at about eight days after conception. Most of the urine pregnancy testing kits that you can buy are as accurate as those available in hospitals. A blood test for hCG isn't needed unless there are concerns about the viability or site of the developing pregnancy.

The level of hCG in the blood should rise by at least 60 per cent and ideally double every 48 hours in early pregnancy, until it reaches a level of about 1,000–1,200IU/L, which is usually around 5–6 weeks' gestation. A pregnancy is usually first visible on an ultrasound scan at around 5 weeks' gestation when usually only the gestational sac is seen. The embryo itself may be just visible at this stage, but is usually more clearly visible at 6 weeks, when it is about 5–8mm long and a heartbeat should be seen.

Dating of a pregnancy

It is important to remember that a pregnancy is dated by convention from your last period, not from the moment of conception. So assuming that you have a 28–30-day cycle, conception will have occurred about two weeks after your last period, which is also about two weeks before your period was due. Therefore when we say a pregnancy is six weeks' gestation, it is in reality four weeks from conception. If you have a longer cycle, remember that it is the first phase (follicular phase) before ovulation that tends to be the most variable (see page 156) and the luteal phase after ovulation that is about 14 days. So if your pregnancy measures the size expected for 6 weeks' gestation and you have a 35-day cycle, your pregnancy will be dated from your last period and will be actually stated as being 7 weeks by convention – in other words, your pregnancy will measure one week smaller than expected, although there is absolutely nothing wrong. This is why it is important to know the length of your cycle so that appropriate adjustments can be made during pregnancy and a correct dating of the pregnancy given.

Measuring the very tiny structures of an early embryo on an ultrasound scan is difficult, so a variation of a millimetre or two is of no real significance. If there is any doubt about measurements, viability or site of the developing pregnancy, you will usually have a repeat ultrasound scan after 7–14 days. There is little point in having the repeat scan before seven days because a reasonable interval is needed to detect a change. Sometimes you will have hCG blood tests, at least 48 hours apart, to identify the rate of change. Early pregnancy can be a time of uncertainty until viability has been confirmed.

You will usually only have a very early ultrasound scan if you have experienced problems, such as pain or bleeding, or have a past history of miscarriage or ectopic pregnancy. Otherwise, your first scan will be at about 10–12 weeks. If problems are identified at that stage there is a possibility that they may have started much earlier on – in other words, if a pregnancy is found not to be viable on a first scan at 12 weeks, it may well have not been viable had a scan been performed a few weeks earlier.

When there is doubt about the date of a pregnancy because of discrepancy of size and you have a history of a long menstrual cycle or variable cycle length, it can be re-dated. Usually, however, your pregnancy won't be definitively dated until your 12-week scan. In early pregnancy a structure called the yolk sac is seen close to the fetus – it provides nutrition to the fetus and eventually disappears when the placenta takes over this function. From 6 weeks to about 12 weeks the usual measurement is of the length of the fetus (the crown–rump length or CRL). As the fetus gets bigger, it starts to curl and so it is harder to get an accurate measurement of the CRL, which is why from about 14 weeks the femur length, width of the skull and head circumference are measured.

MISCARRIAGE

A miscarriage can happen at any time up to 24 weeks' gestation, which is usually considered to be the age of viability, after which the loss of a pregnancy is termed a stillbirth. Pregnancy is arbitrarily divided into three trimesters: the first up to 12 weeks, the second between 12 and 24 weeks and the third from 24 weeks until 'term', which is usually around 40 weeks. The vast majority of miscarriages (about 85 per cent) occur during the first trimester.

A pre-clinical miscarriage, or biochemical pregnancy, occurs when there is a measurable hCG in your blood, usually less than 50IU/L, which remains high for a few days only and results in a delay to your period of no more than 14 days. A clinical miscarriage occurs after the hCG has continued to rise to a time when an intrauterine gestation sac can be seen by ultrasound, either with or without a fetal pole or heartbeat, but then a miscarriage occurs.

TERMINOLOGY

A miscarriage involves the uterus (womb) expelling the pregnancy and usually starts with pain and bleeding, similar to the start of a period. Sometimes a pregnancy isn't identified as not being viable until the first scan. This is termed a 'missed miscarriage' or, in rather old-fashioned terminology, a 'blighted ovum' (that is literally a non-viable egg). Some use the term spontaneous abortion to signify a miscarriage, as opposed to a therapeutic abortion, to refer to a termination of pregnancy.

Causes of first trimester miscarriage

The causes and management of a single miscarriage tend to be different compared to recurrent miscarriage and don't always mean there is an underlying problem. Understanding this distinction and what might be going on for you can help you avoid unnecessary heartache and a very prolonged journey to parenthood.

One of the main factors leading to miscarriage is increasing age – particularly of the mother, which relates to the fact that the eggs have been there since birth and, as they get older, so does their ability to develop into a genetically normal embryo. The egg is the largest cell in the body and contains all the machinery that controls normal and even division of the cells in the embryo after fertilisation. When this process goes wrong it leads to an imbalance of the genetic material in the dividing cells, which is then either incompatible with life or may result in a viable pregnancy with a baby that has a genetic (or chromosomal) abnormality, such as Down syndrome (also known as Down's syndrome) when there is an extra chromosome 21. This is why the risk of having a child with Down syndrome also increases with maternal age.

While it is thought that at least half of miscarriages are a result of a chromosomal (genetic) problem, this has usually developed within the pregnancy itself and is not a reflection of either mother or father having abnormal chromosomes themselves (either in their bodies or in their eggs or sperm). In other words, it occurs when something has gone wrong after the sperm has fertilised the egg.

While the overall rate of miscarriage is about 25 per cent (1:4) of all pregnancies, for women under 30 years of age the risk is about 10 per cent (1:10), for those aged 35–40 it rises to 20 per cent (1:5), and over the age of 45 it is about 50 per cent (1:2).

The risk of miscarriage is also increased in women who are overweight and those who smoke, so lifestyle and general health are very important, not only for fertility but also in sustaining a pregnancy (see Part 1). There are certain conditions that have been associated with an increased risk of miscarriage, such as polycystic ovary syndrome (PCOS) (see Chapter 15), although in reality this appears to be associated more with the increased likelihood of being overweight in women with PCOS.

Miscarriage may also occur if there are problems with the developing placenta and the way that it attaches to the inside of the uterus and links in with the maternal blood supply. This is still an area where a lot more research is required (see also page 288).

Male factor contribution

There is debate about the degree to which male factors may influence the risk of miscarriage. If there are abnormal semen parameters severe enough to affect fertility (such as a low count or motility), there does not appear to be a correlation with an increased risk of miscarriage. However, genetically abnormal sperm that achieve fertilisation may lead to the development of an abnormal fetus, and the risk also increases with advancing paternal age. There is also evidence to suggest that DNA fragmentation is more common in the partners of women who have had more than three miscarriages (see Chapter 20).

Causes of second trimester miscarriage

Miscarriage after the first 12 weeks of pregnancy may occur if there is an abnormality with the shape or function of the uterus – for example, the cervix may be weak (known as an 'incompetent cervix') and start to open up. This can sometimes be detected on an ultrasound scan and action taken to reduce the risk of miscarriage by inserting a stitch around the cervix (cervical cerclage). The use of a stitch may be of benefit when the cervix has started to open up; however, a large scientific review has failed to find evidence of a benefit for cervical cerclage in reducing recurrent miscarriage.[1] A typical cause of cervical weakness is past treatment for an abnormal smear, so discuss this with your doctor if you conceive and this applies to you. There is also increased risk if the size of the uterus is smaller than average because it has developed abnormally or is distorted by fibroids (see page 236).

Some medical conditions also increase the risk of miscarriage including poorly controlled diabetes, high blood pressure, kidney disease, thyroid problems and coeliac disease.

Infections during pregnancy

Infection may also get through the cervix and affect the pregnancy, causing a miscarriage to occur. Everybody has bacteria throughout their body and on the surface of the skin that don't cause any problems and can even be good for general health (see page 91), but sometimes they can migrate to parts of the body where they shouldn't be and cause problems. The bacteria that can do this to cause miscarriage include E. coli and group B streptococcus. Other infections that can be implicated include sexually transmitted infections such as bacterial vaginosis, chlamydia, trichomonas, gonorrhoea and syphilis. Urinary tract infections may also be problematic, especially if associated with a fever. Infection can also rarely get into the womb via the fallopian tubes or after an invasive procedure such as an amniocentesis, which is when a needle is passed into the womb to collect some fluid in order to see if the baby has a chromosomal abnormality.

Certain infections such as listeriosis can cause miscarriage and may be acquired from cooked chilled foods that have not been adequately reheated. Cold meat pies, ready-to-eat poultry, unpasteurised milk and soft ripened cheeses (Brie, Camembert and blue-vein types) should be avoided by women who may be pregnant. When pregnant, women should also avoid contact with sheep at lambing time and handling silage because of the risk of contracting listeriosis, toxoplasmosis or chlamydiosis. Toxoplasmosis can be caught from cats and dogs, and so women should make sure that they wash their hands thoroughly after handling pets or their food bowls and litter trays.

Miscarriage after fertility treatment

Fertility treatments on the whole don't appear to increase the likelihood of miscarriage over and above the age-related risk. One exception appears to be the use of clomiphene citrate, which is used to stimulate ovulation for women with PCOS (see page 227): those who respond by having high levels of luteinising hormone (LH) during the follicular phase have both a reduced chance of conception and an increased risk of miscarriage. Therefore if LH levels are found to be elevated it is sensible to use alternative treatments.

It should be remembered that hCG is administered in most assisted conception regimens in order to mimic the mid-cycle LH surge. This is needed to initiate oocyte (egg) maturation prior to a timed oocyte collection procedure. The injected hCG should have cleared from the circulation by 9–10 days after ovulation or oocyte retrieval, so an hCG level of greater than 10IU/L on luteal days 11–13 indicates that an embryo has implanted. You will need luteal support after assisted conception, provided in the form of either progesterone or hCG (see page 266), although these days progesterone alone is used in most treatments. If hCG is used, a pregnancy can only be diagnosed by a rising concentration of serum hCG. When the serum hCG concentration is measured 12 days after embryo transfer, a value of greater than 50IU/L predicts a high likelihood of a normal ongoing pregnancy, while lower values suggest either miscarriage or ectopic pregnancy.

The phenomenon of the 'vanishing embryo' has come to light since the advent of early pregnancy monitoring after assisted conception therapies. This is when a twin pregnancy reduces to a singleton, usually with the absorption of the non-viable twin gestation sac into the uterus, where it gradually shrinks as the pregnancy progresses. This has been reported to occur in as many as 25–30 per cent of twin and 50 per cent of triplet pregnancies. The 'vanishing embryo' can apply equally to naturally- or artificially-conceived pregnancies, although the risk of multiple pregnancy is of course greater after ovulation induction or assisted conception (depending upon the number of eggs ovulated or embryos transferred).

What happens if I have a miscarriage?

If you find yourself in the heartbreaking situation of experiencing a miscarriage you may be offered either expectant or active management, depending upon how much you are bleeding and your wishes. Expectant management – waiting for bleeding to stop and a natural and complete resolution of the miscarriage – does not affect future fertility any more than medical management or surgery to empty the womb. If bleeding has already started, then it is more likely you will miscarry without the need for treatment than if a non-viable pregnancy is detected on ultrasound scan in the absence of any symptoms. Active management is often offered if you have a non-viable pregnancy after fertility treatment as the problem is usually detected before signs of impending miscarriage (e.g. bleeding or pain) and expectant management could involve a wait of days or even weeks.

The options for active management include surgery or drugs to empty the womb. The latter is often preferred because you don't need to have an anaesthetic or instruments in the uterus. Medical management usually involves the administration of the drug miso-prostol and sometimes also mifepristone, given as tablets that either dissolve under the tongue or alternatively can be placed inside the vagina. Approximately two hours later, your womb will start to cramp and very sadly start to expel the pregnancy. The pain is usually worse than period pains and so you will need to take painkillers. The process is usually completed within four hours but can sometimes take two to three days. In about 5 per cent of cases a second course of medication is needed, or alterna-tively a surgical procedure can be performed to empty the uterus. This can be done either using local anaesthetic injected around the cervix or with you asleep under a light general anaesthetic. A tube is then inserted into the womb through which the pregnancy is aspirated by vacuum suction (also known as 'evacuation of retained products of conception', ERPC; sometimes also referred to as 'dilation and curettage', D&C). Some women prefer the pro-cedure to the use of drugs, although the insertion of instruments into the womb always brings with it the small risk of infection, damage to the cervix or scarring within the womb (Asherman's syndrome, see page 240).

Whatever treatment you have, it is a very difficult experience, so the decision as to how best to manage things is very personal to you. It's also important to take the time to recover emotionally as well as physically: remember also that the majority of miscar-riages are a 'one-off' occurrence and the likelihood of a second miscarriage is very low. Nonetheless, it goes without saying that if you experience miscarriage you should be offered support and counselling as the loss of a pregnancy is heartbreaking for you and your partner. The Miscarriage Association provides support for people who have experienced miscarriage (see Resources, pages 371).

ECTOPIC PREGNANCY

As we've described, after the egg is released from the ovary at the time of ovulation it should be picked up by the fallopian tube, within which fertilisation then takes place. The fertilised egg develops into an embryo and is then propelled along the tube and into the uterus a few days later (see page 11). An ectopic pregnancy may occur if this process goes wrong, resulting in the pregnancy developing within the fallopian tube, where it will start to grow. As an ectopic pregnancy enlarges it cannot survive and so will start to bleed within the pelvis, causing pain and serious problems if it ruptures.

Ectopic pregnancies occur in approximately 0.5–1 per cent of all pregnancies, but this figure rises to about 5 per cent after IVF and to about 20–30 per cent in women with tubal damage or a past history of ectopic pregnancy.

While most ectopic pregnancies occur within the fallopian tube, a pregnancy can also develop within the 'cornual region' of the uterus – the very first part of the tube as it passes through the upper corner within the muscular layers of the uterus – and is known as a 'cornual ectopic'. An ectopic pregnancy may also develop in other sites, such as on the cervix as it leaves the uterus or within the abdominal cavity, where it might attach to the ovary or even the bowel. This can cause difficulties making the diagnosis.

Diagnosis

It is important to make the diagnosis of an ectopic pregnancy as early as possible so as to treat it before it ruptures. A ruptured ectopic pregnancy is an emergency and can be a potentially life-threatening situation. If you have a history of tubal damage or previous ectopic pregnancy, or after fertility therapy, you should have an ultrasound scan at five weeks' gestation. Transvaginal ultrasound should detect a gestational sac in the womb at about 35 days from the previous menstrual period. If the picture is unclear and you are well a repeat scan should be arranged for one week later. Ultrasound scans should then be performed on a weekly basis until the location and viability of the pregnancy are confirmed. Sometimes an ectopic pregnancy can be seen clearly in the fallopian tube, although this is the exception rather than the rule, as the tube is hard to see by ultrasound.

If you experience pain or bleeding or if there are concerns about the possibility of an ectopic pregnancy, you should have a blood test to measure hCG. An ectopic pregnancy should be suspected if a gestational sac cannot be seen in the uterus by transvaginal ultrasound scan (and the serum hCG level is greater than 1,000IU/L) or a transabdominal scan (and the serum hCG level is greater than 1,500IU/L). Serum hCG concentrations are higher in multiple pregnancy, and this is particularly relevant after fertility therapy when the risk of multiple gestation is increased. The gestational age is known fairly precisely after ovulation induction and even more accurately after IVF. In these cases, an intrauterine sac, or sacs, should be visible on a transvaginal ultrasound 24 days after conception.

It is also important to remember the possibility of heterotopic pregnancy (the combination of an ectopic with a normal intrauterine pregnancy), particularly after IVF when two or, rarely, three embryos may have been transferred.

We can understand more about the pregnancy by monitoring the rate of rise of hCG levels. In a normal pregnancy, the serum hCG concentration doubles every two to three days from six weeks' gestation (see above). If the rise in hCG is less than 66 per cent in a 48-hour period, a non-viable pregnancy (ectopic or miscarriage) is likely in 80 per cent of cases.

What happens if I have an ectopic pregnancy?

If you have signs of a ruptured ectopic pregnancy, it is essential to have an urgent laparoscopy (see page 177). As well as bleeding, symptoms to look out for include fainting and pain in the tip of your shoulder. While the vast majority of ectopic pregnancies can be managed by laparoscopic surgery (also known as minimal access or 'keyhole' surgery), occasionally it is necessary to do a bigger operation to open up the abdomen (laparotomy).

If the tubal ectopic pregnancy is unruptured, it may be possible to remove it and preserve the fallopian tube. Often, however, it is necessary to remove the whole tube (salpingectomy), particularly if it looks unhealthy or there is a past history of pelvic infection. A salpingectomy should certainly be performed if there is extensive damage to the fallopian tube from a ruptured ectopic pregnancy or if there are signs of pre-existing tubal damage that suggest a high risk of loss of function. Following an ectopic pregnancy, the chance of having a healthy natural intrauterine pregnancy in the future is about 40–50 per cent and of a future ectopic pregnancy about 20 per cent.

If the pregnancy occurred after IVF for tubal disease, it is worthwhile considering either sterilisation or removal of both tubes (bilateral salpingectomies) in order to prevent further ectopic pregnancies. However, we do appreciate how hard it is to decide to have the tubes removed if you have become pregnant after extensive investigations and treatment, so sometimes salpingectomy is best left for a later date, although this means another operation.

Medical treatment

If you are pregnant and there is no sign of anything developing in the womb and you are well, it is reasonable to perform measurements of hCG at 48-hour intervals and a follow-up ultrasound scan after one week. If the hCG concentration is falling and you remain well it is sometimes possible to avoid surgery altogether, although rarely the tube can still rupture after conservative treatment even when the hCG levels are falling.

You may alternatively have drug therapy to prevent an ectopic pregnancy from growing and causing problems if you are stable with minimal symptoms. The drug methotrexate has been used successfully. The hCG level has to be monitored carefully and often rises before it begins to fall. It is essential to measure hCG levels until they are undetectable and this can take 30–90 days. Methotrexate therapy is suitable when the serum hCG level is less than 3,000IU/L and the diameter of the ectopic pregnancy less than 3cm, if you are otherwise well.

Sometimes you will need a second dose of methotrexate if hCG levels do not fall satisfactorily after 10–14 days. In our experience, this is necessary in less than 5 per cent of cases. If the ectopic pregnancy is more advanced and in a place that makes safe surgery more difficult (e.g. cornual ectopic or cervical ectopic), it is possible to give a higher dose of methotrexate, although this brings with it possible side effects and has to be monitored carefully. The main side effects are: nausea or vomiting, stomach pain or upset, diarrhoea, tiredness, headache and chills. It is also unsafe to get pregnant for at least three months after methotrexate therapy (some recommend six months) and it is important to be taking folic acid during this time as methotrexate lowers folate levels in the body.

It is reassuring that the chance of your tubes remaining open is similar after medical and surgical management of ectopic pregnancy.

PREGNANCY OF UNKNOWN LOCATION

Sometimes it can be difficult to determine whether a pregnancy is ectopic or may have started within the uterus and failed to develop to a size that can be seen by ultrasound. This is termed 'pregnancy of unknown location' (PUL). There can sometimes be a week or two of uncertainty while things are monitored with a combination of ultrasound and hCG blood tests. Treatment has to be tailored to how the woman is feeling, and if the hCG levels have either plateaued or are rising, it may be necessary to administer methotrexate (see above).

MOLAR PREGNANCY

A molar pregnancy is a pregnancy that develops abnormally from the outset. It is very uncommon, affecting about 1 in 600 pregnancies, and most people won't have heard of it. Essentially the placental tissue, also known as the trophoblast, develops abnormally into what is known as a 'hydatidiform mole'. This is usually identified on an ultrasound scan with a characteristic appearance, whereby the trophoblastic tissue has developed out of control and there are also lots of cystic areas within the pregnancy. This is also known as gestational trophoblastic disease and it can sometimes be a challenge to treat.

A molar pregnancy cannot be viable and occurs when either two sperm fertilise one egg (partial mole) or a sperm fertilises an egg which doesn't have any genetic material (complete mole). Because the trophoblast grows so rapidly, levels of hCG in the blood climb very high early in pregnancy and exaggerate all the symptoms of pregnancy, especially nausea. If a miscarriage starts to occur, some of the small cystic structures may be passed at the same time.

If the diagnosis hasn't been made on the scan then it is likely to be made after a miscarriage has occurred by the appearance of what has been passed. If you need surgery to clear the uterus, then the tissue will be sent for examination in the pathology laboratory where the diagnosis will be made. It is important that the uterus is completely emptied and that tests are done every one to two weeks to ensure that hCG levels have returned to normal. Once levels have dropped to normal, pregnancy should be avoided for six months. If levels of hCG don't fall then it will be necessary to use methotrexate (see above), sometimes in multiple doses, and then pregnancy should be avoided for a year. The risk of recurrence is about 1 per cent.

Very rarely the trophoblastic tissue can become deeply embedded into the womb and turn into a type of cancer, known as choriocarcinoma. The tissue can be difficult to remove and the use of chemotherapy (methotrexate, combined with actinomycin D and etoposide) is required and is usually very effective. A pregnancy should then again be avoided for a year.

We appreciate how difficult it is to lose a pregnancy and support is available through your clinic, counsellors, local and national support organisations (see Resources, page 371). Remember that you are not alone, even though it may feel like it. For most people the sad loss of a pregnancy is a single event and the greatest likelihood is that your next pregnancy will be fine. Talk to your doctor next time you get pregnant so that you are monitored carefully and supported during what will naturally be an anxious time.

Chapter 20

Recurrent Miscarriage

I F YOU HAVE experienced a miscarriage it is unlikely that it will happen again (see Chapter 19). Some couples, however, experience repeated or recurrent miscarriage/recurrent pregnancy loss (RPL), which usually means at least three miscarriages occurring at the same stage in pregnancy. There are different (though sometimes overlapping) causes for recurrent miscarriage, and understanding the distinction will help you get the medical care that you need. Most couples with recurrent miscarriage are fertile as they will have experienced at least three consecutive miscarriages. Some, however, have coexistent subfertility and so the repeated loss of long-awaited pregnancies adds to the trauma that they have already experienced.

We covered the common causes of a single miscarriage in the last chapter (pages 279–284). If you have experienced a miscarriage and the factors that we have already discussed don't explain why it might have happened, it's important to be thoroughly investigated. In the UK, current guidelines stipulate that women have to have experienced three miscarriages to have extended testing, and many other countries have similar criteria, but we believe this needs to change.

After one miscarriage the risk of another miscarriage has been estimated as approximately 23 per cent; after two consecutive miscarriages this increases to 29 per cent; and after three the risk is about 33 per cent if a cause is found and about 25 per cent if no cause is found – in other words, there is still a 66–75 per cent chance of having a live birth in the next pregnancy after three miscarriages have occurred.

Relatively few couples (approximately 1 per cent) will experience recurrent miscarriages and this is when further investigations should be performed.

While up to a third of couples with recurrent miscarriage have experienced fertility problems at some time, we are often faced with couples attending the fertility clinic who have experienced one or two miscarriages. They might have undergone extensive fertility investigations and received various fertility therapies and so are naturally concerned that their next pregnancy is viable should they conceive after further treatment. Using the above criteria, they do not have 'recurrent' miscarriage and so would not usually warrant investigation, yet because their concerns are understandable, it is our view that all women who have experienced one or more miscarriages should also have the following tests, without having to wait to have three miscarriages:

TEST	PURPOSE
TSH, T3, T4 and TPO antibody tests	To identify any problems with the thyroid gland.
Vitamin D test	To identify vitamin D deficiency.
Ferritin test	To identify iron deficiency (at risk at 30ng/mL and below).
Coeliac disease screen – TTG antibody test	To investigate autoimmune serology, whereby healthy cells inside the body may be attacked by abnormal cells.
HbA1C test	To investigate for diabetes.

Couples who lose a pregnancy, whether through miscarriage or ectopic, need support and counselling, as the loss of a pregnancy is a heartbreaking experience. Your GP can refer you to counselling and all fertility clinics have counsellors too. The Miscarriage Association in the UK (see Resources, page 371) also provides support in a number of ways, including local support groups and contact with others who have had similar experiences.

INVESTIGATIONS FOR RECURRENT MISCARRIAGE

FIRST TRIMESTER MISCARRIAGES:
· Chromosomal analysis of both partners (not always available through the NHS in certain parts of the UK)
· Endocervical swabs for bacterial vaginosis (BV)
· Measurement of lupus anticoagulant and anticardiolipin antibodies and thrombophilia profile
· Factor V Leiden and prothrombin gene mutations
· Possible assessment of haemostatis activated protein C resistance and thromboelasticity
SECOND TRIMESTER MISCARRIAGES:
· Chromosomal analysis of both partners
· Measurement of lupus anticoagulant and anticardiolipin antibodies and thrombophilia profile
· Ultrasound of the uterus followed by hysteroscopy and/or hysterosalpingogram if an abnormality is detected

CAUSES OF RECURRENT MISCARRIAGE

A tremendous amount of research has been undertaken in recent years in order to try to unravel the causes and treatment of recurrent miscarriage and to demystify some of the traditional remedies, which were of unproven benefit.

An underlying cause is most likely to be found if the repeated miscarriages occur at a similar stage in pregnancy. First trimester (the first 12 weeks of pregnancy) losses account for 75 per cent of recurrent miscarriages and second trimester losses the remaining 25 per cent. Even if a cause is found there is always the possibility that future miscarriages might be due to another cause. Miscarriages are of a sporadic nature and so any treatment that is offered has to allow for the fact that future miscarriages may not be due to the condition that has been treated.

The causes of recurrent miscarriage may have genetic, anatomical, infective, hormonal or immune origins. While often no cause is found, it may be that with future research currently unknown issues may be identified.

Factors that are common causes of single miscarriage, and sometimes of recurrent miscarriage, include:

- **Environmental factors**: exposures such as radiation (but not working with visual display units), occupational exposure to chemicals (toluene, xylene, formalin, some chemical disinfectants, glues, paints) and pollution may lead to an increased rate of sporadic miscarriage, but there is no evidence that they are implicated in recurrent pregnancy loss. Alcohol and smoking also increase the risk of sporadic and possibly recurrent miscarriage.

- **Infection**: intrauterine infection is a common cause of sporadic miscarriage (see page 292), but not recurrent miscarriage. Despite recent interest in the association of **BV** with very early miscarriage after *in vitro* fertilisation (**IVF**), second trimester miscarriage and premature delivery, no studies have found a link and therefore you will not be offered routine screening for **BV**.

- **Hormonal abnormalities**: poorly controlled diabetes and thyroid disease are associated with miscarriage, but should be treated and therefore not a cause of recurrent pregnancy loss. Sometimes thyroid disease is associated with a generalised underlying autoimmune disturbance, which could then predispose to recurrent miscarriage.

Factors that may cause or contribute to the risk of recurrent miscarriage include:

- genetic cause

- anatomical abnormalities

- luteal phase defects

- immunological factors

- coeliac disease when not managed with a gluten-free diet

- sperm DNA fragmentation

Genetic causes

An abnormal chromosomal or genetic make-up in the fetus is found in about 60 per cent of sporadic miscarriages and in about 30 per cent of recurrent miscarriages. The most common abnormalities are when there is a duplication or absence of one or more chromosomes. As we've seen, all bodily cells should have 46 chromosomes – there are only 23 in egg cells and 23 in sperm, so that when the two combine the complete set of 46 is formed (see page 15). Each chromosome contains the messages for how we develop, which are contained in thousands of genes, all of which need to work in harmony. The genes determine our individual characteristics, how we vary and also our risk for certain diseases.

During the early cell divisions of the embryo, the chromosomes and genetic material have to divide evenly and this process may go wrong (see Chapter 21). This usually occurs out of the blue, but the risk increases with the age of both the father and mother.

Sometimes one or both parents have an underlying genetic abnormality, which may not affect their health but may lead to problems in a developing embryo. However, only 3–5 per cent of couples with recurrent miscarriage are found to have an obvious chromosomal abnormality themselves. The abnormalities that are sometimes found in parental chromosomes are usually what are known as balanced Robertsonian or reciprocal translocations (often between chromosomes 14 and 21). While carriers of balanced translocations are healthy, they have a 50–70 per cent risk of having an unbalanced embryo.

Parental chromosomal abnormalities cannot be treated, so you should have genetic counselling and be offered prenatal diagnosis for future pregnancies. This involves a sample being taken from the pregnancy for genetic analysis, either from the placenta (chorion villus sampling, CVS) or fluid from the pregnancy sac (amniocentesis). If the abnormality is so severe as to result in a very low chance of a healthy pregnancy, it may be necessary to consider the use of donated eggs or sperm. Pre-implantation genetic screening may also be considered in some circumstances (see page 301).

Anatomical abnormalities

Sometimes abnormalities within the inside of the uterus may prevent a pregnancy from developing normally. For example, the uterus may develop with an abnormal shape or size (see page 240), or may have a bridge of muscle (septum) separating it into two. Other problems may develop over time, such as adhesions or scar tissue following a miscarriage, termination of pregnancy or other operations (also known as Asherman's syndrome – see page 240), or fibroids may develop and restrict the capacity of the uterus to enable a pregnancy to grow properly (see Chapter 16). These, however, are uncommon causes of repeated pregnancy losses. Detailed three-dimensional ultrasonography may help with the full assessment of the uterus. On the other hand, there is no evidence that the surgical treatment of uterine anomalies improves the chance of conception or the risk of miscarriage. Many specialists advocate the removal of a uterine septum or large fibroids that distort the inner part of the uterus, although there is no firm evidence of benefit.

A weak cervix (cervical incompetence) may cause a second trimester miscarriage, but needs to be carefully assessed and is thought to be overdiagnosed. Cervical incompetence is associated with painless cervical dilatation before a miscarriage and few women with recurrent miscarriage experience this, with most having pain and bleeding as a miscarriage is starting. A weak cervix can be treated with a stitch (see page 281).

Luteal phase defects

Opinions on the role of a defective luteal phase (the second part of the cycle after ovulation, when progesterone is released from the ovary to sustain implantation and an early pregnancy) in both infertility and miscarriage vary. Our view is that a defective luteal phase is a reflection of inadequate follicular function and a 'poor-quality' ovulation. Luteal phase hormone concentrations do not correlate with the risk of miscarriage and luteal deficiency does not appear to be a recurrent phenomenon so is unlikely to cause recurrent miscarriage.

There is mixed evidence for the use of human chorionic gonadotrophin (hCG) injections, which stimulate progesterone production by the ovary, with some evidence of benefit, although the treatment is largely considered to be empirical – that is, of uncertain benefit but unlikely to cause harm.[1] A recent large study has suggested that progesterone supplementation may be beneficial for reducing miscarriage rates for women with recurrent miscarriage, and so this is a treatment that we now recommend from the time of the positive pregnancy test.[2]

Immunological factors

Immunology is a controversial topic – like much in the field of reproductive medicine! Essentially, the immune system is designed to help the body to deal with external threats, such as infection. So, when exposed to viruses or bacteria, the immune defences produce antibodies, which are complex proteins that help to combat disease. Sometimes we may also produce antibodies that can affect healthy organs, which is as a result of autoimmune disease – for example, rheumatoid arthritis involves the joints, thyroid disease affects the thyroid gland, and so on. Women with autoimmune disease have an increased risk of developing reproductive problems too, such as premature ovarian insufficiency (POI – see chapter 24, page 329), which can sometimes also be due to antibodies against the ovaries. It has been suggested that recurrent miscarriage may result from a breakdown in the normal immune mechanisms, because of either autoimmune disease or the failure of the mother to produce a protective immune response for enabling the pregnancy to develop.

Because a developing embryo has been considered by some to be partly 'foreign' material, as genetically half is formed from the sperm, there is much debate about how the uterine environment behaves towards it and the way that the endometrium receives and becomes receptive to the embryo during implantation. This process may go wrong, secondary to problems within the endometrium and the uterus itself, and sometimes this may be due to lack of coordination of the immune system. This is of relevance for recurrent miscarriage, which is also known as recurrent pregnancy loss, and for many women is thought to be a very similar process to that seen in recurrent implantation failure, which is the earliest stage in the process whereby an embryo doesn't implant and develop.

Autoimmunity

Approximately 2 per cent of normal pregnant women and 15 per cent of women with recurrent miscarriage have the lupus anticoagulant (LA) or anticardiolipin (aCL) antibody, both of which are antiphospholipid antibodies (aPL). The primary antiphospholipid syndrome (PAPS) relates to recurrent miscarriage and/or a tendency to arterial and venous thrombosis (blood clots). Women with aPL who haven't experienced pregnancy problems before have a miscarriage rate of 50–75 per cent, while those with recurrent miscarriage and aPL lose 90 per cent of their pregnancies, and the miscarriage rate is even higher if the patient has a condition known as systemic lupus erythematosus (SLE). Testing for these conditions can be difficult and positive results may sometimes be due to viral and other infections.

The majority of miscarriages in women with antiphospholipid syndrome occur in the first trimester (first third of pregnancy, conventionally 12 weeks) and are thought to be caused by antibodies directed to the trophoblast (placenta) that disrupt implantation. Second trimester miscarriages are probably caused by earlier abnormal placental development leading to clots in and loss of blood supply to the placenta. Low-dose aspirin (75–150mg) combined with heparin injections may reduce the risk of miscarriage from 90 to 30 per cent. The treatment is continued until 34 weeks' gestation.

Thrombophilia

Women with thrombophilia – an increased likelihood of forming blood clots in vessels – may be at increased risk of recurrent miscarriage. Thrombophilic conditions include deficiencies of antithrombin III, protein C and protein S, and activated protein C resistance caused by a mutation in the factor V Leiden gene (G1691A). There are two other thrombophilic gene mutations: factor II pro-thrombin G20210A and methylene tetrahydrofolate reductase C677T. There is limited evidence for the use of heparin or aspirin in women with thrombophilia and recurrent miscarriage.

Natural killer (NK) cells

NK cells are blood cells that are part of the immune system and thought to have an impact on your risk of miscarriage. NK cells are found in both peripheral blood circulating in the body (PBNK) and the lining of the uterus (uNK). Measurement of peripheral blood NK cell numbers/activity doesn't tell us what is happening in the uterus as there are important differences between NK cells in the blood and NK cells in the womb – in other words, a blood test doesn't appear to be helpful and instead a sample should be taken from the lining of the uterus (endometrium).

There is a lot of contentious debate in this area and no agree-ment on what a raised NK cell level is or, for that matter, what it means in practice. We feel that promising research on the assess-ment of uterine NK cells will help us better understand any potential association with miscarriage and, if so, the right treat-ment to use. Currently there is a vogue to prescribe corticosteroids (e.g. prednisiolone), which also bring with them some risks and side effects and so need to be used with caution. Furthermore, there is no conclusive evidence of their benefit. If you are found to have these problems it is important to have a careful discussion with an experienced reproductive medicine specialist in order to discuss your options.

Other contributors to miscarriage risk

Sperm DNA fragmentation, undiagnosed coeliac disease (when not managed with a gluten-free diet), MTHFR (methylenetetrahy-drofolate reductase) mutations leading to low folate and high homocysteine (see page 103) and multiple nutrient deficiencies including iron and vitamin D (see Chapter 4) may also contribute to the risk of recurrent miscarriage. Following the guidance and recommendations for nutrient testing outlined in Chapter 4 along with the necessary medical investigations will help ensure you give yourself the best chance of conceiving and having a healthy pregnancy and a healthy baby.

Couples with repeated pregnancy losses need support within a specialised recurrent miscarriage clinic, which at the very least will be able to perform comprehensive investigations, ensure reproductive health is optimised and provide counselling and psychological support. Supportive care and serial ultrasound scans of future pregnancies has been shown to increase the chance of a live birth to about 80 per cent.

Chapter 21

Genetics

MANY NEW TECHNOLOGIES have developed on the back of the scientific techniques used in the *in vitro* fertilisation (IVF) laboratory. Some of these can then be used for the treatment of infertility and others for helping people with other problems, such as genetically inherited diseases, even if they don't have infertility themselves.

GENETIC TESTING

If you or your partner have a serious inherited (genetic) condition running through the family, you may be offered pre-implantation genetic testing (PGT). This is also sometimes suggested for older women with a history of repeatedly unsuccessful IVF treatments. PGT involves the removal of one or more cells from an embryo in order to perform genetic testing to allow specialists to select genetically healthy embryos to transfer. The technology has developed considerably in recent years and there are a number of different ways in which it is performed and also different applications.

PGT may be separated into two main categories of assessment:

1. Pre-implantation genetic *testing* for single gene (monogenic) conditions (PGT-M) or for structural genetic anomalies (PGT-SR) – formerly known collectively as pre-implantation genetic *diagnosis* (PGD)

This is used for couples who have had previous children/ pregnancies affected by life-threatening or major genetic disease, who otherwise would have to conceive naturally and undergo antenatal testing of the pregnancy (e.g. chorionic villus sampling (CVS) or amniocentesis) and face the possibility of a subsequent termination of the pregnancy if tested positive and, of course, only if they wish to.

There are two main categories of genetic defects that cause inherited disease: those that affect chromosomes and those that affect single genes. Common conditions are listed on pages 303–5. These will include different modes of inheritance such as autosomal dominant conditions (e.g. Huntington's disease), autosomal recessive conditions (e.g. cystic fibrosis) and X-linked conditions (e.g. Duchenne muscular dystrophy). It is also possible to test for hereditary cancer syndromes (e.g. BRCA1 and 2).

Somewhat more controversial is the possibility to perform what's known as HLA matching in order to 'create' a sibling who is matched to an existing child who is suffering with a life-threatening condition that requires a bone marrow transplant, in order to avoid the rejection of the transplant. The creation of a 'saviour sibling' in this way is considered by some as the commodification of life by creating a child who otherwise wouldn't have been desired or conceived naturally. Others deem this to be a perfectly acceptable way to use IVF technology in order to save the life of an existing child, even if the new sibling may not have initially been planned for.

2. **Pre-implantation genetic *testing* for aneuploidy (PGT-A) – formerly known as pre-implantation genetic *screening* (PGS)**
   This can be performed to ensure that only genetically normal embryos are transferred during routine IVF in couples without a history of genetic disease – a potentially attractive option for older women, who have a significantly increased risk of genetically imbalanced (aneuploidy) embryos. PGT-A has also been proposed as an option for women who have experienced recurrent miscarriage or recurrent implantation failure (several cycles of IVF in which a pregnancy hasn't

occurred for no apparent reason). This is still controversial and by no means a guarantee, as we shall explain further down.

The technology of pre-implantation testing has moved forward in leaps and bounds and now uses a technique known as 'next generation sequencing' to assess the genetic profile of the embryo.

Controversial and ethical issues concern what constitutes a 'major genetic disorder' and the possibility of 'designer babies' now that the human genome has been mapped and so, theoretically, all genes can be assessed. Also, there is a high frequency of chromosome or genetic abnormalities (40–50 per cent) in human embryos, which increases with female age and explains why many embryos that look healthy down the microscope don't go on to develop into a pregnancy after they have been put in the womb.

If you find yourself in this position, it is essential to have counselling so that you understand the process, its limitations, the risk of false results and also what to do if unexpected genetic abnormalities are detected – or even whether they should be disclosed if they are not being actively looked for. This is therefore still a highly controversial area that is very challenging ethically.

In the UK, the Human Fertilisation & Embryology Authority (HFEA) has restricted licenses for PGT to a handful of centres and then for specified and clearly defined conditions. Elsewhere in the world, however, aneuploidy screening is becoming more widespread and largely unregulated. To date, there is no convincing evidence that routine PGT-A in IVF is of value, despite the promise that this technology has suggested.

The process of PGT

Embryos are created in an IVF cycle together with intracytoplasmic sperm injection (ICSI) to prevent contamination of the subsequent genetic analysis with surplus sperm that would otherwise be in left in the dish during standard IVF. The success of PGT relies upon the ability to culture embryos for up to five days *in vitro* and to use micromanipulation techniques to remove a few cells (blastomeres).

A blastocyst embryo comprises the inner cell mass, which will eventually form the baby, and an outer layer of cells – the trophectoderm – which will develop into the placenta. During PGT, between five and ten blastomeres will be removed from the trophectoderm for assessment. Each blastomere is thought to be pluripotent (that is, has the ability to develop into any cell type for the future embryo) and so those that remain have the potential to develop normally. There is, however, the risk that one or more cells aren't representative of the true genetic health of the embryo as there can be variation in the genetic make-up of cells within the embryo – so called mosaicism – and so the cells tested may each be different. There is also evidence that the transfer of mosaic embryos may not be detrimental and furthermore that some embryos may 'fix' themselves; in other words, have a mechanism for getting rid of genetically abnormal cells. So it's not nearly as straightforward as it initially seems.

Once the biopsy has been taken, the embryos are then usually frozen while the genetic testing takes place, and a genetically healthy embryo is then selected for transfer in a subsequent frozen embryo replacement cycle (see page 271).

The inheritance of genetic conditions is complex and doesn't always follow defined rules. For example, there can be what is known as variable penetrance with not all individuals carrying the abnormal genes being affected to the same degree. This is a crucial issue to discuss with an experienced genetic counsellor who can advise you on both risk and the prospects for PGT.

Common inherited conditions that can be screened for

There are many conditions that can be screened for, but below are those that may impact on your fertility. We have listed them in order of most often tested.

Single gene defects

- cystic fibrosis (autosomal recessive, AR)

- myotonic dystrophy type 1 (autosomal dominant, AD)

- Huntington's disease (AD)

- beta thalassemia (AR)

- sickle cell anaemia (AR)

- fragile X syndrome (X-linked)

- spinal muscular atrophy (AR)

- Duchenne muscular dystrophy (X-linked recessive)

- neurofibromatosis type 1 (AD)

- haemophilia A (X-linked recessive)

- human leukocyte antigen for acquired diseases

- familial adenomatous polyposis (AD or AR)

- Charcot-Marie-Tooth disease type 1 (AD)

- familial amyloidotic polyneuropathy (AD)

- Marfan syndrome (AD)

- tuberous sclerosis (AD)

- Von Hippel-Lindau syndrome (AD)

- Tay–Sachs disease (AR)

- severe combined immune deficiency (AR or X-linked recessive)

Chromosomal disorders

- structural chromosome aberrations

- translocations

- inversions

- deletions

Aneuploidy risk

- trisomy syndromes: 21 (Down); 18 (Edwards); XXY (Klinefelter)

- monosomy syndromes: XO (Turner)

- tetraploidy

The technology and science of PGT are advancing at a pace and there is a danger in this field that anything written will be outdated by the time it is published! Therefore, it is important to seek the advice of an experienced reproductive specialist and genetic counsellor to discuss your personal situation in appropriate detail.

NEW TECHNOLOGIES: GENE THERAPY AND CLONING

We have already described how every cell in the body should have 23 pairs of chromosomes, except the egg and sperm cells, which have one set of 23 – so that when combined to create an embryo there are 23 pairs (see page 15). Each chromosome contains thousands of genes, each of which provides the messages for the way cells behave to enable the body to develop and function normally. Some use the analogy of each person being like a book, with the chromosomes being the chapters and the genes being the words that make up the sentences. The sentences have to occur in the correct sequence in order for everything to be understood and work properly – if a word is missing, or even a letter within a word, then the whole sequence and balance is disturbed. Genes will code for similarities and differences between individuals and also for when things go wrong and result in illness or disease. Some genetic conditions lead to problems from birth, while others may not come to light until later in a large variety of ways.

The more we understand about genetic conditions the more we can identify, predict and potentially modify outcomes. The use of modern genetic technologies opens all sorts of possibilities, but at the same time raises numerous ethical concerns and conundrums, which may vary around the world due to cultural, religious and philosophical differences.

We all have some genetic factors that predispose us to developing particular diseases, whether this is a well-defined condition, such as certain cancers or forms of dementia, or an increased risk for developing illness, for example heart disease or diabetes. As well as being possible to test embryos to see if they are at risk of carrying life-threatening problems that affect children and may limit duration and quality of life, such as muscular dystrophy or cystic fibrosis, it is also possible to test for certain genes that may not cause immediate problems during childhood but may nonetheless have far-reaching consequences. This raises the whole debate about eugenics and 'How far should we go?'

In the last few years it has become possible to alter genes and change the way they behave. The technology, known as CRISPR-Cas9, is rapidly expanding and again highly controversial. It is possible to alter a genetic abnormality that leads to a condition in a particular type of cell – for example, sickle cell anaemia that affects the way red blood cells carry oxygen around the body. Furthermore, gene therapies have been used to try to improve the development of the endometrium to aid implantation.

With respect to sickle cell disease (sickle cell anaemia), the genetic make-up of the stem cells in the bone marrow has been changed to ensure that they start making healthy blood cells rather than the abnormal sickle cells. This has been successfully achieved and has been heralded as a cure for this condition for the affected individual. However, they will still have the genetic abnormality in their make-up and so this can still be passed down to their children – unless, of course, their 'germline' is edited, which essentially means editing embryos created during IVF to remove the genetic abnormality. There is currently an international ban on so-called genome editing because of the huge uncertainties about safety and also the concern that this will affect all subsequent generations, with unknown consequences.

There are a number of other possible uses for this technology – from the prevention of genetic conditions that affect certain cell types, to the protection of an individual against the risk of developing certain cancers or infections, such as HIV.

Another emerging treatment that has developed more quickly as a result of reproductive technologies is stem cell therapy. The stem cells are the 'factories' that produce cells throughout life – and can be cultured in the laboratory to create new cells, such as blood, nerve and muscle cells, which can then be used therapeutically, for example to try to cure blindness or spinal cord injury.

While there is an international consensus among responsible countries that these technologies should be used with great caution, as they are still experimental and of uncertain safety, there are maverick scientists in some countries who are already working outside the international agreements, with potentially unpredictable and alarming consequences. Indeed this has already happened in China, with a resultant outcry among the more responsible international scientific community.

Mitochondrial donation and mitochondrial disease

Mitochondria are tiny structures within cells that are often referred to as the energy source or 'batteries' of the cells. The health of the mitochondria is critical for the normal functioning of all cells and there has been much interest recently in looking at mitochondrial function in embryos as a way of predicting embryo health. It has also been suggested that it may be possible to improve the health of an older egg by transferring more or younger mitochondria into it. However, this controversial technology is not permissible in most countries and has not been proven to achieve the benefits that were initially hoped for.

Some families are affected by genetic diseases of mitochondria function, which may lead to children having a number of severely debilitating problems and reduced life expectancy. The mitochondria are inherited from your mother and it is thought that these mitochondrial diseases can be prevented by performing IVF using the father's sperm to fertilise his partner's egg (with the abnormal mitochondria) and a donated egg, with healthy mitochondria. The fertilised nucleus of the single cell embryo is then removed from each embryo and the nucleus created from the mother's egg is transferred into that created from the donated egg. This exciting advance opens up further possibilities for curing severely debilitating disease, but again has to be very tightly regulated.

Chapter 22

Building Modern Families: Disability, Single Parenting, LGBTQ+ Parenting, Surrogacy and After Sterilisation

T HE TERM 'MODERN families' has become a popular term that encapsulates the numerous ways that families are configured and formed, both naturally and using modern fertility technologies. Single women can use donated sperm, as will lesbian couples; gay men require egg donation and surrogacy; transgender people may wish fertility preservation before they transition and then subsequently may require assistance in a variety of ways. Surrogacy is also available for women without a womb or for whom getting pregnant would be unsafe. People who have been sterilised may undergo reversal surgery or may require assisted conception treatments. And people with disabilities can be supported in a variety of ways to become parents. In this chapter we will give a brief overview of all these situations.

I HAVE A DISABILITY AND WANT TO CONCEIVE

If you have a disability this shouldn't prevent you from having a family. Disabilities do, of course, vary greatly from one person to another and even different medical conditions may vary in how they affect individuals. Important considerations include whether your condition may impact your fertility and reproductive health, the effects and risks during pregnancy to both you and baby, the potential risk of transmitting a problem to the child and how you will care for your child after they are born. These issues relate to both women and men with disability, although the latter, of course, do not have to worry about the pregnancy side of things.

It is beyond the scope of this book to deal with every medical condition that can lead to problems with fertility and parenting, and so we shall discuss the issues in general terms. If you have a long-term medical condition, then it is important that you seek the advice of the doctors who care for you and an expert in a fertility clinic. Modern medicine has enabled many people with severe disability to survive through childhood to an age where parenting is possible. Some conditions, such as chronic heart, lung, kidney or liver disease, may affect general health to the extent that fertility is impaired. While steps may then be taken to enhance fertility or provide assisted conception such as *in vitro* fertilisation (IVF), there are then risks to be considered during pregnancy that may sometimes even put the life of the mother in jeopardy and also have an impact on the development of the baby. A multi-disciplinary assessment is required, which should fully involve the individual concerned together with all healthcare professionals involved in her care.

Sometimes the medical problems are so severe that it is unsafe to carry a pregnancy, in which case other options, such as surrogacy or adoption (see pages 315 and 355), may be suggested.

Passing on a condition

Some conditions that result in disability may occur out of the blue, while others may have a genetic origin, with potential risk of transmission to future children. Genetic counselling is important for both parents in order to understand those risks so as to be able to make the right decision as to whether to try to conceive naturally, possibly have screening tests during pregnancy or use IVF technologies to screen for healthy embryos (see Chapter 18). There is a huge range of genetically transmissible conditions and occasionally the use of donated sperm or eggs may be suggested as a way of preventing genetic transmission.

There are also ethical debates regarding the rights of individuals with disability opting to have children with the same/similar disabilities rather than having to go down the route of embryo selection and/or screening. In our opinion, there are no right or wrong answers and it has to be a matter for the informed choice of the individual.

Freya and Ahmed: Disability and conception

Freya and Ahmed each had different disabilities and used wheelchairs for mobility. They were both in their late twenties and met at their local sports club. Ahmed was involved in an accident while riding his bicycle and was paralysed from the waist down. He had lost all sensation in his 'saddle area' and so needed to self-catheterise to empty his bladder. He was unable to maintain an erection or to ejaculate without the assistance of an external vibrator, which was used to obtain some sperm that was then frozen. Freya had meningitis as a child, which led to her legs being amputated just below her hips. Because her mobility was restricted there were potential increased risks during pregnancy and so we arranged a preconception assessment to make a plan for her care during pregnancy. Freya responded well to ovarian stimulation for IVF and, despite Ahmed's frozen sperm being of very low quality (low numbers, poor motility and morphology), there was a good rate of fertilisation. The fresh cycle didn't result in a pregnancy. They then conceived with the second of their frozen embryo replacement cycles. Freya's pregnancy was uneventful, but she did require a caesarean section to deliver a healthy baby girl.

I'M SINGLE AND WANT TO HAVE A BABY

If you are a single woman, either through choice or because you haven't met the right person, you can still seek medical help to start a family. If you think that you might find yourself in this situation, it may be sensible to consider having some eggs frozen as a future insurance against ovarian ageing (see page 324) – although in the UK eggs can only be frozen for so-called social reasons for a maximum of ten years.

Deciding whether or not to freeze your eggs is something more and more women are facing. It's impossible to see into the future and know whether or not you will need to use any eggs you freeze – indeed most women do not. However, given that freezing techniques have improved and survival rates of eggs that are then thawed has improved significantly, it is worth considering if you feel you may end up delaying parenthood for whatever reason. It's important to remember that freezing your eggs does not guarantee you will have a baby with those eggs and it should be seen as one part of your reproductive life plan not a cast-iron solution by itself.

Your chance of pregnancy from future treatment will depend on the age at which you froze your eggs, as egg quality and age of the eggs are the main things that impact IVF success (see page 10). An older uterus will have little impact on how likely you are to conceive from donated or your own previously frozen eggs, though risks during pregnancy do increase with age.

Another thing to consider when deciding whether or not to freeze your eggs is your natural fertility and when you are likely to reach the menopause. Your mother's age at menopause can give a good indication of your genetic predisposition. Your periods can also provide information – longer regular cycles (more than 26 days) are associated with better ovarian reserve and a good blood flow during your period means it is likely you have good levels of oestrogen. Both these things are indicators of reproductive age and monitoring whether they are changing over time can also tell you how quickly you are ageing in terms of your fertility. Cycles that get shorter with age and periods that get lighter indicate that there are meaningful changes in your ovarian reserve. This shouldn't happen until you are in your forties, but can happen earlier. By the time these changes are noticeable, it may be too late to successfully freeze your eggs, but certainly if you have shorter cycles to begin with, a mother who had an early menopause or if your periods are very light, it may be more worthwhile to consider egg-freezing.

You can also have hormone testing and ultrasound scans to assess your ovarian reserve (see page 159), though this doesn't tell you a great deal about your future natural fertility, and paying attention to the above signs may be more useful in practical terms. Having repeat tests over time can provide information on how things are changing with time and indicate how quickly your fertility is declining.

Most fertility clinics can also offer egg-freezing services and this is always on a self-funded basis when done for social reasons. Costs can vary and include treatment costs for stimulating the ovaries and egg collection. You may need several rounds of treatment to have enough eggs to ensure you have enough for fertility treatment later. The current recommendation is to have 20 eggs frozen if you are over 37, which is likely to take at least two rounds of safe stimulation (see page 256). Freezing eggs overseas can be cheaper, but you always have to bear in mind that you will then have to travel for fertility treatment when the time comes to use those eggs and possibly multiple times for repeat egg collections initially.

If you don't have a partner, it is possible to consider the use of donated sperm (see page 205).

I'M LGBTQ+ AND WANT TO START A FAMILY

If you're gay, lesbian, bisexual, gender fluid or transgender, modern medicine and assisted conception treatments now enable you to have children. While pregnancies can be achieved without the use of a fertility clinic, it is important to be aware of the possible risks and we advocate that you seek the advice of fertility specialists who can both advise about the safest way to conceive and have a healthy pregnancy, and also provide implications counselling and guidance about any legal considerations. Furthermore, regulations may vary considerably between different countries – here we deal with the British perspective.

If you are gay and wish to have a family this would need to be by surrogacy (see page 315) or adoption (see page 355). Furthermore, surrogacy may be either straight (using sperm from the intended parent to inseminate the surrogate, which then fertilises the surrogate's own eggs so your surrogate is the biological mother) or with IVF (either using the surrogate's eggs or donated eggs). Sometimes private arrangements for straight surrogacy are made without linking in with a clinic – this can be fraught with difficulty when it comes to agreeing a legal contract and so we advise against this, even if at initial glance it may seem more attractive and less medicalised. For all surrogacy arrangements it is important that all involved have received detailed counselling about both the implications and legal issues and that a clear contract is signed at the outset (see page 316).

Lesbian women can conceive with the use of donated sperm (see page 313). Again, this may be achievable by private arrangements, whereby friends provide sperm that can then be 'inseminated' at home, using simple syringe devices that are available online. It is even possible these days to obtain sperm online and get it delivered directly to your home. It is our advice to be very careful if you're thinking of doing things for yourselves. While it may seem attractive, it is important to appreciate the need for careful counselling from a trained fertility counsellor and both emotional and clinical support. Sperm needs to be carefully screened (see page 206) in order to ensure that the donor is healthy, fertile and that there is no risk of transmission of infection or genetic conditions. Furthermore, donor insemination only works if the recipient of the sperm has been carefully checked to ensure that she is healthy, ovulating and has open fallopian tubes.

Transgender pregnancies

Transgender individuals may have children, but this will depend upon where they are in the process of transitioning. If you are born female ('natal females'), you may conceive and carry a pregnancy if you are ovulating, not taking transitioning hormone therapy and still have a womb. Alternatively, eggs can be taken from the ovaries after ovarian stimulation, as during IVF treatment, and frozen (cryopreserved) for use in the future (see page 324). The frozen eggs would need to be thawed, fertilised with sperm from a future natal male, trans partner or sperm donor, and the resultant embryos implanted in a future natal female, trans partner or surrogate. For natal males, sperm can be frozen prior to the use of transitioning hormone therapy and definitive surgery and used in the future with a natal female, trans partner or surrogate. Careful thought and professional fertility counselling via your fertility clinic or treating doctor is therefore required to explore all these possibilities.

SURROGACY

If you have ovaries but no uterus either because of a congenital absence (e.g. Rokitansky syndrome) or after hysterectomy (e.g. after severe obstetric haemorrhage or cervical cancer), or if pregnancy would be a medical risk for you (e.g. severe heart or lung disease), surrogacy is an option. There are two types of surrogacy: host (gestational) surrogacy, in which IVF is used to create embryos that are then transferred into the surrogate, or straight (traditional) surrogacy, in which the surrogate conceives with her own eggs.

Surrogacy should only be provided within the context of a licensed fertility clinic. Sperm must be frozen and quarantined for six months to reduce the risk of infection with HIV.

With host (gestational) surrogacy, a standard IVF regimen is used and the surrogate host prepared as for a frozen embryo replacement cycle (see page 271). The surrogate will not have a genetic link to the conceived child as her eggs are not being used. Usually the eggs are obtained from the commissioning woman (or intended parent, IP), who has her ovaries stimulated, as would anyone undergoing IVF. Egg collection can sometimes be difficult, however, if the ovaries are high in the abdomen, in which case a transabdominal approach may be needed (with the needle going through the skin of the abdominal wall rather than through the vagina). You may need to use donated eggs – for example, if you are the commissioning woman and have no ovarian function or in the case of gay men commissioning surrogacy. Occasionally donated sperm may be needed. However, in the UK, it is not permissible to use both donated sperm and eggs. This is because in order to apply for a parental order, which is the way that legal parenthood is transferred from the surrogate to the IPs, at least one of the IPs in a couple must be a genetic parent of the child born to them through surrogacy.

Straight surrogacy is less commonly performed. Some people attempt this treatment at home using home insemination kits, but we advise against this because of the risks of using unquarantined sperm and the need for careful support and counselling during such treatment, and so it should be offered within the context of a fertility clinic (see page 150).

In the UK, the birth mother is legally the mother of the baby until a parental order has been signed and submitted to the family court in order to transfer legal parenthood from the surrogate (and her spouse or civil partner if she has one) to the IPs. If the surrogate is married or in a civil partnership, their spouse or civil partner will be the child's second parent at birth, unless they did not give their permission. The surrogate has to give her consent to the parental order and it has to be submitted after six weeks and within six months of the birth of the baby, although there are currently attempts to change a number of the laws that apply to surrogacy in order to make it an easier and more streamlined process. For example, until recently single people were unable to have children through surrogacy, but they may do so now and apply for a parental order. Surrogacy agreements are not enforceable by UK law, even if there is a signed document between the commissioning couple (IPs) and the surrogate and they have paid their expenses. If there is disagreement about who the child's legal parents should be, the courts will decide based on the best interests of the child. Laws may vary considerably around the world and so it is essential to seek expert advice if you are thinking about pursuing surrogacy overseas.

There are strict regulations concerning surrogacy arrangements and few clinics offer this treatment because of ethical concerns and the complexities of the arrangements. It is our experience that surrogacy can work extremely well and we strongly advise that all surrogacy arrangements should be carried out by licensed assisted conception clinics, who will be able to provide safe treatment and appropriate counselling and direct patients as to where to obtain the right legal advice. In the UK there are surrogacy charities that help to link commissioning couples with potential surrogates (see Resources, page 371). While these are charitable organisations, they may charge a registration fee to cover costs. Furthermore, while surrogates themselves are considered to be altruistic in their offer to 'host' a pregnancy, they may claim legitimate 'expenses' to cover the costs of attending hospital appointments, time off work, etc. In some countries, surrogates are allowed to be paid and surrogacy has become a highly commercialised business (as indeed has egg donation in these countries too). We caution against people going overseas for treatment, because of both the commercialised nature and the lack of tight regulation. In addition, the laws vary around the world regarding surrogacy and taking babies conceived in this way from one country to another.

Uterine transplantation

We mention the possibility of uterine transplantation in order to complete the picture for those who may not have a uterus and are wondering whether it is possible to receive a uterus from another woman. While the transplantation of a uterus is technically feasible and has now been successfully performed in a number of countries, it is an extremely complicated procedure and so by no means routine. First a uterus has to be donated by either a living donor, who would have to undergo an extremely lengthy and complex operation to have her uterus removed intact with all its blood vessels, or from a donor who is 'brain dead' and on a ventilator, for example after a catastrophic accident. The recipient would also need to undergo a very long and complex operation and then take immunosuppressive medication to prevent the transplant from being rejected. Prior to surgery it is recommended that she has eggs removed for IVF and embryos frozen to be transferred into the transplanted uterus once the operation has been deemed successful. A uterine transplant may be an option to consider in countries where surrogacy is illegal or for those who may have ethical or religious objections to undergoing surrogacy, yet it is still a very new technique and not without potentially very significant risks and complications.

I'VE BEEN STERILISED: WHAT CAN I DO?

These days we see many couples in whom one partner has been sterilised having thought that they had completed their family in a previous relationship. In the UK if you've been sterilised you will not be eligible for NHS funding for either reversal surgery or IVF and so all treatment will have to be self-funded.

Men

It is the length of time since vasectomy that is the key determinant as to whether it is worthwhile considering a reversal operation (see also page 200). The breach of the blood–testis barrier at the time of the vasectomy may result in antisperm antibody (ASAB) production and the levels rise with time, causing the sperm to be adherent to each other and so less likely to fertilise an egg when released in the ejaculate. Surgical reconstruction of the vasa in a man who requests reversal of vasectomy is associated with a significant rate of ASABs. The success of surgery declines with increasing time beyond five years after the initial vasectomy operation – and probably shouldn't be attempted after ten years. The procedure should be performed by an appropriately skilled urological surgeon, and preferably one who works in conjunction with an IVF clinic so that sperm can be obtained for freezing at the time of the attempt at reversal in case the procedure is unsuccessful.

If vasectomy reversal results in too few viable, motile sperm in the ejaculate, then the sperm should be used for IVF/intracytoplasmic sperm injection (ICSI) and a sample frozen as a back-up in case the reversal site seals over in the future. If the procedure is unsuccessful or it is considered too long since the vasectomy, sperm may be obtained by percutaneous epididymal sperm aspiration (PESA – see page 201), frozen and then used for IVF/ICSI.

It is essential prior to seeking vasectomy reversal to ensure that your partner has been thoroughly assessed by a fertility specialist too, as there may be female factors that suggest the need for IVF, in which case a PESA should be performed and the sperm frozen. There are very few risks from these procedures and sperm can usually be obtained by PESA in about 95 per cent of cases.

Women

Reversal of sterilisation may be considered if the original procedure was performed using clips across the fallopian tubes and can be performed by either laparoscopy or open laparotomy surgery. However, if the tubes were tied, particularly at the time of a caesarean section, there is unlikely to be a sufficient length of normal tube to enable reversal to be a viable option. It is essential to check your ovarian function and your new partner's semen analysis before embarking on surgery.

Pregnancy rates are between 60 and 80 per cent, with ectopic pregnancy rates usually less than 5 per cent. The cumulative chance of delivery over 72 months after reversal of sterilisation has been reported as 72 per cent for women under the age of 37 years – this is still lower than with IVF and so the pros and cons need careful discussion. When taking cost-effectiveness into consideration, it is recommended that older women may be better proceeding straight to IVF.

Chapter 23

Fertility Preservation

THE TECHNOLOGY FOR the freezing of gametes (eggs and sperm) is quite extraordinary if you think about it, as 'life' itself is placed in a state of suspended animation for the duration of the freezing. When we freeze meat or fish, we don't require it to spring into life when it is thawed, whereas we require sperm to start moving again, and the mechanisms for fertilisation and controlling cell division to remain viable in both sperm and eggs.

It is now possible to successfully freeze gametes and maintain their viability for future fertility. The main reason for doing this is to preserve fertility before someone has treatment that would render them infertile – usually chemotherapy or radiotherapy for cancers and some other serious medical conditions. Fertility preservation is also offered to young people with gender dysphoria (transgender) before they start the process of transition. There is also a vogue for considering the freezing of eggs and sperm for 'social reasons' – to protect against the effects of ageing on fertility and as an insurance for the future.

Usually eggs and sperm are frozen on their own, but it is also possible to freeze parts of the ovary (ovarian tissue), which contains the eggs and also testicular tissue – although the latter is more experimental.

After freezing, embryos, eggs and sperm are all stored in liquid nitrogen at -196°C. Cryopreservation (freezing) of sperm is relatively straightforward and has been available for many years. Cryopreservation of oocytes (eggs) has become much more successful in the last five years, particularly with the development of a newer technique (vitrification) as an alternative to slow freezing. This approach is also used for the freezing of surplus embryos from *in vitro* fertilisation (IVF) treatment (see page 271), with better success rates than previously. Many pregnancies have now been achieved with the use of frozen eggs, albeit with a lower overall return rate for the number of oocytes frozen compared with outcomes after embryo freezing.

Chemotherapy and radiotherapy

When a life-threatening disease such as cancer is diagnosed in a young person, fertility is seldom at the front of their mind. It is the responsibility of the physician to advise the patient of the possibility of fertility-preserving techniques prior to embarking upon potentially sterilising therapy. Not all treatments for cancer affect fertility, and there are also ways to try to reduce the effects of treatment on the developing sperm and eggs. There is clear guidance on which treatments have the greatest effect and when fertility preservation should be offered. Also, as a general rule, the fertility of younger patients is more resilient to toxic challenges. If fertility remains after chemotherapy, it is usually lower than expected for women of a similar age, and pregnancies that occur are more likely to deliver prematurely. Reassuringly, however, there appears to be no increased risk of congenital anomalies in the resultant children.

If radiotherapy is required over the pelvis, the uterus (womb) is likely to be affected as well as the ovaries. Therefore, if the treatment is required prepubertally it may not develop and grow normally or, if later in life, the uterine blood supply and endometrium may be affected such that implantation may not be possible even if there is residual ovarian function (or if donor eggs are required).

There are a number of conditions in young women that may require potentially sterilising treatment – not only malignant conditions such as breast cancer, Hodgkin's disease, sarcomas, germ cell tumours, lymphomas and leukaemias, but also some systemic conditions such as severe connective tissue diseases (e.g. systemic lupus erythematosus). There are an estimated 1 in 1,000 young adults who are survivors of childhood malignancy and this figure is expected to rise. Furthermore, as women are deferring childbearing there are more young women who may require chemotherapy before they have had a chance to start trying for a family.

Treatments that are most likely to cause damage to the germ cells (eggs and sperm) include:

- total body irradiation, prior to bone marrow or stem cell transplantation, for example, in the treatment of both malignant (leukaemias) and benign haematological conditions (thalassemia and sickle cell anaemia)

- localised pelvic irradiation; sometimes surgery is performed to try to move the ovaries away from the target field of the radiation exposure (ovarian transposition)

- chemotherapy: alkylating agents (cyclophosphamide, procarbazine, cisplatin, lomustine, etc.), vinblastine, cytosine arabinoside

Many regimens are evolving and so it is difficult to predict the long-term effects on fertility of some of the newer protocols. After treatment it is generally advisable to wait a few years – usually five – to be given the 'all clear' before trying to conceive. Some conditions, such as certain types of breast cancer, require the long-term use of hormonal medication (such as tamoxifen), which may be recommended for up to ten years. Given the age-related decline in fertility (if residual ovarian function remains) and the rise in risks during pregnancy, some women take a break in treatment to try for a pregnancy. The risks of cancer recurrence therefore have to be balanced very carefully with the prospects of having a healthy pregnancy and often these are difficult to accurately quantify or predict.

There are also some genetic conditions that place young women at increased risk of an early menopause (known as premature ovarian insufficiency, POI – see Chapter 24) for whom oocyte or ovarian tissue cryopreservation may be suggested. These include mosaic Turner syndrome (the incomplete form of the condition where there is some ovarian function as opposed to the complete form when puberty doesn't occur and there is no activity within the ovaries at all), galactosaemia and fragile X pre-mutations. Some women only have one ovary, for example having lost the other as a result of surgery for a cyst – if surgery is then required on the remaining ovary because of the development of another cyst, there is a risk of compromise to future fertility and the freezing of eggs should be discussed either prior to or after such surgery.

CRYOPRESERVATION OF SPERM

The ability to freeze sperm has been available for many decades for a number of animals including humans – the latter both after donation for the treatment of women requiring donor insemination and as an insurance before chemotherapy or vasectomy. Sperm freezes well and the laboratory will usually split one sperm sample into a number of small tubes, with the aim of each one having sufficient sperm for a single treatment when required in the future. Sometimes men are asked to produce several times in order to build up a sufficient store to provide a viable prospect for future fertility. The future treatment may be an insemination procedure or IVF (often with intracytoplasmic sperm injection – ICSI) depending upon the concentration of sperm in the sample.

Men with debilitating conditions that necessitate freezing are often very unwell and may find it difficult to produce a sample of sperm by masturbation. Also prepubertal boys will not have the sexual maturity to be able to masturbate. There is therefore the possibility of freezing tissue removed surgically from the testes, although this is still very much an experimental procedure. Furthermore, the tissue that is frozen will not contain viable sperm but rather the spermatogonial stem cells (SSCs) from which sperm develop and so the cryopreserved tissue would need to be reimplanted at a later date in order to re-establish spermatogenesis after cancer therapy.

The freezing of sperm for 'social reasons' has also been suggested for young men as fertility declines with age in both women and men, and older men are more at risk of having children with health conditions such as autism. The elective freezing of sperm as an insurance for the future is, however, somewhat more controversial than the freezing of eggs (see below), and so is seldom performed.

CRYOPRESERVATION OF EGGS

In recent times there has been immense public interest in the potential for the freezing of oocytes and ovarian tissue, predominantly for young women about to undergo sterilising chemo-/radiotherapy.

Until recently, the most realistic prospect of achieving future pregnancy for women has been the cryopreservation of embryos generated during a quick IVF protocol (for example, using gonadotrophins and a gonadotrophin-releasing hormone (GnRH) antagonist), which should usually be complete within 12–14 days. However, relatively few embryos are likely to be generated in this way (on average ten).

Sometimes it is feasible to undergo two rapid cycles in succession if the woman is well enough and there isn't too much of a time pressure on the need to commence treatment for the cancer. Furthermore, it is possible to start the treatment at any stage in the woman's menstrual cycle in order to avoid delays.

The creation of embryos does, of course, require sperm and so the freezing of embryos would require the woman to be in a stable relationship with a partner with whom she would wish to have a family in the future. However, sadly some couples separate and there have been many cases when this has happened and embryos have had to be destroyed as the former male partner has withdrawn his consent for their use (as he would be the legal father). In more recent times, the technology for freezing eggs (vitrification) has improved considerably such that survival of eggs after vitrification is as good as embryos and so consideration should be made to freeze eggs in preference to embryos. These factors obviously have to be carefully discussed, which can be difficult considering that it is a time of great distress, when having to confront a recent diagnosis of cancer and its treatment and also think about fertility preservation at the same time.

Chemotherapy can usually commence 48 hours after egg collection, providing the woman is well and not experiencing problems such as ovarian hyperstimulation syndrome (OHSS). There are increased risks of thrombosis after ovarian stimulation, which may be compounded by the underlying cancer diagnosis, and so anticoagulant prophylaxis may be required.

Until recently the returns from oocyte cryopreservation have not been as good as for embryos but with improvements in technology, at least 80–90 per cent of oocytes are expected to survive and achieve similar fertilisation rates to standard IVF. The oocyte is the largest single cell in the human body and is very sensitive to external insults, and the outer surface of the oocyte may harden as a result of the freezing process and so ICSI is usually used in order to achieve fertilisation.

Caution may be required for women with hormonally sensitive tumours, for example oestrogen receptor positive breast cancer, when low-dose stimulation combined with the drug letrozole may be used (which aims to keep oestrogen levels as low as possible). Furthermore, if it is felt that there is either insufficient time or too great a risk with the stimulation of the ovaries, it is possible to collect eggs from a small, unstimulated follicle and mature them in the laboratory (*in vitro* maturation, IVM), although this technique has limited success and is only performed in a few specialised centres (see page 231).

Worldwide, several hundred babies have been born from previously frozen eggs with no evidence of an increased risk of congenital anomalies. Once a patient embarks upon chemotherapy there is some evidence that the prolonged use of a GnRH agonist might help protect the ovary, although there are the associated downsides of oestrogen deficiency with such treatment. There is also research into the use of new agents that may inhibit the early development of the follicle before it becomes hormonally sensitive, although these are not yet available outside of research studies.[1]

When the woman comes back later to use the eggs it is common practice to thaw them all, fertilise them and watch them develop into embryos with a view to transferring one (or at the most two) and then freezing any remaining good-quality embryos for future use.

Cryopreservation of eggs for social reasons

There is increasing use of this oocyte cryopreservation as an insurance against ovarian ageing for career women who wish to delay childbearing. While fertility preservation before cancer treatment is usually funded by the NHS in the UK, cryopreservation for 'social reasons' needs to be self-funded.

Social egg freezing is a controversial subject as the issue concerns healthy women and choices to have children during fertile years – that is, during the years in which women are deemed to be naturally equipped and ready for bearing and bringing up children – or deferring to a later time, when natural fertility has declined. It has been debated that moving childbearing from its natural place in a woman's life and putting it artificially late in life brings risks, difficulties and disadvantages, and means forgoing the many advantages that belong to having children in the years of natural fertility. Many women who freeze eggs expect to be trying by their forties; however, this is often not the case.

Despite the huge improvements in the technology, egg freezing still gives a lower chance of conceiving a biological child later in life and certainly no guarantee. As might be expected, the younger the woman when her eggs are frozen the greater the chance of them being able to achieve a pregnancy in the future. A woman younger than 37 is expected to have a good chance of having a baby in the future if she has one cycle of egg freezing, with the cryopreservation of 12–15 eggs. Indeed your eggs are at their best quality when you are in your twenties, so we always recommend freezing early if this is something you are considering. Once older than 37 the prospects decrease, coupled with the need for an increased number of eggs to be frozen (maybe 20 or more, requiring 2 or more cycles of ovarian stimulation) to give a viable chance of future success.

There is no evidence that there is any deterioration of frozen eggs, sperm or embryos over time. Children conceived from cryopreserved eggs and embryos have similar rates of minor and major congenital abnormalities to children conceived normally. Furthermore, the rates of pregnancy, miscarriage and congenital anomalies do not appear to be related to the duration of embryo storage.

There is an increased risk of medical complications for the mother associated with pregnancy in older women, particularly over the age of 50, which is the usual cut-off for treatment in the UK (either with cryopreserved or donor eggs), while in North America the suggested cut-off is 54 years. There have, however, been some high-profile and controversial cases of women being treated, usually using donated eggs, in their late sixties, which we consider to be beyond the bounds of what modern technology should be offering, even if technically feasible, because of the significant implications for the potential welfare of any children conceived in this way.

We feel it is vitally important to educate young people about the key issues that affect reproductive health, in particular the decline in fertility that occurs with age (in both women and men). Indeed we have led a very successful national campaign in the UK (the Fertility Education Initiative). Society needs to change in order to support young people to develop their careers, relationships and families when they are young and not one to the exclusion of the other. For while egg freezing may offer an opportunity for some to delay, there is no guarantee and there is a danger of giving false hope for the future, which may then stop women with frozen eggs trying naturally before it's too late.

LEGAL TIME LIMITS

In the UK it is possible to store frozen sperm, eggs and embryos for up to 55 years for those who require preservation for medical reasons that will have an effect on their fertility. However, if freezing is for social reasons the legal time limit is only 10 years and so a woman who freezes her eggs as an insurance policy at the age of 25 would need to use them by the time she is 35. Many feel this law is obsolete and there are currently calls to try to change it.

OVARIAN TISSUE CRYOPRESERVATION

Cryopreservation of ovarian tissue is now a therapeutic reality, although it is only available in a few centres worldwide. The surface of the ovary (ovarian cortex) contains the primordial follicles, the number of which declines progressively through a woman's reproductive years. The number of primordial follicles at a given age varies considerably between individuals and it is this number that constitutes a woman's 'ovarian reserve' (see page 11) and also reflects the ovaries' ability to withstand the insult of chemo-/radio-therapy in the treatment of cancer. Thus, young women are more likely to retain fertility than older women. If it is considered that the risk of POI is greater than 50 per cent, then ovarian tissue cryopreservation is a viable option for women under the age of 35 years.

Cryopreservation of ovarian tissue generally requires the removal of an entire ovary, usually by laparoscopy, after which the outer cortex (surface) is removed and then frozen in strips. To date there have been a number of pregnancies after the reimplantation of frozen–thawed ovarian tissue.

A concern with the reimplantation of ovarian tissue is the re-introduction of malignant cells, for example if the underlying condition was a lymphoma. An alternative approach is to culture the ovarian tissue in the laboratory in order to obtain eggs from follicles that have been stimulated to grow in an incubator. This technology is still some way from being perfected. Furthermore, concerns have been expressed about the possible adverse effects of culture on the overall genetic health of the egg ('genetic imprinting'). It is anticipated that there are still many years of research before this technology becomes a reality.

Chapter 24

Premature Ovarian Insufficiency (POI)

THE CONTROL OF ovarian ageing is still one of the biggest enigmas in reproductive biology. It is difficult to predict when you might go through the menopause, and sometimes this can occur much earlier than expected. If you find that you are not having regular periods or your periods have stopped altogether, your doctor will perform the tests that we outline in Chapter 14 and may advise you that your ovaries have either run out of eggs or are close to running out of eggs. You may also have symptoms of being low in oestrogen, such as experiencing hot flushes, mood changes and vaginal dryness.

Premature ovarian insufficiency (POI, formerly known as premature ovarian failure, POF, or a 'premature menopause') is defined as the cessation of ovarian function under the age of 40 years. The function of the ovary depends upon the total number of eggs (oocytes) contained within the microscopic primordial follicles, which develop during the time that a female fetus is growing in her mother's womb. The eggs have stopped being produced by the time a girl is born and they are then lost progressively throughout life, as explained on page 328.

The rate of ovarian ageing appears to be influenced by both genetic and environmental factors. The age of a woman's mother's own menopause is the best predictor for an individual. Environmental factors may include the nutrition that a developing female fetus is exposed to in her mother's womb and then later on by the exposure to toxic chemicals, the best known of which being cigarette smoking.

The age of menopause appears to be similar in all Western communities (approximately 51 years), although women in developing countries appear to have a menopause 5 or 6 years earlier, and this may be a reflection of undernutrition during fetal life as nutritional status during infant or adult life does not appear to have a direct bearing on ovarian ageing.

The loss of one ovary, through surgery for a large cyst for example, is thought to bring forward the age of the menopause by a maximum of about 7 years, depending upon the age that the operation occurred.

The exact incidence of POI is unknown as many cases go unrecognised, but estimates vary between 1 and 5 per cent of women. In one large study the incidence of POI was 1:1,000 by the age of 30 and 1:100 by the age of 40.[1]

Occult/incipient (early) ovarian failure

For any woman, as you age, your antral follicle count (AFC) will go down, as will the blood levels of anti-Müllerian hormone (AMH – see page 160) and oestradiol (oestrogen). This decline happens more quickly as you approach the menopause. At the same time, your levels of follicle-stimulating hormone (FSH) and luteinising hormone (LH) in the blood will start to rise. The first signs of reproductive ageing that you may notice are your cycles getting shorter, more irregular (from on average 28 to 23 days) and periods getting lighter as oestrogen declines, as discussed in Chapter 14. You will also have more cycles where you don't ovulate, which in itself can cause shorter cycles.

For women with POI, changes start to happen at a younger age. Before periods stop completely, you may experience an intermittent return of the menstrual cycle, interspersed with variable periods of amenorrhea (an absent cycle). Your gonadotrophin (FSH and LH) levels will usually remain fairly high during these natural cycles and the AMH will be lower than the level expected for your age. During the early stages of this occult/incipient ovarian failure (previously known as 'resistant ovary syndrome' because the ovaries are resistant to FSH), you may still ovulate occasionally and have infrequent periods. Some women do also conceive naturally during this phase. Treatment to stimulate the ovaries with a view to collecting eggs, however, is rarely successful as the ovaries are usually resistant to gonadotrophin injections – just as they are to your natural hormones that trigger the development of follicles.

Another early sign of POI is missing just one period, and this should not be ignored. If this happens where previously your cycles have been regular and it cannot be explained, it should be taken seriously and investigated by your GP, especially if you have a family history of early menopause. This should include having hormone blood tests including oestrogen and FSH. If caught early, an elevated FSH will give advance warning of POI, so having this awareness could rescue your ability to freeze your eggs and have your own biological children before it is too late as it is sometimes possible to retrieve some eggs following stimulation treatment when caught in the early stages.

DIAGNOSIS

Premature menopause is defined as stopping your periods by 45 years and POI as stopping your periods by 40 years, although some people use the two terms interchangeably and define the cutoff as 40 years for both. The first hormonal change is an isolated increase in FSH (hence the importance of testing this hormone as soon as possible if POI is suspected), followed by elevation of FSH and LH, with a fall in oestrogen (oestradiol) levels that coincides with the development of amenorrhea. Over the next year oestrogen continues to fall. If you have an ultrasound, the scan will first show your ovaries to be normal, then they appear smaller with few follicles. In the advanced stages, the ovaries have a volume of less than 2ml with no follicles. AMH levels also fall and become undetectable when tested.

If your periods have stopped and you have high FSH (> 20IU/L) on more than two tests, it is likely that you have POI. The longer the period of amenorrhea, the higher the FSH level and the lower the AMH, the greater the likelihood that the ovarian failure is permanent. A single elevated FSH level, even if greater than 40IU/L, should be treated with caution as spontaneous ovulation and pregnancy have still been observed, but it is a warning sign and you should not delay fertility treatment or natural conception if you want to have a baby.

Additional investigations you may need include checking chromosomes (known as the karyotype) as sometimes there can be a genetic cause of POI and screening for autoantibodies – as if you have autoimmune conditions, such as thyroid problems and pernicious anaemia, you have an increased risk of developing POI (in fact, between 20 and 40 per cent of women with POI have a history of other autoimmune disorders, most commonly thyroid disease). You will also need a bone density scan, as low oestrogen causes progressive thinning of the bones. Assessing your heart health is also important, which includes a blood pressure and cholesterol check.

CAUSES

In approximately two-thirds of cases, the cause of POI cannot be identified. It is unknown whether these cases are truly idiopathic (unexplained) or caused by genetic, immunological or environmental factors that we don't yet understand. When the cause has been identified, one of the commonest reasons for POI is Turner syndrome (see below), followed by a past history of chemotherapy, pelvic surgery, pelvic irradiation, or other rare genetic problems (such as galactosaemia or 46, XY gonadal dysgenesis). Viral and bacterial infection may also rarely lead to ovarian failure, so infections such as mumps, cytomegalovirus or HIV in adult life can cause your ovaries to work less well in the long term, as can severe pelvic inflammatory disease (infection).

Ovarian failure before puberty is usually caused by genetic chromosomal abnormalities or childhood cancer that needed chemotherapy or radiotherapy (see below). Environmental toxins might be a factor in causing POI. The best-known toxin is of course smoking, which has been shown to lower the age of menopause.

Genetic causes

A female fetus usually has two active X chromosomes that make her genetically a girl. Both are needed when you are in your mother's womb in order to make a normal number of eggs. POI, therefore, is often caused when something goes wrong with these chromosomes. Turner syndrome is the most common cause where a female fetus only has one of the two X chromosomes and so development of the ovaries and follicles is affected. This means puberty doesn't happen as the ovaries don't have any eggs and can't function. Another condition is partial Turner syndrome ('Turner mosaic') where there is an extra X chromosome. This often causes periods to stop soon after entering adolescence.

With Turner syndrome, because women only have one X chromosome, this means the total number of chromosomes is also lower, which causes other changes in the body. Instead of the normal 46 chromosomes, women have 45 in total and this is known as a 45X profile (instead of the usual 46XX or in men 46XY). This usually causes short stature, other changes in appearance such as a broad neck, heart and kidney problems, and a higher risk of various other conditions such as diabetes and thyroid disease. Sometime the aorta, which is one of the main arteries from the heart, may be narrowed. If you have Turner, it is therefore very important to have a scan of your heart and vessels, as it is not safe to get pregnant by egg donation unless such problems have been properly checked and treated where needed.

Fragile X syndrome

Fragile X syndrome is a condition where genes on the X chromosome that are needed for nerve development don't work properly. It is the commonest way a learning disability can be passed from parent to child and affects 1 in 4,000 boys and 1 in 8,000 girls. It causes a mixture of physical, behavioural and cognitive symptoms. It also increases the risk of developing POI in women.

Medical causes

There are many medical treatments (iatrogenic) that cause periods to stop (amenorrhea), which may be either temporary or permanent. These include cancers that need either radiation to the abdomen/pelvis or chemotherapy. Both these treatments may result in permanent damage to the ovaries. It's difficult to predict how much cancer treatments will impact future fertility, but age is a significant factor – the younger a girl is, the more follicles she has and the better her chances of the ovaries continuing to work well after treatment. The dose and type of chemotherapy are also important. It is estimated that 1 in every 1,000 adults is now a survivor of childhood cancer and for these women the freezing of ovarian tissue before treatment is now offering a real chance of restoring fertility (see page 321).

Gynaecological operations such as removing the ovaries and uterus (oophorectomy and hysterectomy) inevitably result in amenorrhea. Hormone replacement therapy (HRT) should be prescribed, but fertility is only achievable with either egg donation or surrogacy – depending upon what has been lost.

MANAGEMENT

If you are diagnosed with POI, you will be referred to a counsellor to discuss the implications for your fertility and whether you might wish to consider the use of egg donation. In terms of your medical treatment, you will be advised to take HRT to give your body what it is missing with medication containing both oestrogen and progesterone if you still have a uterus (if not, oestrogen alone can be used as there is no risk of abnormal development of the womb lining). Oestrogen deficiency has a number of effects on the body including hot flushes, mood swings, vaginal dryness and, over time, circulatory problems and thinning of the bones (osteoporosis), and HRT will minimise these problems.

HRT medications prescribed for menopausal women are also preferred for young women rather than the low-dose combined oral contraceptive preparations, which contain at least twice the amount of oestrogen that is recommended for HRT. HRT also contains 'natural' oestrogens rather than the synthetic ethinyloestradiol that is found in most oral contraceptives.

The beneficial effects of HRT in reducing osteoporosis and the cardiovascular risks that come with the loss of oestrogen are thought to outweigh the small potential risk of breast cancer, particularly in women with POI. In essence, the hormones being given are designed to replace the hormones that your ovaries should be making and so should provide greater benefit than risk up to the age of 50. You will only need an annual breast examination if you are at high risk, for example if you have a family history of breast cancer.

If you would like to conceive, it's best to take a more 'natural' form of HRT, which will not inhibit ovulation (or adversely affect a pregnancy) and so shouldn't prevent conception in the rare cases where this is possible, but will still provide you with sufficient oestrogen. If, on the other hand, you don't want to conceive it makes sense to use a contraceptive for the provision of oestrogen to ensure you don't unintentionally get pregnant.

In terms of treatments to enhance fertility, there have been some experimental immunosuppressive drugs, but this is not something we can recommend without evidence from proper clinical trials. It is likely that pregnancies reported in women with POI or 'resistant ovary syndrome' are due to the occasional ovulation described above rather than successes of treatment.

Oocyte (egg) donation

Whatever the cause, if you have POI, or do not wish to use your own eggs for genetic reasons, you always have the option of oocyte (egg) donation. Oocyte donation may also have a place for women who do not respond to ovarian stimulation during IVF or whose oocytes repeatedly fail to fertilise in the presence of apparently normal sperm.

Your chance of success with treatment largely depends on the age of the woman donating the eggs, and implantation rates are usually about 30–40 per cent per treatment cycle. The upper age limit for egg donation treatment in the UK is 50.

The highest pregnancy rates in women having egg donation are seen in women with POI who have an anatomically normal uterus, whereas women who have any problems with the uterus do less well. Women with Turner syndrome who have not had a spontaneous puberty and women who have had radiotherapy to the pelvis, have reduced uterine blood flow and whose endometrium doesn't respond well to oestrogen therapy (sometimes radiotherapy destroys any subsequent endometrial function) have a lower chance of success. Furthermore, it's important to be aware that if you use eggs donated by a sister when you have POI, you are likely to do less well than if you use an anonymous fertile donor.

When it comes to IVF with donated eggs, your treatment will be similar to that during a normal frozen embryo cycle (see page 271) with increasing doses of oral oestrogens, with the addition of progesterone four days before embryo transfer. The only difference is that your natural cycle doesn't usually need to be switched off when you have POI. If, on the other hand, you have been diagnosed early and you still have a natural cycle, you will need down-regulation before starting treatment (see page 256). Close synchrony is needed between your cycle and the donor's IVF cycle if fresh embryos are to be transferred.

As with sperm donation, careful counselling is important for you, your partner and the donor (see page 275). The donor should be under the age of 35 in order to reduce the chance of age-related chromosomal problems.

Egg sharing has become more popular in recent years, whereby a woman having IVF who can't afford her own treatment donates some of her eggs in return for free treatment. With appropriate counselling, egg sharing appears to work well, without having a negative affect psychologically if the donor doesn't conceive. A strict protocol is needed to prevent overstimulation of the donor's ovaries and also to ensure that surplus oocytes are donated only if a prerequisite number (usually six to ten) has been collected for the donor's own use.

The ethics of egg donation and egg sharing is discussed in Chapter 26.

Egg freezing

If you know that you are at increased risk of developing POI then you might consider egg freezing (see page 324), although the prospects for success are more limited than if you have completely normal ovarian function.

Embryo donation

Embryo donation is an option in a few, relatively uncommon scenarios. For example, if you need IVF and either you have no sperm and eggs or have very poor-quality sperm and eggs that result in embryos that are not viable, and so need to consider using both donated sperm and donated eggs, an option then is to use embryos that have been donated by couples who have completed their family through IVF and have surplus frozen embryos that they wish to donate for treatment rather than be destroyed or used for research.

It goes without saying that careful counselling is important for you, your partner and also the donors (see page 275). In the UK single women cannot receive donated embryos as the man whose sperm was used to create the embryos is considered to be the legal father – which is a different scenario to the use of donated sperm and one of the vagaries of UK fertility law.

Having treatment with embryo donation is technically very easy and simply requires undergoing a frozen embryo replacement cycle (see page 271).

Chapter 25

Alternative Therapies

I N THIS BOOK we have provided a thorough appraisal of an evidence-based approach to the management of fertility problems. We are aware that a huge industry has developed around the field of fertility and that many 'therapies' and alternative approaches have been suggested to enhance fertility, but often without sufficient evidence of benefit.

There are a number of therapies that are not bound by the same degree of regulation and scrutiny as *in vitro* fertilisation (IVF) and so we have to be cautious when considering them. Furthermore, as we stress repeatedly throughout this book, fertility declines with age and so if you are experiencing difficulties in conceiving it is important to seek the advice of an appropriately qualified medical specialist without delay, rather than turning to alternative therapies that may not help you and could cause harm by delaying your opportunity to access the right treatment.

There is no doubt that methods that aid relaxation may provide additional benefit while undergoing the stresses of fertility therapy, although there is no firm evidence that they increase the chance of having a baby. Anything that you feel helps you to relax and improves your general well-being, and that of your partner, is likely to be beneficial. Furthermore, this can be beneficial for your overall health. Doing simple things together, like gardening or listening to music, as way of relaxing while you're trying to conceive or going though fertility treatment can help bring you closer.

We have discussed exercise and other approaches including meditation therapies and all forms of yoga in Part 1 (see pages 84, 128 and 129), along with the rationale for their inclusion in a preconception care programme. Other approaches to improve psychological well-being include acupuncture and reflexology. Both involve regular sessions with a therapist and this in itself may enable you to feel better supported as you progress through fertility treatments. We are well aware that visits to the fertility clinic can be stressful and often relatively brief – dealing more with the practical issues than providing all the emotional support that you need. All clinics should have counsellors who you can access for additional support, but there is no doubt that finding your own means of extra help and support can certainly be beneficial.

There has been much research on the use of acupuncture in the context of fertility – both natural and assisted.[1] It is difficult to draw firm conclusions from the numerous scientific studies that have been conducted because of differences in approach, poor study design and the many differing underlying causes of infertility in women leaving the possibility that some categories of patient may benefit, while others do not. Nonetheless, a number of studies have been carried out, particularly during different stages of the IVF process.[2] Some have shown benefit and some have demonstrated a negative effect. A recent review of studies looking at acupuncture conducted on the day of embryo transfer, for instance, showed that acupuncture did have an effect, but one that actually reduced the chance of ongoing pregnancy.[3] Anecdotally, many patients report improvements in symptoms and regularisation of the menstrual cycle after having acupuncture. Overall, we do not feel that there is likely to be any harm in pursuing acupuncture with an appropriately qualified practitioner but, on balance, we would not encourage treatment on the day of embryo transfer itself. Whether treatment in the run-up to IVF or during stimulation will improve the chance of you having a baby overall is far from certain.

There are some therapies that we advise against, for example the use of Chinese herbal medicines, which can be very strong, bring with them potential side effects and occasionally do harm. Furthermore, the market for herbal medicines is unregulated and the purity of these products is difficult to verify; they may not contain the ingredients claimed and may be contaminated with unwanted ingredients, including heavy metals. We have certainly seen patients encounter problems with their use and so, while traditional Chinese medicine (TCM) has its foundations in history and has been practised for hundreds of years, we urge caution in the context of modern, Western fertility therapy.

PART 3

Ethics, the Law and Options If Treatment Doesn't Work

In the final part of the book we discuss important issues that underpin the whole of fertility treatment – namely ethical considerations and legal frameworks that encompass what we do. We also offer options to consider for those who may not wish to pursue treatment or for when treatment doesn't work, such as adoption and fostering.

Chapter 26

The Ethics of Fertility Treatments

THERE ARE MANY ethical issues that may arise when treating infertility. Indeed, we have seen a great many ethically challenging scenarios in our own clinical practice that would not have arisen from natural conception, even though real life outside the laboratory can also bring moral dilemmas in terms of relationships and families in the context of having children. Understanding some of these issues can explain and give context to some of the things that happen during your treatment.

One of the most important principles when it comes to medical ethics is respect for the autonomy of the individual patient. This means you should be fully informed and the confidentiality of all consultations is guaranteed. Beneficence and justice are also key. Beneficence involves considering the welfare of others and doing no harm. Here we are talking principally about the welfare of those undergoing treatments and the potential welfare of any children conceived as a result of treatment. We tend to balance the physical harm risked by a potential mother or parent against the psychological benefit that a successful outcome of treatment will bring to either her or a couple.

A postcode lottery

There is no doubt that in the UK, with its current 'postcode lottery' of health service funding, many funding authorities regard *in vitro* fertilisation (IVF) as a luxury form of treatment, on a parallel with the removal of tattoos and other cosmetic procedures.

This is something that we have argued against and campaigned to change for many years.

Assisted conception treatments are highly regulated in the UK by the Human Fertilisation & Embryology Authority (HFEA), which has facilitated progress and research within the confines of tight yet permissive regulation that allows us doctors and scientists to continue to innovate and improve the chances of success from fertility treatment. Despite public opposition to the concept of IVF babies in the early days, it is now very well accepted as a medical treatment for infertility. Furthermore, any changes or advances have been the subject of public consultation and wide debate (for example mitochondrial donation, see page 307).

Does everyone have a right to treatment?

Two issues that will always be central to any consideration of the ethics of reproduction are who has the right to reproduce and to what extent this right has to be balanced against the welfare of a child born as a result of the treatment. Generally speaking, in most societies a married heterosexual couple in a stable relationship is considered to provide an appropriate environment for rearing children. On the other hand, most people recognise that legal marriage offers no guarantee of a suitable environment, and that couples and, we would argue, even individuals who are not married may not only assert a moral right to be parents but in fact provide a satisfactory environment in which to bring up children. While many people feel that some of the advanced technologies now used in fertility treatments challenge the meaning of 'family', the challenge does not really come from technology but rather from social changes that, in parts of the Western world, have resulted in the concept of 'modern families'. The experience, therefore, of an increasing proportion of our population is of a family life that has not included all the traditional components, leading to many single women, same-sex couples and transgender individuals choosing to have families both with and without medical assistance (see Chapter 22). This isn't always available with funding from the NHS, although in Yorkshire Adam successfully campaigned for

NHS funding for lesbian couples to be treated equally when seeking treatments with donated sperm.

As we have stated elsewhere in this book, we are firm believers in providing safe and regulated treatment through properly licensed fertility clinics rather than people 'doing it themselves', for example by home insemination with unscreened sperm. In the UK, the view of the HFEA has been that, providing the medical team considers that the usual criteria in relation to the welfare of the child can be met, there need be no restriction of fertility treatments for unmarried couples, single women and same-sex female and male couples. There is plenty of good evidence now that children born into 'modern families' aren't at any risk for psychological or other problems.[1] And indeed, it is the quality of parenting and a loving environment that are of greatest importance. Furthermore, any child born as a result of fertility treatments, which by their very nature are often complex, time-consuming and costly, is likely to be a much-wanted child and therefore well cared for.

Is IVF ethical?

So far as the major religions are concerned, IVF and embryo transfer are acceptable within the framework of a marital relationship to Judaism, Islam, part of Christianity, Hinduism and Buddhism. The Roman Catholic Church considers that IVF involves a disregard for the sanctity of human life, which is defined as starting at the moment of fertilisation. Moreover, the IVF procedure separates procreation from sexual union – it takes it away from an act of love. Other objections that have been raised to the IVF procedure are that it involves the possibility of harm to the progeny, i.e. it involves exposing others (the embryo) to a risk of harm for which consent has not (could not have) been obtained.

It has been argued that IVF is but one step down a slippery slope that will permit strange forms of treatment that will not prove acceptable. 'Slippery slope' arguments are, of course, the very stuff of philosophy and, in our opinion, do not constitute a very powerful argument against IVF. They do, though, emphasise the importance of thinking through its implications. It has also been argued that since infertility is not life-threatening, we should not permit medicalisation of what is not seen as a medical problem. In our opinion, the view that medical therapy is only to be used for life-threatening conditions is nonsense. Few medical interventions are life-saving, although it is to be hoped that all bring comfort. A general objection often raised is that IVF involves the use of medical resources to provide more offspring to an overpopulated world. In our view, this sets a perceived need of that vague entity, the world, to have fewer people against the immediate and actual right of an individual to have the children they desire.

In accord with the major professional bodies that have offered opinions on the subject, most regions of the world and the majority of religions, IVF is ethically acceptable, until it comes to donations.

Donor ethics

Many of the major religions object to third-party involvement in fertility therapy – that is, the use of donated eggs, sperm and surrogacy.

Donor sperm, donor oocytes and donor embryos have become an integral part of the modern management of infertility. People who need these treatments are not simply those with infertility but now include families with genetic disorders. The interests of the child, the recipients and the donors must all be considered. In some countries, donation of genetic material to single women is forbidden and, where the practice is allowed, regulations cover the relationships between biological and social parents, the banking and disposal of genetic material, the interests of the child and the maintenance of medical records. Furthermore, the issue of donor anonymity varies around the world – in the UK, for example, donation may be anonymous at the time of donation, but any child born as a result of donation has the right to know the identity of the donor when they themselves become an adult (aged 18 years) provided, of course, that they are aware that they have been conceived with the use of donated sperm or eggs.

An important issue concerning third-party involvement in infertility treatment is that of payment to donors or, indeed, to surrogates. In some countries such donations are seen as genuine gifts, a public service performed with no thought of compensation either in the form of a reward or even for expenses. An alternative is payment for expenses but not for the donation itself – as happens in the UK. Another possibility is that the donor receives a reasonable reward as recompense for the time, pain (for example, egg donors) and inconvenience of the donation, processes that clearly vary between men, women and surrogates. Proposals have even been made that a reward be given for gametes, for embryos or, indeed, for infants. While it is unlikely that anyone would have difficulty in rejecting the idea of payment for an infant, payment for an embryo implies no respect for its humanity and payment for eggs and sperm dehumanises them and turns them into a commodity.

Egg sharing

'Egg sharing' is another aspect of fertility treatment that raises ethical questions, where a woman has free or subsidised IVF treatment in return for donating a certain number of her eggs. The procedure, which has been fuelled by a lack of egg donors, has allowed more women who need egg donation to be treated in the UK. Its supporters argue that since the donor is already undergoing treatment, egg sharing avoids the need for healthy volunteers to undergo ovarian stimulation and oocyte retrieval. This means they are not at risk from these procedures. The arrangement usually works well, although careful counselling is needed and the donor needs to consider the possibility that she may not conceive while the recipient could (see page 336). With the rules on anonymity this could create challenges for the future. This all needs to be carefully managed as the donor provides her eggs in return for receiving a service she would otherwise have to pay for, raising straight away concern about the potential exploitation of those who are desperate for treatment they cannot afford. Nonetheless, those clinics that offer 'egg sharing' report good outcomes for all involved.

Sex selection

Many patients would like the opportunity to select the sex of their baby when going through IVF. This is possible during both fertility treatment and pregnancy, but usually only considered ethical when it is done for medical reasons. This is where a disease is linked to the X chromosome and a male child is more likely to be affected, though females can be carriers. There are hundreds of genetic diseases that affect only males in this way.

Prenatal sex selection may be undertaken by sorting sperm (not 100 per cent reliable), by pre-implantation identification of the sex of the embryo (see Chapter 21) or by antenatal screening and aborting a fetus of the sex that carries the disorder. While most people find sex selection for medical reasons acceptable, there are issues to be considered, such as the severity of the condition to be prevented.

Prenatal sex selection for non-medical reasons is a very different matter. The major religions oppose the procedure because it is seen to interfere with a divine plan. Two sets of non-religious arguments may also be considered. The first is: who has the right to decide what sort of people there should be? The second considers the consequences of sex selection: would it, for example, unbalance the sex ratio of the next generation? It would certainly have to be applied on a very wide scale to do so. In Western society, more pressing arguments concern the commodification of life. Treating one sex as more desirable than another, to the point of prenatal sex selection, is to value one sex (the commodity) above life itself. It breaches the fundamental concept of equality for men and women.

Sex selection has been proposed for 'family balancing'; when a couple have, for example, many children (say more than four) of one sex and wish for a child of the opposite sex. This is not permitted in the UK, although we can see the argument for justifying its use.

Fetal reduction

The chances of successfully delivering all the babies from a multiple pregnancy falls dramatically as the number of fetuses increases. Selective reduction of high-order multiple pregnancy (triplets or more) is where an attempt is made to save some of the fetuses by destroying the others. It is usually done at about 12 weeks' gestation. The associated rate of losing the whole pregnancy is about

10–15 per cent. This is controversial in terms of risk–benefit for triplet pregnancies, but it very clearly improves the perinatal outcome for women carrying four or more fetuses.

With fetal reduction, or 'selective abortion', the principle is to sacrifice one or more potentially normal lives so that the others will have a better chance of survival and lead healthy lives. This is obviously fraught with emotional and ethical concerns and is very challenging if you personally find yourself in this situation. In the context of IVF, the number of multiple pregnancies has been greatly reduced by the policy to try to transfer a single embryo (see page 264). However, some embryos may split into identical twins, leading to triplet or quadruplet pregnancies when only two have been transferred. It is with ovulation induction, however, when there is less 'control' over the number of eggs released, that high-order multiple pregnancies unfortunately still occur.

Should older women be offered IVF?

The biggest thing that affects the chance of a successful outcome from fertility treatment is age, so IVF becomes, like all other forms of treatment for infertility, less effective as the woman gets older. The most important reason, therefore, for not offering older women IVF has little to do with ethics and everything to do with the very poor outcome of treatment.

The next debate about infertility treatment for older women concerns the issue of egg (oocyte) donation. Here the impact of ageing on fertility is avoided because that impact is predominantly exerted on the egg. The excellent results of egg donation in general have encouraged clinicians, and indeed patients, to believe that there need be no upper biological age limit to pregnancies achieved in this way. And many pregnancies have now been achieved by egg donation in women past the usual age of the menopause, that is, 50–51 years old. Broadly speaking, the risks to mother and baby seem to be relatively small until the age of 54 when obstetrical problems start to rise. In the UK, most clinics will not treat women over the age of 50 with donated eggs, as is our practice, and in North America the cut-off is usually 54 years, while in some parts of the world there are no limits – with occasional reports of women being treated well into their sixties. The use of donated eggs for postmenopausal women in their fifties and sixties is more controversial and it is a matter of ethical debate as to who should determine an individual couple's right to parenthood. So far as the child is concerned, the point is sometimes made that the life expectancy of its parents will be less than a child should normally expect. This argument should be seen in the context of children born into families of a more usual age, in which one or other of the parents dies. Furthermore, the broader issue of the available support within an 'extended family' needs to be considered.

A complicated issue

Many other ethical issues frequently arise in infertility practice and we have touched upon just a few of the very many ethical judgements that face us in everyday clinical practice. A few more examples include:

- Who owns gametes and embryos and who should decide their fate?

- What are the implications of the advances in pre-implantation testing?

- Are there limits to the extent that we should change nature by genome editing?

- Are there indeed limits to parental choice; what is our attitude, for example, to patients with congenital deafness, or other genetic conditions, who wish to have a child with the same condition?

- Should women be inseminated with their dead husband's sperm?

All of these questions and many more have been discussed in detail, and clinics working within the legislative framework that exists in countries such as the UK will have to abide both by the

350

law (in the UK, the Human Fertilisation and Embryology Act) and ethics committees that exist within hospitals. Multi-disciplinary case conferences are often held to discuss complex cases and reach an agreement that fits within both the ethical and legal framework, and supports the welfare of all of those involved in the proposed treatment.

THE LEGAL SITUATION: HOME AND AWAY

Assisted conception procedures are tightly regulated in the UK, which should provide reassurance for anyone seeking treatment. There are strict laws concerning the use of donated eggs, sperm and embryos (see page 208) and surrogacy (see page 316). Furthermore, there are clear definitions of what is known as 'legal parenthood', and it is vital that you understand these fully if you are embarking upon treatments such as surrogacy or the use of donated sperm as a same-sex couple or as a single woman. It is our strong advice only to access treatments through a licensed clinic where you will not only be able to obtain appropriate counselling but also, if necessary, be directed to someone who can give you the correct legal advice.

Going overseas for treatment

It is essential to take great care if you plan to travel overseas for treatment – as laws and the level of regulation of fertility treatment vary greatly around the world. Furthermore, laws vary concerning travelling out of a country with a child conceived through donation or surrogacy, and there may be further challenges when returning to the UK with a child. There are several law firms now that have developed great expertise in providing specialist advice for these issues. Receiving treatment using donated eggs is usually fairly straightforward, but more complex treatments such as surrogacy may be fraught with legal complexity. If you consider going overseas for treatment, consider carefully all of these issues and ensure that the clinic is operating to high standards and is under appropriate regulation. Some clinics are linked with UK clinics and offer 'shared-care' packages, which makes the process run more smoothly and also provides reassurance with respect to the standards of care. Also, remember that going overseas for treatment isn't always cheaper, even if the actual treatment costs look to be so – you will have the added costs of travel, hotel bills and the uncertainties over success rates (which are rarely regulated in the way they are in the UK) and potential risks and complications. Inherently we feel it is always preferable to have treatment closer to home, not only because it makes clinic visits easier, but also so that you can be properly cared for if there are any complications.

Chapter 27

Where to Go If Treatment Doesn't Work

THE MOST DIFFICULT part of fertility treatment is knowing when to stop. If there is an absolute cause of infertility, for example premature ovarian insufficiency (POI or early menopause), when there is no possibility of becoming pregnant without treatment, stopping treatment is final. If, on the other hand, there are intermediate factors, such as an extremely low sperm count, partial tubal damage or unexplained infertility, it is more difficult to stop treatment.

First, one can never be certain that the next cycle of treatment will not be the one in which a pregnancy occurs; and second, there is always a chance of a natural conception, albeit usually extremely slim by the time you have reached this stage. Of course, we are generally referring to *in vitro* fertilisation (IVF) here as by now most people are likely to have spent many years going through investigations, simple treatments and then assisted conception. Some couples, however, do not wish to pursue high-tech assisted conception therapies and stop treatment at the point that IVF is advised. Others may discontinue treatment because of the psychological stress, even if funding is still available to carry on.

There are several approaches to dealing with how many treatment cycles you should have. It's important to have a realistic appraisal of your problems before you start and an honest view of your overall chance of having a baby after a certain number of cycles. This will depend upon your circumstances, including age, duration of infertility and your diagnosis. With all of this information, you should have an understanding of what the treatment has to offer at the outset and hence realistic expectations. It's important to appreciate that cumulative conception statistics apply to populations or groups of patients rather than individuals and can only be used to provide a rough guide of the efficacy of treatment. It's natural to feel optimistic, and the doctors and nurses in your fertility clinic will wish to be optimistic and positive too. At the same time, it's necessary to have a realistic idea as to what your chances are, so please talk this through with your specialist to ensure that you fully understand how the statistics relate to your personal situation.

Some couples drop out along the way because they find the treatment too difficult, unpleasant, painful, stressful, disruptive or expensive. While couples who drop out would no doubt benefit from counselling and support, they are a different group from those who persevere and require guidance from the clinic about when to stop. We feel that if treatment is not working satisfactorily it is sensible to discuss its goal; in other words, to suggest how many more cycles the couple should undertake with the agreement to stop definitely after the agreed limit. It is our experience that this policy is generally better accepted than simply stopping treatment at the end of a cycle without prior discussion.

Most couples find discontinuing treatment extremely traumatic and the majority will always be deeply affected by their infertility. There are also those who already have a child but are equally traumatised when they find they are unable to provide them with brothers or sisters and complete their family. If you find yourself in this situation, you absolutely deserve sympathy and support, both when trying to conceive and if you eventually have to stop. This is when accessing counselling through your clinic may be very helpful (see page 275).

After stopping treatment some choose to put their dreams of having a family behind them while others pursue other means of achieving one, such as adoption.

Dom and Zara: When to stop treatment

Dom and Zara had been attending our clinic for four years. They'd been together for 25 years, since they were teenagers, but because of career pressures and money worries didn't start trying for a family until they were in their late thirties. They first came to the clinic when Zara was 40 and Dom was 41. They were fully investigated and no problems were identified, apart from hormone levels compatible with Zara's age. They were both fit and healthy. They also embarked upon a programme to enhance their natural health and fertility. After four unsuccessful rounds of IVF (one funded by the NHS and three self-funded) they were feeling despondent. We discussed the possibility of using donated eggs, but this wasn't a route they wished to go down. They had six sessions together with our counsellors and came to the conclusion that they were not going to proceed with further treatment. This was such a hard decision to make – there is always the 'what if' factor with any treatment, and there is rarely an absolute situation when we say that treatment cannot work at all. Zara and Dom did consider adoption, but decided to have a bit of a break before deciding whether to explore this further.

ADOPTION

It has become very difficult to adopt a baby in the UK, largely because there are few babies available. This is for a number of reasons, principally reliable contraception, legal abortion and the greater acceptability of single motherhood than in the past. There is tremendous geographical variation in how easy it is for you to adopt around Britain. The upper age limits vary from 34 to 40 years. Couples are also asked to stop any fertility treatment as soon as they embark upon the adoption process, because it is thought that, if they were to conceive, the adopted child might be made to feel unwelcome.

Adoption is controlled through adoption agencies that are either part of local authority social services departments or independent voluntary agencies, which may be connected with churches. The local social services adoption agencies often hold information evenings that you can attend. Assuming that the local adoption agency's list is open, you are then allocated a social worker. It is the social worker's duty to ensure that you are suitable and can provide an appropriate family life for the adopted child(ren). You need to obtain a medical record from your GP and a police check is undertaken to ensure that neither partner has a criminal record. You will also need references from friends, employers, etc. The process can take between nine months and two years, or more. By then, the social worker will have prepared a report for the adoption panel, which consists of members of the social services, police and lay representatives. The panel tends to be quite authoritarian and have tight criteria, although there are no set standards around the country and there is some geographical variability. If you are approved by the adoption panel, you then go on a waiting list for a child. The birth parent(s) may express their wishes about the placement of their child(ren), for example with respect to religious upbringing, and this has to be considered by the adoption agency. Most agencies also place children into the same racial background as their birth parents, although controversial decisions have been made in the case of mixed-race children or children of different religious backgrounds.

It is very rare these days to be able to adopt a newborn baby and much easier to adopt an older child who might come from a disturbed background, from a children's home or from a foster home. Also, babies who are put up for adoption may have been born to mothers who are considered unsuitable to be parents because of alcohol or drug dependency, which in turn may have had a major effect on the health of the baby during its development in the womb leaving a lifelong legacy of possible problems. Agencies are more flexible with people who wish to adopt children with special needs, not only because they are harder to place but also because older parents, for example, might be better able to cope with more demanding youngsters than their younger counterparts.

If you adopt, you will be given as much information as possible about the child's background, health and former life, primarily so that this information can be passed on as the child grows and learns to understand their origins. It is considered essential to tell children that they are adopted so that they grow up with this knowledge rather than make the discovery when a lot older. Adopted children are permitted to see their birth certificate once they have reached the age of 18 and some then try to trace their original parents.

Once an adoption order has been granted it cannot be reversed and the adopted child becomes a full member of the new family, losing all legal ties with its birth parents. The child has to have lived with the adopters for at least 13 weeks before an adoption order can be made and this period cannot start until the child is at least 6 weeks old. The court appoints a reporting officer who checks that the birth parents understand what is taking place and both the mother and father (if the father is known) have to sign their agreement to the adoption. If the birth parents do not agree to the adoption but have abandoned their child, the court can, in rare circumstances, make an adoption order without their agreement. It is also possible for the birth parents to transfer parenting rights to the adoption agency, by way of a 'freeing order', which in turn is transferred to the adopting parents at the time of the adoption order.

The cost of going through adoption is relatively low, as the agencies are not allowed to charge a fee and no money is allowed to pass from the adopters to the birth parents. The medical, police and court certificates usually require a small fee. The adopting parents are allowed to claim child benefit from the social services department and other state benefits if the child has special needs.

It is interesting to note that while an immense effort is made in the screening of parents before they can adopt, there is no follow-up by the social workers who have made the decisions. This appears to be a major failing, not only because there is no audit of the selection process, but also because couples who have been trying hard to start a family for many years often need support and guidance once they have their first child; consider, for example, the support provided in the UK by the network of midwives and health visitors who regularly visit parents who go through a normal pregnancy. Nonetheless, it appears that adoption tends to work well both for the adopting parents and the children, most of whom experience good family lives.

Adopting a child from overseas

Many countries have a central agency that coordinates inter-country adoption, although none exists in the UK. The Intercountry Adoption Centre (see Resources, page 371) has published a comprehensive procedural guide. An inspection has to be performed by the local social services department, in the same way as the standard adoption process, although the couple is required to pay for this and the costs can range from £2,000 to £20,000. A detailed 'home study' is performed by a social worker, who visits the home of the prospective adopters on more than one occasion and also speaks to the referees. Local authorities differ greatly with respect to the speed with which they organise the home study and the fees that they charge. Other expenses include travel, legal and translation fees, plus the possibility of donations to an orphanage.

The country from which the child is to be adopted often imposes strict criteria and sometimes communicates with the social services department. Once the inspection process is complete and both health and police certificates have been obtained, an application is submitted to the Department of Health, which in turn puts the application to the Foreign and Commonwealth Office for legislation.

The Department of Health then coordinates the paperwork, which has to be sent to the relevant embassy, which will translate the documents and forward them to the appropriate agency within their country. This local agency has then to approve the application and locate a suitable child, at which point the prospective parents can travel to meet the child. The adopters have then to apply for British entry clearance for the child and go through the relevant requirements for adoption in the child's country before being able to bring the child into Britain. Once home, the adopters have to inform the social services department of their 'intention to adopt' under British law and an adoption order is made by a British court. When the adoption order is granted the child becomes a British citizen, provided that at least one of the adopting parents is British. Some countries stipulate, however, that the child should also retain their original nationality until aged 18 years, although such rules are not binding in Britain. As previously mentioned, it is essential to get full legal advice to ensure that everything goes smoothly.

FOSTERING

It is in some ways easier to become a foster parent, although social services still scrutinise foster parents very carefully. A fostering agency shares the responsibility for the child with the foster parents and an allowance is provided to help care for the child. Many foster parents have children of their own, while some have experienced infertility. Fostering is also often open to older parents and also same-sex couples. Fostering is generally for a limited period of time, until the child is able to return to its own family, be placed for adoption or live independently. The temporary aspect of fostering can be especially emotionally traumatic for the couple who have no other children at home. Its effects on the child can be traumatic too. Nonetheless, it's also very worthwhile and much-needed, and some people find it very rewarding.

Appendix 1: Official Guidance for Female Vitamin and Mineral Intake[1]

The table below lists the important nutrients for fertility, pregnancy and breastfeeding, and the daily amounts you can supplement at each stage if you do not have any deficiencies. You can use this table to check against any supplements you are taking if you are starting without professional supervision.

NUTRIENT	PRECONCEPTION	PREGNANCY	BREASTFEEDING
Vitamin A	700µg	750–770µg	1300µg
Vitamin B_1 (thiamine)	1.0mg	1.4mg	1.4mg
Vitamin B_2 (riboflavin)	1.1mg	1.4mg	1.6mg
Vitamin B_3 (niacin)	1.3mg	1.9mg	2.0mg
Vitamin B_6 (pyridoxine)	1.3mg	1.9mg	2.0mg
Vitamin B_9 (folate)	400µg	400–600µg	600µg
Vitamin B_{12} (cobalamin)	2.4µg	2.6µg	2.8µg
Biotin	25–30µg	30µg	35µg
Vitamin C	75mg	85mg	120mg
Choline	425mg	450mg	550mg

Vitamin D	15µg (600iu) in the absence of deficiency, but our patients usually need more to maintain sufficient levels	15µg (600iu) in the absence of deficiency, but our patients usually need more to maintain sufficient levels	15µg (600iu) in the absence of deficiency, though higher levels may be needed. Seek professional supervision to ensure optimal levels for your baby while breastfeeding
Vitamin E	15mg	15mg	19mg
Vitamin K	90µg/day or in proportion to vitamin D as outlined	75µg/day – may need to increase in proportion to vitamin D. Seek professional advice	90µg/day or in proportion to vitamin D as outlined
Calcium	1,000–1300mg	1,000–1300mg	1,000–1300mg
Copper	900µg	1,300µg	1,000µg
Iodine	150µg	220µg	290µg
Iron	18mg	27mg	9mg
Magnesium	320mg	360mg	320mg
Manganese	1.8mg	2.0mg	2.5mg
Selenium	55µg	60µg	70µg
Zinc	8–9mg	11–12mg	12mg

Note: You may need to supplement at a higher amount if you are deficient. Recent research suggests higher amounts of some nutrients including vitamin D and choline may be beneficial during pregnancy. Always seek the advice of your doctor before taking supplements and test where possible.

Appendix 2: Key Nutrients for Reproductive Health

The table below outlines the key nutrients that are commonly low and the signs and impact of deficiency.

NUTRIENT	NEEDED FOR	POTENTIAL IMPACT OF MATERNAL DEFICIENCY/EXCESS ON REPRODUCTIVE HEALTH OUTCOMES	SYMPTOM OF DEFICIENCY
Iodine	Thyroid function, development of the fetal brain	Deficiency: reduced IVF success, lower IQ in the baby, miscarriage, placental abruption, preterm birth, miscarriage and placental problems, reduced psychomotor skills Excess: damages thyroid and toxic at very high doses	Thyroid problems (deficiency or excess)
Iron	Increased blood supply during pregnancy, fetal brain development, building endometrium	Deficiency: preterm births, anaemia, low birth weight, miscarriage, impaired placental development, 40–50% decrease in brain iron 10 days after birth Excess: gestational diabetes, can be a marker of inflammation if serum levels are significantly raised	Fatigue, learning difficulties and depression
Magnesium	Necessary for the functioning of over 300 enzymes, energy metabolism, nerve functioning, production of vitamin D from sunlight, maintaining adequate potassium levels	Deficiency: disrupted oestrogen and progesterone metabolism, preterm birth, may worsen insulin resistance, resistance to vitamin D supplementation Excess: very rare unless exceeding upper limits of supplementation, high dose supplement may cause diarrhoea	Neuromuscular disturbances (tingling, weakness in limbs), headaches, very severe premenstrual pain, headaches

Zinc	Gene expression, cell growth and division, nerve transmission, overall reproductive function including ovulation, sperm production	Deficiency: impaired synthesis and secretion of FSH and LH, disruption of menstrual cycle, impaired cognitive development, impaired growth, compromised fetal and placental growth, and neural tube closure	Reduced sense of taste and smell, low appetite, frequent infections, ADHD, anorexia, depression, immune system dysfunction, frequent infections, poor nail growth and wound healing
Vitamin A	Male and female reproductive function, oocyte quality and formation of the blastocyst, brain and eye function, growth and development, fat and carbohydrate metabolism, immune function, regulation of thyroid function co-factor for vitamin D	Deficiency: infertility, low birth weight, severe deficiency can cause birth defects and infant blindness Excess: through supplements *or* food – both cause birth defects	Poor vision, dry eyes, night blindness, aversion to light

Vitamin D	Regulator of the immune system and genes, receptors for vitamin D are found throughout the reproductive tract in men and women, important for pathways involved in implantation	Deficiency: reduced IVF success rate, delayed natural conception, pre-eclampsia, low birth weight, increased risk of infection including bacterial vaginosis, fetal skeletal defects, nervous system and immune system dysfunction, gestational diabetes, impaired fetal brain development Excess: elevated calcium in the blood, toxicity with very serious excesses (rare) including kidney damage and nausea	Fatigue, frequent infections, weak bones
Omega-3	Fetal brain development, all cell membranes need DHA (a type of omega-3), essential for vision (30–50% of retina should be made up of omega-3 DHA)	Deficiency: potential impaired fetal vision and cognitive development, higher body fat in child	Poor concentration, insomnia, depressive disorders with long-term deficiency and anxiety

Appendix 3: Potential Antioxidants for Male Fertility

CLINICAL CIRCUMSTANCE	ANTIOXIDANT
Basic semen parameters	
Oligozoospermia	Vitamin E, vitamin C, NAC, carnitines, CoQ10, lycopene, selenium and zinc
Asthenozoospermia	Vitamin E, vitamin C, NAC, carnitines, CoQ10, lycopene, selenium and zinc
Teratozoospermia	Vitamin E, NAC, lycopene, selenium and zinc
Advanced sperm function	
High sperm DNA fragmentation	Vitamin E, vitamin C, zinc, selenium and folic acid
Oxidative stress	Vitamin E, vitamin C, NAC, selenium and zinc
Improving success rate of assisted reproductive techniques	Vitamin E, vitamin C, lycopene, CoQ10, folic acid, selenium, zinc
Live birth rate	Vitamin E, vitamin C, carnitines, coQ10, and zinc

Abbreviations:
NAC: n-acetyl cysteine
CoQ10: co-enzyme Q10
LC: L-carnitine
LAC: L-acetyl carnitineβ-carotene (beta carotene)

Appendix 4: Summary of Investigations and Treatment of Infertility

FOR THE INVESTIGATION OF INFERTILITY:
General practitioner
• Semen analysis – twice if first abnormal
• Confirmation of rubella immunity; infection screening for chlamydia and pelvic infection; general health assessment to ensure normal full blood count, and if possible vitamin D, iron and folate levels • Confirmation of normal cervical smear within last three years
• Baseline hormone profile of the woman (FSH, LH and oestradiol days 1–3 of the cycle plus thyroid function (TSH); ± prolactin, testosterone for those with irregular periods)
• Luteal phase progesterone
• Baseline pelvic ultrasound scan
Infertility clinic
• Baseline pelvic ultrasound scan, if not already done
• Hysterosalpingogram or laparoscopy and dye/hysteroscopy
• More detailed endocrinology if indicated
• Further investigation of endocrine disorders
• More detailed sperm function tests

FOR THE TREATMENT OF INFERTILITY:
General practitioner
• General health and sexual advice
• Folic acid and vitamin D supplements
• Cervical smear
• Rubella immunisation
• Referral for preconception counselling if other health concerns, drug therapy, older age group, family history of genetic disease
Infertility clinic
• All ovulation-inducing agents with appropriate monitoring
• Laparoscopic surgery
• Assisted conception
• Male treatments
• Collaborative clinics with endocrinologist, urologist, psychosexual counsellor
• General counselling

Resources

Useful Websites

We know that it is very tempting to read information online, but some can be excellent, and some can be misleading. We recommend that you use the following websites to get reliable sources of information and support.

Balance Fertility
This is our website, which includes lots of useful information, courses on all aspects of reproductive health and access to tests online. Visit to find out more about:

- *testing for nutrients, minerals and hormones, and how minerals can impact hormones*

- *omega fatty acids and antioxidants*

- *recommendations for supplementation*

- *digestive health and fertility, including bacterial overgrowth and non-coeliac gluten sensitivity, and how to use an elimination process if you experience reactions to certain foods*

- *coping with grief and finding meaning from your experience*

- *genetic testing, sex-linked conditions and patterns of inheritance*

balancefertility.co.uk/the-fertility-book-resources/

Daisy Network
Charity for women with premature ovarian insufficiency.
daisynetwork.org

Donor Conception Network
Supporting donor conception families.
dcnetwork.org

Endometriosis UK
Charity for women with endometriosis.
endometriosis-uk.org

Fertility Network UK
The national patient support group, offering advice, guidance and local support networks on all aspects of infertility and its treatment.
fertilitynetworkuk.org

The Miscarriage Association
The national support organisation for those who experience miscarriage.
miscarriageassociation.org.uk

Verity
The UK national support organisation for women with polycystic ovary syndrome.
verity-pcos.org.uk

Surrogacy charities

Brilliant Beginnings
brilliantbeginnings.co.uk

Childlessness Overcome Through Surrogacy (COTS)
surrogacy.org.uk

Surrogacy UK
surrogacyuk.org

Adoption

Adoption UK
adoptionuk.org

Intercountry Adoption Centre
icacentre.org.uk

Professional bodies

Association of Reproductive and Clinical Scientists (ARCS)
A professional body run by Reproductive Scientists
arcscientists.org

British Association for Counselling and Psychotherapy (BACP)
The professional association for members of the counselling professions in the UK.
bacp.co.uk

British Fertility Society (BFS)
The society for healthcare workers and scientists in the field of fertility care, also provides patient information. Several guidelines are available on the website.
britishfertilitysociety.org.uk

British Infertility Counselling Association (BICA)
Professional association of fertility counsellors
bica.net

European Society for Hyman Reproduction and Embryology
Several guidelines are available on the website.
ESHRE.com

Human Fertilisation and Embryology Authority (HFEA)
The UK's regulatory body of fertility clinics, website contains useful information about clinics and treatments.
hfea.gov.uk

Progress Educational Trust (PET)
Advances public understanding of science, law and ethics in the fields of human genetics, assisted reproduction, embryology and stem cell research.
progress.org.uk

The Royal College of Obstetricians and Gynaecologists (RCOG)
Also has patient information pages and The Women's Voices network with videos from the Fertility Forum, a patient information event. Several guidelines are available on the website.
RCOG.org.uk

Further Reading

Below is some recommended reading on the more detailed aspects of the management of infertility.

Balen, A. H. (2021). *Infertility in Practice*. Informa Healthcare, 5th edition.

Balen, A. H., Casper, R., & Homburg, R. (eds.) (2021). *50 Debates in Reproductive Medicine*. Cambridge University Press.

Infertility guidelines
National Institute for Health and Care Excellence (20 Feb. 2013). Fertility problems: Assessment and treatment: Clinical guideline [CG156]. [Last updated 6 Sep. 2017.]

PCOS guidelines
Balen, A. H., Morley, L. C., Misso, M., Franks, S., Legro, R. S., Wijeyaratne, C. N., Stener-Victorin E., Norman R. J., Fauser B. J. C. M., & Teede, H. (2016). The management of anovulatory infertility in women with polycystic ovary syndrome (PCOS): An analysis of the evidence to support the development of global WHO guidance. *Human Reproduction Update*, 22(6), 687–708.

Teede, H. J., Misso, M. L., Costello, M. F., Dokras, A., Laven, J., Moran, L., Piltonen, T., & Norman, R. J. and the Guideline Development Group including Balen, A.H. (2018). Recommendations from the international evidence-based guideline for the assessment and management of polycystic ovary syndrome. *Human Reproduction*, 33(9), 1602–18.

Fertility preservation
Yasmin, E., Balachandren, N., Davies, M. C., Jones, G. L., Lane, S., Mathur, R. Webber, L., & Anderson, R. A. (2018). Fertility preservation for medical reasons in girls and women: British Fertility Society policy and practice guideline. *Human Fertility*, 21(1), 3–26.

Acknowledgements

We would like to express our gratitude to our family, friends and colleagues who have supported us throughout our careers. Thanks also to the editorial team at Vermilion. In particular, Sam Jackson, Leah Feltham and Julia Kellaway have all offered invaluable support, kindness and guidance as we worked on our manuscript. Thanks to David Woodroffe for drawing clear illustrations of complex subjects.

Most of all, we would like to extend our appreciation to our patients from whom we have learnt so much in so many ways; we admire your courage and perseverance. It has truly been a privilege to help you and be a part of your lives.

Endnotes

Chapter 1: How Fertility Works

1. Jayasena, C. N., Radia, U. K., Figueiredo, M., Revill, L. F., Dimakopoulou, A., Osagie, M., Vessey, W., Regan, L., Rai, R., & Dhillo, W. S. (2019). Reduced testicular steroidogenesis and increased semen oxidative stress in male partners as novel markers of recurrent miscarriage. *Clinical Chemistry*, *65*(1), 161–9; McQueen, D. B., Zhang, J., & Robins, J. C. (2019). Sperm DNA fragmentation and recurrent pregnancy loss: A systematic review and meta-analysis. *Fertility and Sterility*, *112*(1), 54–60.

Chapter 2: Planning for a Healthy Pregnancy

1. Mikkelsen, B., Williams, J., Rakovac, I., Wickramasinghe, K., Hennis, A., Shin, H. R., Farmer, M., Weber, M., Berdzuli, N., Borges, C., & Huber, M. (2019). Life course approach to prevention and control of non-communicable diseases. *BMJ*, *364*; Canipari, R., De Santis, L., & Cecconi, S. (2020). Female fertility and environmental pollution. *International Journal of Environmental Research and Public Health*, *17*(23), 8802; Cherry, N., Moore, H., McNamee, R., Pacey, A., Burgess, G., Clyma, J. A., Dippnall, M., Baillie, H., & Povey, A. (2008). Occupation and male infertility: Glycol ethers and other exposures. *Occupational and Environmental Medicine*, *65*(10), 708–14; Hipwell, A. E., Kahn, L. G., Factor-Litvak, P., Porucznik, C. A., Siegel, E. L., Fichorova, R. N., Hamman, R. F., Klein-Fedyshin, M., Harley, K. G., & program collaborators for Environmental influences on Child Health Outcomes (2019). Exposure to non-persistent chemicals in consumer products and fecundability: A systematic review. *Human Reproduction Update*, *25*(1), 51–71.

2. Stephenson, J., Heslehurst, N., Hall, J., Schoenaker, D. A., Hutchinson, J., Cade, J. E., Poston, L., Barrett, G., Crozier, S. R., Barker, M., & Kumaran, K. (2018). Before the beginning: Nutrition and lifestyle in the preconception period and its importance for future health. *The Lancet, 391*(10132), 1830–41; Fleming, T. P., Watkins, A. J., Velazquez, M. A., Mathers, J. C., Prentice, A. M., Stephenson, J., Barker, M., Saffery, R., Yajnik, C. S., Eckert, J. J., & Hanson, M. A. (2018). Origins of lifetime health around the time of conception: Causes and consequences. *The Lancet, 391*(10132), 1842–52; Barker, M., Dombrowski, S. U., Colbourn, T., Fall, C. H., Kriznik, N. M., Lawrence, W. T., Norris, S. A., Ngaiza, G., Patel, D., Skordis-Worrall, J., & Sniehotta, F. F. (2018). Intervention strategies to improve nutrition and health behaviours before conception. *The Lancet, 391*(10132), 1853–64.

3. Rossi, B. V., Berry, K. F., Hornstein, M. D., Cramer, D. W., Ehrlich, S., & Missmer, S. A. (2011). Effect of alcohol consumption on in vitro fertilization. *Obstetrics and Gynecology, 117*(1), 136.

4. Bu, F. L., Feng, X., Yang, X. Y., Ren, J., & Cao, H. J. (2020). Relationship between caffeine intake and infertility: A systematic review of controlled clinical studies. *BMC Women's Health, 20*(1), 1–9; Í Soylu, L., Jensen, A., Juul, K. E., Kesmodel, U. S., Frederiksen, K., Kjaer, S. K., & Hargreave, M. (2018). Coffee, tea and caffeine consumption and risk of primary infertility in women: A Danish cohort study. *Acta Obstetricia Et Gynecologica Scandinavica, 97*(5), 570–6; Ricci, E., Noli, S., Cipriani, S., La Vecchia, I., Chiaffarino, F., Ferrari, S., Mauri, P. A., Reschini, M., Fedele, L., & Parazzini, F. (2018). Maternal and paternal caffeine intake and ART outcomes in couples referring to an Italian fertility clinic: A prospective cohort. *Nutrients, 10*(8), 1116; Qian, J., Zhang, Y., Qu, Y., Zhang, L., Shi, J., Zhang, X., Liu, S., Kim, B. H., Hwang, S. J., Zhou, T., & Chen, Q. (2018). Caffeine consumption during early pregnancy impairs oviductal embryo transport, embryonic development and uterine receptivity in mice. *Biology of Reproduction, 99*(6), 1266–75.

5. Lyngsø, J., Ramlau-Hansen, C. H., Bay, B., Ingerslev, H. J., Hulman, A., & Kesmodel, U. S. (2017). Association between coffee or caffeine consumption and fecundity and fertility: A systematic

review and dose–response meta-analysis. *Clinical Epidemiology,* 9, 699.

6. Chen, L. W., Wu, Y., Neelakantan, N., Chong, M. F. F., Pan, A., & van Dam, R. M. (2016). Maternal caffeine intake during pregnancy and risk of pregnancy loss: a categorical and dose–response meta-analysis of prospective studies. *Public Health Nutrition,* 19(7), 1233–44; James, J. E. (2021). Maternal caffeine consumption and pregnancy outcomes: A narrative review with implications for advice to mothers and mothers-to-be. *BMJ Evidence-Based Medicine,* 26(3), 114–15.

7. Twigt, J. M., Bolhuis, M. E. C., Steegers, E. A. P., Hammiche, F., Van Inzen, W. G., Laven, J. S. E., & Steegers-Theunissen, R. P. M. (2012). The preconception diet is associated with the chance of ongoing pregnancy in women undergoing IVF/ICSI treatment. *Human Reproduction,* 27(8), 2526–31.

8. Stephenson, J., Heslehurst, N., Hall, J., Schoenaker, D. A., Hutchinson, J., Cade, J. E., Poston, L., Barrett, G., Crozier, S. R., Barker, M., & Kumaran, K. (2018). Before the beginning: Nutrition and lifestyle in the preconception period and its importance for future health. *The Lancet,* 391(10132), 1830–41; Fleming, T. P., Watkins, A. J., Velazquez, M. A., Mathers, J. C., Prentice, A. M., Stephenson, J., Barker, M., Saffery, R., Yajnik, C. S., Eckert, J. J., & Hanson, M. A. (2018). Origins of lifetime health around the time of conception: Causes and consequences. *The Lancet,* 391(10132), 1842–52; Barker, M., Dombrowski, S. U., Colbourn, T., Fall, C. H., Kriznik, N. M., Lawrence, W. T., Norris, S. A., Ngaiza, G., Patel, D., Skordis-Worrall, J., & Sniehotta, F. F. (2018). Intervention strategies to improve nutrition and health behaviours before conception. *The Lancet,* 391(10132), 1853–64.

9. Braun, J. M., Messerlian, C., & Hauser, R. (2017). Fathers matter: Why it's time to consider the impact of paternal environmental exposures on children's health. *Current Epidemiology Reports,* 4(1), 46–55.

Chapter 3: Diet and Optimising Fertility

1. Karayiannis, D., Kontogianni, M. D., Mendorou, C., Mastrominas, M., & Yiannakouris, N. (2018). Adherence to the Mediterranean diet and IVF success rate among non-obese women attempting fertility. *Human Reproduction, 33*(3), 494–502.

2. Grieger, J. A., Grzeskowiak, L. E., Bianco-Miotto, T., Jankovic-Karasoulos, T., Moran, L. J., Wilson, R. L., Leemaqz, S. Y., Poston, L., McCowan, L., Kenny, L. C., & Myers, J. (2018). Pre-pregnancy fast food and fruit intake is associated with time to pregnancy. *Human Reproduction, 33*(6), 1063–70.

3. Sun, H., Lin, Y., Lin, D., Zou, C., Zou, X., Fu, L., Meng, F., & Qian, W. (2019). Mediterranean diet improves embryo yield in IVF: A prospective cohort study. *Reproductive Biology and Endocrinology, 17*(1), 1–7; Silvestris, E., Lovero, D., & Palmirotta, R. (2019). Nutrition and female fertility: An interdependent correlation. *Frontiers in Endocrinology, 10,* 346.

4. Gaskins, A. J., & Chavarro, J. E. (2018). Diet and fertility: A review. *American Journal of Obstetrics and Gynecology, 218*(4), 379–89.

5. Heiman, M. L., & Greenway, F. L. (2016). A healthy gastro-intestinal microbiome is dependent on dietary diversity. *Molecular Metabolism, 5*(5), 317–20.

6. McDonald, D., Hyde, E., Debelius, J. W., Morton, J. T., Gonzalez, A., Ackermann, G., Aksenov, A. A., Behsaz, B., Brennan, C., Chen, Y., DeRight Goldasich, L., & Knight R. (2018). American Gut: An open platform for citizen science microbiome research. *mSystems, 3*(3), e00031–18.

7. Amati, F., Hassounah, S., & Swaka, A. (2019). The impact of Mediterranean dietary patterns during pregnancy on maternal and offspring health. *Nutrients, 11*(5), 1098; H. Al Wattar, B., Dodds, J., Placzek, A., Beresford, L., Spyreli, E., Moore, A., Gonzalez Carreras, F. J., Austin, F., Murugesu, N., Roseboom, T. J., & Bes-Rastrollo, M. (2019). Mediterranean-style diet in pregnant women with metabolic risk factors (ESTEEM): A pragmatic multicentre randomised trial. *PLoS Medicine, 16*(7), e1002857.

8. Curtis, P. J., van der Velpen, V., Berends, L., Jennings, A., Feelisch, M., Umpleby, A. M., Evans, M., Fernandez, B. O., Meiss, M. S.,

Minnion, M., & Potter, J. (2019). Blueberries improve biomarkers of cardiometabolic function in participants with metabolic syndrome – results from a 6-month, double-blind, randomized controlled trial. *The American Journal of Clinical Nutrition*, *109*(6), 1535–45.

9. Opara, E. I., & Chohan, M. (2014). Culinary herbs and spices: Their bioactive properties, the contribution of polyphenols and the challenges in deducing their true health benefits. *International Journal of Molecular Sciences*, *15*(10), 19183–202; Ulewicz-Magulska, B., & Wesolowski, M. (2019). Total phenolic contents and antioxidant potential of herbs used for medical and culinary purposes. *Plant Foods for Human Nutrition*, *74*(1), 61–7.

10. Vázquez-Fresno, R., Rosana, A. R. R., Sajed, T., Onookome-Okome, T., Wishart, N. A., & Wishart, D. S. (2019). Herbs and spices-biomarkers of intake based on human intervention studies – a systematic review. *Genes and Nutrition*, *14*(1), 1–27.

11. Delimaris, I. (2013). Adverse effects associated with protein intake above the recommended dietary allowance for adults. *International Scholarly Research Notices*, *2013*.

12. Chavarro, J. E., Rich-Edwards, J. W., Rosner, B. A., & Willett, W. C. (2009). A prospective study of dietary carbohydrate quantity and quality in relation to risk of ovulatory infertility. *European Journal of Clinical Nutrition*, *63*(1), 78–86.

13. Studies presented by the Delaware Institute for Reproductive Medicine (DIRM) at the American Society for Reproductive Medicine, 2013 and the European Society for Human Reproduction and Embryology, 2017; McGrice, M., & Porter, J. (2017). The effect of low carbohydrate diets on fertility hormones and outcomes in overweight and obese women: A systematic review. *Nutrients*, *9*(3), 204; Noli, S. A., Ricci, E., Cipriani, S., Ferrari, S., Castiglioni, M., La Vecchia, I., Somigliana, E., & Parazzini, F. (2020). Dietary carbohydrate intake, dietary glycemic load and outcomes of in vitro fertilization: Findings from an observational Italian cohort study. *Nutrients*, *12*(6), 1568.

14. ScienceDaily (1 Feb. 2016). The benefits of chocolate during pregnancy. Retrieved from www.sciencedaily.com/releases/2016/02/160201214629.htm (accessed 2 Jun. 2021); Saftlas, A. F., Triche, E. W., Beydoun, H., & Bracken, M. B. (2010). Does

chocolate intake during pregnancy reduce the risks of preeclampsia and gestational hypertension?. *Annals of Epidemiology, 20*(8), 584–91; Latif, R. (2019). Maternal and fetal effects of chocolate consumption during pregnancy: A systematic review. *The Journal of Maternal-Fetal & Neonatal Medicine, 32*(17), 2915–27.

15. Grieger, J. A., Grzeskowiak, L. E., Bianco-Miotto, T., Jankovic-Karasoulos, T., Moran, L. J., Wilson, R. L., Leemaqz, S. Y., Poston, L., McCowan, L., Kenny, L. C., & Myers, J. (2018). Pre-pregnancy fast food and fruit intake is associated with time to pregnancy. *Human Reproduction, 33*(6), 1063–70.

16. Ibid.

17. Hatch, E. E., Wesselink, A. K., Hahn, K. A., Michiel, J. J., Mikkelsen, E. M., Sorensen, H. T., Rothman, K. J., & Wise, L. A. (2018). Intake of sugar-sweetened beverages and fecundability in a North American preconception cohort. *Epidemiology (Cambridge, Mass.), 29*(3), 369; Borges, M. C., Louzada, M. L., de Sá, T. H., Laverty, A. A., Parra, D. C., Garzillo, J. M. F., Monteiro, C. A., & Millett, C. (2017). Artificially sweetened beverages and the response to the global obesity crisis. *PLoS Medicine, 14*(1), e1002195; Malik, V. S., & Hu, F. B. (2019). Sugar-sweetened beverages and cardiometabolic health: An update of the evidence. *Nutrients, 11*(8), 1840.

18. Setti, A. S., Braga, D. P. D. A. F., Halpern, G., Rita de Cássia, S. F., Iaconelli Jr, A., & Borges Jr, E. (2018). Is there an association between artificial sweetener consumption and assisted reproduction outcomes?. *Reproductive Biomedicine Online, 36*(2), 145–53.

19. Souter, I., Chiu, Y. H., Batsis, M., Afeiche, M. C., Williams, P. L., Hauser, R., Chavarro, J. E., & EARTH Study Team (2017). The association of protein intake (amount and type) with ovarian antral follicle counts among infertile women: Results from the EARTH prospective study cohort. *BJOG: An International Journal of Obstetrics & Gynaecology, 124*(10), 1547–55.

20. Afeiche, M. C., Chiu, Y. H., Gaskins, A. J., Williams, P. L., Souter, I., Wright, D. L., Hauser, R., & Chavarro, J. E. (2016). Dairy intake in relation to *in vitro* fertilization outcomes among women from a fertility clinic. *Human Reproduction, 31*(3), 563–71.

21. Chavarro, J. E., Rich-Edwards, J. W., Rosner, B., & Willett, W. C. (2007). A prospective study of dairy foods intake and anovulatory infertility. *Human Reproduction*, 22(5), 1340–7.

22. Hyland, C., Bradman, A., Gerona, R., Patton, S., Zakharevich, I., Gunier, R. B., & Klein, K. (2019). Organic diet intervention significantly reduces urinary pesticide levels in US children and adults. *Environmental Research*, 171, 568–75; Nicolopoulou-Stamati, P., Maipas, S., Kotampasi, C., Stamatis, P., & Hens, L. (2016). Chemical pesticides and human health: The urgent need for a new concept in agriculture. *Frontiers in Public Health*, 4, 148; Vigar, V., Myers, S., Oliver, C., Arellano, J., Robinson, S., & Leifert, C. (2020). A systematic review of organic versus conventional food consumption: Is there a measurable benefit on human health? *Nutrients*, 12(1), 7.

23. Chiu, Y. H., Williams, P. L., Gillman, M. W., Gaskins, A. J., Mínguez-Alarcón, L., Souter, I., Toth, T. L., Ford, J. B., Hauser, R., Chavarro, J. E., & EARTH Study Team (2018). Association between pesticide residue intake from consumption of fruits and vegetables and pregnancy outcomes among women undergoing infertility treatment with assisted reproductive technology. *JAMA Internal Medicine*, 178(1), 17–26.

24. Chavarro, J. E., Rich-Edwards, J. W., Rosner, B., & Willett, W. C. (2007). A prospective study of dairy foods intake and anovulatory infertility. *Human Reproduction*, 22(5), 1340–7.

25. Bordoni, A., Danesi, F., Dardevet, D., Dupont, D., Fernandez, A. S., Gille, D., Nunes dos Santos, C., Pinto, P., Re, R., Rémond, D., & Shahar, D. R. (2017). Dairy products and inflammation: A review of the clinical evidence. *Critical Reviews in Food Science and Nutrition*, 57(12), 2497–525.

26. Lordan, R., & Zabetakis, I. (2017). Invited review: The anti-inflammatory properties of dairy lipids. *Journal of Dairy Science*, 100(6), 4197–212.

27. Jianqin, S., Leiming, X., Lu, X., Yelland, G. W., Ni, J., & Clarke, A. J. (2015). Effects of milk containing only A2 beta casein versus milk containing both A1 and A2 beta casein proteins on gastrointestinal physiology, symptoms of discomfort, and cognitive behavior of people with self-reported intolerance to traditional cows' milk. *Nutrition Journal*, 15(1), 1–16.

28. Vanegas, J. C., Afeiche, M. C., Gaskins, A. J., Mínguez-Alarcón, L., Williams, P. L., Wright, D. L., Toth, T. L., Hauser, R., & Chavarro, J. E. (2015). Soy food intake and treatment outcomes of women undergoing assisted reproductive technology. *Fertility and Sterility*, *103*(3), 749–55; Cooper, A. R. (2019). To eat soy or to not eat soy: The ongoing look at phytoestrogens and fertility. *Fertility and Sterility*, *112*(5), 825–6.

29. De Punder, K., & Pruimboom, L. (2013). The dietary intake of wheat and other cereal grains and their role in inflammation. *Nutrients*, *5*(3), 771–87.

30. Niland, B., & Cash, B. D. (2018). Health benefits and adverse effects of a gluten-free diet in non–celiac disease patients. *Gastroenterology & Hepatology*, *14*(2), 82; Lerner, B. A., Green, P. H., & Lebwohl, B. (2019). Going against the grains: Gluten-free diets in patients without celiac disease – worthwhile or not? *Digestive Diseases and Sciences*, *64*(7), 1740–7.

31. Braga, D. P. A. F., Halpern, G., Setti, A. S., Figueira, R. C. S., Iaconelli Jr, A., & Borges Jr, E. (2015). The impact of food intake and social habits on embryo quality and the likelihood of blastocyst formation. *Reproductive Biomedicine Online*, *31*(1), 30–8.

32. Borel, P., & Desmarchelier, C. (2017). Genetic variations associated with vitamin A status and vitamin A bioavailability. *Nutrients*, *9*(3), 246.

33. Leung, W. C., Hessel, S., Meplan, C., Flint, J., Oberhauser, V., Tourniaire, F., Hesketh, J. E., Von Lintig, J., & Lietz, G. (2009). Two common single nucleotide polymorphisms in the gene encoding β-carotene 15, 15'-monoxygenase alter β-carotene metabolism in female volunteers. *The FASEB Journal*, *23*(4), 1041–53; Lietz, G., Oxley, A., Leung, W., & Hesketh, J. (2012). Single nucleotide polymorphisms upstream from the β-carotene 15, 15'-monoxygenase gene influence provitamin A conversion efficiency in female volunteers. *The Journal of Nutrition*, *142*(1), 161S–5S.

Chapter 4: Nutrients and Supplements

1. Public Health England (11 Dec. 2020). NDNS: results from years 9 to 11 (2016 to 2017 and 2018 to 2019). Retrieved from

https://www.gov.uk/government/statistics/ndns-results-from-years-9-to-11-2016-to-2017-and-2018-to-2019 (accessed 2 Jun. 2021).

2. Stephenson, J., Heslehurst, N., Hall, J., Schoenaker, D. A., Hutchinson, J., Cade, J. E., Poston, L., Barrett, G., Crozier, S. R., Barker, M., & Kumaran, K. (2018). Before the beginning: Nutrition and lifestyle in the preconception period and its importance for future health. *The Lancet, 391*(10132), 1830–41; Fleming, T. P., Watkins, A. J., Velazquez, M. A., Mathers, J. C., Prentice, A. M., Stephenson, J., Barker, M., Saffery, R., Yajnik, C. S., Eckert, J. J., & Hanson, M. A. (2018). Origins of lifetime health around the time of conception: Causes and consequences. *The Lancet, 391*(10132), 1842–52; Barker, M., Dombrowski, S. U., Colbourn, T., Fall, C. H., Kriznik, N. M., Lawrence, W. T., Norris, S. A., Ngaiza, G., Patel, D., Skordis-Worrall, J., & Sniehotta, F. F. (2018). Intervention strategies to improve nutrition and health behaviours before conception. *The Lancet, 391*(10132), 1853–64.

3. Li, W., Xu, B., Cao, Y., Shao, Y., Wu, W., Zhou, J., Tan, X., Wu, X., Kong, J., Hu, C., & Xie, K. (2019). Association of maternal folate intake during pregnancy with infant asthma risk. *Scientific Reports, 9*(1), 1–8; Colapinto, C. K., O'Connor, D. L., Sampson, M., Williams, B., & Tremblay, M. S. (2016). Systematic review of adverse health outcomes associated with high serum or red blood cell folate concentrations. *Journal of Public Health, 38*(2), e84–97.

4. Zhao, J., Huang, X., Xu, B., Yan, Y., Zhang, Q., & Li, Y. (2018). Whether vitamin D was associated with clinical outcome after IVF/ICSI: A systematic review and meta-analysis. *Reproductive Biology and Endocrinology, 16*(1), 1–7.

5. Fung, J. L., Hartman, T. J., Schleicher, R. L., & Goldman, M. B. (2017). Association of vitamin D intake and serum levels with fertility: Results from the Lifestyle and Fertility Study. *Fertility and Sterility, 108*(2), 302–11.

6. Aguayo-Ruiz, J. I., García-Cobián, T. A., Pascoe-González, S., Sánchez-Enríquez, S., Llamas-Covarrubias, I. M., García-Iglesias, T., López-Quintero, A., Llamas-Covarrubias, M. A., Trujillo-Quiroz, J., & Rivera-Leon, E. A. (2020). Effect of supplementation

with vitamins D3 and K2 on undercarboxylated osteocalcin and insulin serum levels in patients with type 2 diabetes mellitus: A randomized, double-blind, clinical trial. *Diabetology & Metabolic Syndrome*, *12*(1), 1–10; DiNicolantonio, J. J., Bhutani, J., & O'Keefe, J. H. (2015). The health benefits of vitamin K. *Open Heart*, *2*(1).

7. Ma, H., Zhang, B. L., Liu, B. Y., Shi, S., Zhang, T. C., Shi, H. J., Li, Z., & Shum, W. W. (2019). Vitamin K2-Dependent GGCX and MGP are required for homeostatic calcium regulation of sperm maturation. *Iscience*, *14*, 210–25.

8. F. A. O., & World Health Organization (2–6 May 2005). A model for establishing upper levels of intake for nutrients and related substances [context paper]. Retrieved from https://www.who.int/ipcs/highlights/context_paper.pdf?ua=1 (accessed 2 Jun. 2021).

9. Bastos Maia, S., Rolland Souza, A. S., Costa Caminha, M. D. F., Lins da Silva, S., Callou Cruz, R. D. S. B. L., Carvalho dos Santos, C., & Batista Filho, M. (2019). Vitamin A and pregnancy: A narrative review. *Nutrients*, *11*(3), 681; Hammouda, S. A. I., Abd Al-Halim, O. A. F., & Mohamadin, A. M. (2013). Serum levels of some micronutrients and congenital malformations: A prospective cohort study in healthy Saudi-Arabian first-trimester pregnant women. *International Journal for Vitamin and Nutrition Research*, *83*(6), 346–54.

10. Nasiadek, M., Stragierowicz, J., Klimczak, M., & Kilanowicz, A. (2020). The role of zinc in selected female reproductive system disorders. *Nutrients*, *12*(8), 2464; ScienceDaily (24 Apr. 2018). Preconception zinc deficiency could spell bad news for fertility. Retrieved from https://www.sciencedaily.com/releases/2018/04/180424133639.htm (accessed 2 Jun. 2021); Lo, M. N., Damon, L. J., Tay, J. W., Jia, S., & Palmer, A. E. (2020). Single cell analysis reveals multiple requirements for zinc in the mammalian cell cycle. *Elife*, *9*, e51107; Severo, J. S., Morais, J. B. S., de Freitas, T. E. C., Andrade, A. L. P., Feitosa, M. M., Fontenelle, L. C., de Oliveira, A. R. S., Cruz, K. J. C., & do Nascimento Marreiro, D. (2019). The role of zinc in thyroid hormones metabolism. *International Journal for Vitamin and Nutrition Research*, *89*(1–2), 80–8.

11. Böckerman, P., Bryson, A., Viinikainen, J., Viikari, J., Lehtimäki, T., Vuori, E., Keltikangas-Järvinen, L., Raitakari, O., & Pehkonen, J. (2016). The serum copper/zinc ratio in childhood and educational attainment: A population-based study. *Journal of Public Health, 38*(4), 696–703.

12. Wakeman, M. P. (2019). A review of the effects of oral contraceptives on nutrient status, with especial consideration to folate in UK. *Journal of Advances in Medicine and Medical Research*, 1–17.

13. Showell, M. G., Mackenzie-Proctor, R., Jordan, V., & Hart, R. J. (2020). Antioxidants for female subfertility. *Cochrane Database of Systematic Reviews*, (8).

14. Yang, Y., Xu, P., Zhu, F., Liao, J., Wu, Y., Hu, M., Fu, H., Qiao, J., Lin, L., Huang, B., & Jin, H. (2021). The potent antioxidant MitoQ protects against preeclampsia during late gestation but increases the risk of preeclampsia when administered in early pregnancy. *Antioxidants & RedoxSsignaling, 34*(2), 118–36.

15. Florou, P., Anagnostis, P., Theocharis, P., Chourdakis, M., & Goulis, D. G. (2020). Does coenzyme Q 10 supplementation improve fertility outcomes in women undergoing assisted reproductive technology procedures? A systematic review and meta-analysis of randomized-controlled trials. *Journal of Assisted Reproduction and Genetics, 37*(10), 2377–87; Xu, Y., Nisenblat, V., Lu, C., Li, R., Qiao, J., Zhen, X., & Wang, S. (2018). Pretreatment with coenzyme Q10 improves ovarian response and embryo quality in low-prognosis young women with decreased ovarian reserve: A randomized controlled trial. *Reproductive Biology and Endocrinology, 16*(1), 29.

16. Moon, R. J., Harvey, N. C., Robinson, S. M., Ntani, G., Davies, J. H., Inskip, H. M., Godfrey, K. M., Dennison, E. M., Calder, P. C., Cooper, C., & SWS Study Group (2013). Maternal plasma polyunsaturated fatty acid status in late pregnancy is associated with offspring body composition in childhood. *The Journal of Clinical Endocrinology & Metabolism, 98*(1), 299–307.

Chapter 5: Trying to Conceive Naturally

1. Martinez-Perez, O., Rodriguez, P. P., Hernandez, M. M., Pardilla, M. B. E., Perez, N.P., Hernandez, M. R. V., Yarza, A. V., Velasco, O. N., Fernandez, P. G. D. B., Acebal, L. F., & Lago, C. M. O. (2021). The association between SARS-CoV-2 infection and preterm delivery: A prospective study with a multivariable analysis. *BMC Pregnancy and Childbirth*, *21*(1), 1–11.

2. Subramanian, A., Anand, A., Adderley, N. J., Okoth, K., Toulis, K. A., Gokhale, K., Sainsbury, C., O'Reilly, M. W., Arlt, W., & Nirantharakumar, K. (2021). Increased COVID-19 infections in women with polycystic ovary syndrome: A population-based study. *European Journal of Endocrinology*, *184*(5), 637–45.

3. Alexander, J., Tinkov, A., Strand, T. A., Alehagen, U., Skalny, A., & Aaseth, J. (2020). Early nutritional interventions with zinc, selenium and vitamin D for raising anti-viral resistance against progressive COVID-19. *Nutrients*, *12*(8), 2358.

4. Bousquet, J., Anto, J. M., Czarlewski, W., Haahtela, T., Fonseca, S. C., Iaccarino, G., Blain, H., Vidal, A., Sheikh, A., Akdis, C. A., Zuberbier, T., & Constantinidis, J. (2021). Cabbage and fermented vegetables: From death rate heterogeneity in countries to candidates for mitigation strategies of severe COVID-19. *Allergy*, *76*(3), 735–50.

5. Segal, J. P., Mak, J. W., Mullish, B. H., Alexander, J. L., Ng, S. C., & Marchesi, J. R. (2020). The gut microbiome: An under-recognised contributor to the COVID-19 pandemic? *Therapeutic Advances in Gastroenterology*, *13*, 1756284820974914.

6. Shimabukuro, T. T., Kim, S. Y., Myers, T. R., Moro, P. L., Oduyebo, T., Panagiotakopoulos, L., Marquez, P. L., Olson, C. K., Liu, R., Chang, K. T., & Ellington, S. R. (2021). Preliminary findings of mrna covid-19 vaccine safety in pregnant persons. *New England Journal of Medicine*.

Chapter 6: Fertility, Weight and Metabolism

1. Dhillon, J., Craig, B. A., Leidy, H. J., Amankwaah, A. F., Anguah, K. O. B., Jacobs, A., Jones, B. L., Jones, J. B., Keeler, C. L., Keller, C. E., & McCrory, M. A. (2016). The effects of increased protein

intake on fullness: A meta-analysis and its limitations. *Journal of the Academy of Nutrition and Dietetics, 116*(6), 968–83; Roberts, J., Zinchenko, A., Mahbubani, K. T., Johnstone, J., Smith, L., Merzbach, V., Blacutt, M., Banderas, O., Villasenor, L., Vårvik, F. T., & Henselmans, M. (2019). Satiating effect of high protein diets on resistance-trained individuals in energy deficit. *Nutrients, 11*(1), 56.

2. Hu, F. B., & Malik, V. S. (2010). Sugar-sweetened beverages and risk of obesity and type 2 diabetes: epidemiologic evidence. *Physiology & Behavior, 100*(1), 47–54.

3. Franquesa, M., Pujol-Busquets, G., García-Fernández, E., Rico, L., Shamirian-Pulido, L., Aguilar-Martínez, A., Medina, F. X., Serra-Majem, L., & Bach-Faig, A. (2019). Mediterranean diet and cardiodiabesity: A systematic review through evidence-based answers to key clinical questions. *Nutrients, 11*(3), 655.

4. Gardner, C. D., Kim, S., Bersamin, A., Dopler-Nelson, M., Otten, J., Oelrich, B., & Cherin, R. (2010). Micronutrient quality of weight-loss diets that focus on macronutrients: Results from the A TO Z study. *The American Journal of Clinical Nutrition, 92*(2), 304–12.

5. Study presented at the European Society for Human Reproduction and Embryology, 2017 by Delaware Institute for Reproductive Medicine (DIRM).

6. Müller, M. J., Bosy-Westphal, A., & Heymsfield, S. B. (2010). Is there evidence for a set point that regulates human body weight? *F1000 Medicine Reports, 2.*

7. Drazen, D. L., Vahl, T. P., D'Alessio, D. A., Seeley, R. J., & Woods, S. C. (2006). Effects of a fixed meal pattern on ghrelin secretion: Evidence for a learned response independent of nutrient status. *Endocrinology, 147*(1), 23–30.

8. Friedman, J. M., & Halaas, J. L. (1998). Leptin and the regulation of body weight in mammals. *Nature, 395*(6704), 763–70; Jansson, J. O., Palsdottir, V., Hägg, D. A., Schéle, E., Dickson, S. L., Anesten, F., Bake, T., Montelius, M., Bellman, J., Johansson, M. E., & Cone, R. D. (2018). Body weight homeostat that regulates fat mass independently of leptin in rats and mice. *Proceedings of the National Academy of Sciences, 115*(2), 427–32.

9. Ahrens, K., Mumford, S. L., Schliep, K. C., Kissell, K. A., Perkins, N. J., Wactawski-Wende, J., & Schisterman, E. F. (2014). Serum leptin levels and reproductive function during the menstrual cycle. *American Journal of Obstetrics and Gynecology,* *210*(3), 248-e1; Kumari, P., Jaiswar, S. P., Shankhwar, P., Deo, S., Ahmad, K., Iqbal, B., & Mahdi, A. A. (2017). Leptin as a predictive marker in unexplained infertility in north Indian population. *Journal of Clinical and Diagnostic Research: JCDR,* *11*(3), QC28.

10. Chaput, J. P., McNeil, J., Despres, J. P., Bouchard, C., & Tremblay, A. (2013). Seven to eight hours of sleep a night is associated with a lower prevalence of the metabolic syndrome and reduced overall cardiometabolic risk in adults. *PloS One,* *8*(9), e72832; Wild, C. J., Nichols, E. S., Battista, M. E., Stojanoski, B., & Owen, A. M. (2018). Dissociable effects of self-reported daily sleep duration on high-level cognitive abilities. *Sleep,* *41*(12), zsy182; Mills, J., & Kuohung, W. (2019). Impact of circadian rhythms on female reproduction and infertility treatment success. *Current Opinion in Endocrinology, Diabetes and Obesity,* *26*(6), 317–21.

11. Sharma, S., & Kavuru, M. (2010). Sleep and metabolism: An overview. *International Journal of Endocrinology,* *2010*; Kim, T. W., Jeong, J. H., & Hong, S. C. (2015). The impact of sleep and circadian disturbance on hormones and metabolism. *International Journal of Endocrinology,* *2015*; Stamatakis, K. A., & Punjabi, N. M. (2010). Effects of sleep fragmentation on glucose metabolism in normal subjects. *Chest,* *137*(1), 95–101.

12. Chowdhury, E. A., Richardson, J. D., Holman, G. D., Tsintzas, K., Thompson, D., & Betts, J. A. (2016). The causal role of breakfast in energy balance and health: A randomized controlled trial in obese adults. *The American Journal of Clinical Nutrition,* *103*(3), 747–56.

13. Lopez-Minguez, J., Dashti, H. S., Madrid-Valero, J. J., Madrid, J. A., Saxena, R., Scheer, F. A., Ordoñana, J. R. & Garaulet, M. (2019). Heritability of the timing of food intake. *Clinical Nutrition,* *38*(2), 767–73; Dashti, H. S., Merino, J., Lane, J. M., Song, Y., Smith, C. E., Tanaka, T., McKeown, N. M., Tucker, C., Sun, D., Bartz, T. M., & Li-Gao, R. (2019). Genome-wide association

study of breakfast skipping links clock regulation with food timing. *The American Journal of Clinical Nutrition, 110*(2), 473–84.

14. Miller, B. H., & Takahashi, J. S. (2014). Central circadian control of female reproductive function. *Frontiers in Endocrinology, 4,* 195.

15. Baker, F. C., & Driver, H. S. (2007). Circadian rhythms, sleep, and the menstrual cycle. *Sleep Medicine, 8*(6), 613–22; Shechter, A., & Boivin, D. B. (2010). Sleep, hormones, and circadian rhythms throughout the menstrual cycle in healthy women and women with premenstrual dysphoric disorder. *International Journal of Endocrinology, 2010.*

16. Warren, M. P., & Perlroth, N. E. (2001). Hormones and sport – the effects of intense exercise on the female reproductive system. *Journal of Endocrinology, 170*(1), 3–12; De Souza, M. J., Van Heest, J., Demers, L. M., & Lasley, B. L. (2003). Luteal phase deficiency in recreational runners: Evidence for a hypometabolic state. *The Journal of Clinical Endocrinology & Metabolism, 88*(1), 337–46; Foucaut, A. M., Faure, C., Julia, C., Czernichow, S., Levy, R., Dupont, C., & ALIFERT collaborative group. (2019). Sedentary behavior, physical inactivity and body composition in relation to idiopathic infertility among men and women. *PLoS One, 14*(4), e0210770.

17. Wise, L. A., Rothman, K. J., Mikkelsen, E. M., Sørensen, H. T., Riis, A. H., & Hatch, E. E. (2012). A prospective cohort study of physical activity and time to pregnancy. *Fertility and Sterility, 97*(5), 1136–42; Tobias, D. K., Zhang, C., Van Dam, R. M., Bowers, K., & Hu, F. B. (2011). Physical activity before and during pregnancy and risk of gestational diabetes mellitus: A meta-analysis. *Diabetes Care, 34*(1), 223–9; Hakimi, O., & Cameron, L. C. (2017). Effect of exercise on ovulation: A systematic review. *Sports Medicine, 47*(8), 1555–67.

18. Schumacher, L. M., Thomas, J. G., Raynor, H. A., Rhodes, R. E., & Bond, D. S. (2020). Consistent morning exercise may be beneficial for individuals with obesity. *Exercise and Sport Sciences Reviews, 48*(4), 201–8.

19. Willis, E. A., Creasy, S. A., Honas, J. J., Melanson, E. L., & Donnelly, J. E. (2020). The effects of exercise session timing on weight

loss and components of energy balance: Midwest exercise trial 2. *International Journal of Obesity*, 44(1), 114–24.

20. Romero-Moraleda, B., Del Coso, J., Gutiérrez-Hellín, J., Ruiz-Moreno, C., Grgic, J., & Lara, B. (2019). The influence of the menstrual cycle on muscle strength and power performance. *Journal of Human Kinetics*, *68*, 123.

21. Rosa-Caldwell, M. E., & Greene, N. P. (2019). Muscle metabolism and atrophy: Let's talk about sex. *Biology of Sex Differences*, *10*(1), 1–14.

22. Klump, K. L., Keel, P. K., Culbert, K. M., & Edler, C. (2008). Ovarian hormones and binge eating: Exploring associations in community samples. *Psychological Medicine*, *38*(12), 1749.

Chapter 7: Other Factors that Affect Fertility

1. Manor, O., Dai, C. L., Kornilov, S. A., Smith, B., Price, N. D., Lovejoy, J. C., Gibbons, S. M., & Magis, A. T. (2020). Health and disease markers correlate with gut microbiome composition across thousands of people. *Nature Communications*, *11*(1), 1–12.

2. Grembi, J. A., Nguyen, L. H., Haggerty, T. D., Gardner, C. D., Holmes, S. P., & Parsonnet, J. (2020). Gut microbiota plasticity is correlated with sustained weight loss on a low-carb or low-fat dietary intervention. *Scientific Reports*, *10*(1), 1–14; Aoun, A., Darwish, F., & Hamod, N. (2020). The influence of the gut microbiome on obesity in adults and the role of probiotics, prebiotics, and synbiotics for weight loss. *Preventive Nutrition and Food Science*, *25*(2), 113.

3. Berry, S. E., Valdes, A. M., Drew, D. A., Asnicar, F., Mazidi, M., Wolf, J., Capdevila, J., Hadjigeorgiou, G., Davies, R., Al Khatib, H., & Bonnett, C. (2020). Human postprandial responses to food and potential for precision nutrition. *Nature Medicine*, *26*(6), 964–73.

4. Alcock, J., Maley, C. C., & Aktipis, C. A. (2014). Is eating behavior manipulated by the gastrointestinal microbiota? Evolutionary pressures and potential mechanisms. *Bioessays*, *36*(10), 940–9.

5. López-Moreno, A., & Aguilera, M. (2020). Probiotics dietary supplementation for modulating endocrine and fertility microbiota dysbiosis. *Nutrients*, *12*(3), 757.

6. Barrientos-Durán, A., Fuentes-López, A., de Salazar, A., Plaza-Díaz, J., & García, F. (2020). Reviewing the composition of vaginal microbiota: Inclusion of nutrition and probiotic factors in the maintenance of Eubiosis. *Nutrients*, *12*(2), 419.

7. Robertson, S. A., Care, A. S., & Moldenhauer, L. M. (2018). Regulatory T cells in embryo implantation and the immune response to pregnancy. *The Journal of Clinical Investigation*, *128*(10), 4224–35.

8. Soldati, L., Di Renzo, L., Jirillo, E., Ascierto, P. A., Marincola, F. M., & De Lorenzo, A. (2018). The influence of diet on anti-cancer immune responsiveness. *Journal of Translational Medicine*, *16*(1), 1–18.

9. Mazidi, M., Valdes, A. M., Ordovas, J. M., Hall, W. L., Pujol, J. C., Wolf, J., Hadjigeorgiou, G., Segata, N., Sattar, N., Koivula, R., Spector, T. D., Franks, P. W., & Berry, S. E. (2021). Meal-induced inflammation: Postprandial insights from the Personalised REsponses to DIetary Composition Trial (PREDICT) study in 1000 participants. *The American Journal of Clinical Nutrition*, nqab132.

10. Asnicar, F., Berry, S. E., Valdes, A. M., Nguyen, L. H., Piccinno, G., Drew, D. A., Leeming, E., Gibson, R., Le Roy, C., Al Khatib, H., & Francis, L. (2021). Microbiome connections with host metabolism and habitual diet from 1,098 deeply phenotyped individuals. *Nature Medicine*, *27*(2), 321–32.

11. Marcho, C., Oluwayiose, O. A., & Pilsner, J. R. (2020). The preconception environment and sperm epigenetics. *Andrology*, *8*(4), 924–42.

12. Wu, H., Estill, M. S., Shershebnev, A., Suvorov, A., Krawetz, S. A., Whitcomb, B. W., Dinnie, H., Rahil, T., Sites, C. K., & Pilsner, J. R. (2017). Preconception urinary phthalate concentrations and sperm DNA methylation profiles among men undergoing IVF treatment: A cross-sectional study. *Human Reproduction*, *32*(11), 2159–69.

13. Waterland, R. A., Kellermayer, R., Laritsky, E., Rayco-Solon, P., Harris, R. A., Travisano, M., Zhang, W., Torskaya, M. S., Zhang, J., Shen, L., & Manary, M. J. (2010). Season of conception in rural Gambia affects DNA methylation at putative human metastable epialleles. *PLoS Genetics*, *6*(12), e1001252.

14. Chen, Y., Michalak, M., & Agellon, L. B. (2018). Focus: Nutrition and food science: Importance of nutrients and nutrient metabolism on human health. *The Yale Journal of Biology and Medicine*, 91(2), 95.

Chapter 8: Hormone Balance

1. Mosconi, L., Berti, V., Dyke, J., Schelbaum, E., Jett, S., Loughlin, L., Jang, G., Rahman, A., Hristov, H., Pahlajani, S., & Andrews, R. (2021). Menopause impacts human brain structure, connectivity, energy metabolism, and amyloid-beta deposition. *Scientific Reports*, 11(1), 10867.

2. Abdi, F., Ozgoli, G., & Rahnemaie, F. S. (2019). A systematic review of the role of vitamin D and calcium in premenstrual syndrome. *Obstetrics & Gynecology Science*, 62(2), 73; Draper, C. F., Duisters, K., Weger, B., Chakrabarti, A., Harms, A. C., Brennan, L., Hankemeier, T., Goulet, L., Konz, T., Martin, F. P., & Moco, S. (2018). Menstrual cycle rhythmicity: Metabolic patterns in healthy women. *Scientific Reports*, 8(1), 1–15.

3. Andrews, M. A., Schliep, K. C., Wactawski-Wende, J., Stanford, J. B., Zarek, S. M., Radin, R. G., Sjaarda, L. A., Perkins, N. J., Kalwerisky, R. A., Hammoud, A. O., & Mumford, S. L. (2015). Dietary factors and luteal phase deficiency in healthy eumenorrheic women. *Human Reproduction*, 30(8), 1942–51.

4. Li, J., Huang, D., Sun, X., Li, X., & Cheng, C. H. (2019). Zinc mediates the action of androgen in acting as a downstream effector of luteinizing hormone on oocyte maturation in zebrafish. *Biology of Reproduction*, 100(2), 468–78; Kim, A. M., Vogt, S., O'halloran, T. V., & Woodruff, T. K. (2010). Zinc availability regulates exit from meiosis in maturing mammalian oocytes. *Nature Chemical Biology*, 6(9), 674–81; Chakraborty, P., Ghosh, S., Goswami, S. K., Kabir, S. N., Chakravarty, B., & Jana, K. (2013). Altered trace mineral milieu might play an aetiological role in the pathogenesis of polycystic ovary syndrome. *Biological Trace Element Research*, 152(1), 9–15; Zagrodzki, P., & Ratajczak, R. (2008). Selenium status, sex hormones, and thyroid function in young women. *Journal of Trace Elements in Medicine and Biology*, 22(4), 296–304.

5. Wactawski-Wende, J., Schisterman, E. F., Hovey, K. M., Howards, P. P., Browne, R. W., Hediger, M., Liu, A., & Trevisan, M. (2009). BioCycle study: Design of the longitudinal study of the oxidative stress and hormone variation during the menstrual cycle. *Paediatric and Perinatal Epidemiology, 23*(2), 171–84.

6. Pizzorno, L. (2015). Nothing boring about boron. *Integrative Medicine: A Clinician's Journal, 14*(4), 35.

7. Williams, C. L., Ybarra, A. R., Meredith, A. N., Durrant, B. S., & Tubbs, C. W. (2019). Gut microbiota and phytoestrogen-associated infertility in southern white rhinoceros. *MBio, 10*(2).

8. Qi, X., Yun, C., Pang, Y., & Qiao, J. (2021). The impact of the gut microbiota on the reproductive and metabolic endocrine system. *Gut Microbes, 13*(1), 1–21; Baker, J. M., Al-Nakkash, L., & Herbst-Kralovetz, M. M. (2017). Estrogen–gut microbiome axis: Physiological and clinical implications. *Maturitas, 103*, 45–53.

9. Kwa, M., Plottel, C. S., Blaser, M. J., & Adams, S. (2016). The intestinal microbiome and estrogen receptor–positive female breast cancer. *JNCI: Journal of the National Cancer Institute, 108*(8).

10. Ibid.

11. Baker, J. M., Al-Nakkash, L., & Herbst-Kralovetz, M. M. (2017). Estrogen–gut microbiome axis: Physiological and clinical implications. *Maturitas, 103*, 45–53.

12. Hullar, M. A., Burnett-Hartman, A. N., & Lampe, J. W. (2014). Gut microbes, diet, and cancer. *Advances in Nutrition and Cancer*, 377–99; Kwa, M., Plottel, C. S., Blaser, M. J., & Adams, S. (2016). The intestinal microbiome and estrogen receptor–positive female breast cancer. *JNCI: Journal of the National Cancer Institute, 108*(8).

13. Abbott, R. D., Sadowski, A., & Alt, A. G. (2019). Efficacy of the autoimmune protocol diet as part of a multi-disciplinary, supported lifestyle intervention for Hashimoto's thyroiditis. *Cureus, 11*(4).

14. Wahls, T. L., Chenard, C. A., & Snetselaar, L. G. (2019). Review of two popular eating plans within the multiple sclerosis community: Low saturated fat and modified Paleolithic. *Nutrients, 11*(2), 352.

15. Rayman, M. P. (2019). Multiple nutritional factors and thyroid disease, with particular reference to autoimmune thyroid disease. *Proceedings of the Nutrition Society*, 78(1), 34–44; van Zuuren, E. J., Albusta, A. Y., Fedorowicz, Z., Carter, B., & Pijl, H. (2013). Selenium supplementation for Hashimoto's thyroiditis. *Cochrane Database of Systematic Reviews*, (6).

16. Lee, J. H., Kwon, S. Y., Chang, J., & Yuk, J. S. (2019). Machine learning approach to find the relation between endometriosis, benign breast disease, cystitis and non-toxic goiter. *Scientific Reports*, 9(1), 1–7; Ghent, W. R., Eskin, B. A., Low, D. A., & Hill, L. P. (1993). Iodine replacement in fibrocystic disease of the breast. *Canadian Journal of Surgery*, 36(5), 453–60; Murshid, K. R. (2011). A review of mastalgia in patients with fibrocystic breast changes and the non-surgical treatment options. *Journal of Taibah University Medical Sciences*, 6(1), 1–18.

Chapter 9: Stress, the Mind and Fertility

1. Boivin, J., Griffiths, E., & Venetis, C. A. (2011). Emotional distress in infertile women and failure of assisted reproductive technologies: Meta-analysis of prospective psychosocial studies. *BMJ*, 342.

2. Matthiesen, S. M. S., Frederiksen, Y., Ingerslev, H. J., & Zachariae, R. (2011). Stress, distress and outcome of assisted reproductive technology (ART): A meta-analysis. *Human Reproduction*, 26(10), 2763–76.

3. Massey, A. J., Campbell, B. K., Raine-Fenning, N., Pincott-Allen, C., Perry, J., & Vedhara, K. (2016). Relationship between hair and salivary cortisol and pregnancy in women undergoing IVF. *Psychoneuroendocrinology*, 74, 397–405.

4. Lynch, C. D., Sundaram, R., Maisog, J. M., Sweeney, A. M., & Buck Louis, G. M. (2014). Preconception stress increases the risk of infertility: Results from a couple-based prospective cohort study – the LIFE study. *Human Reproduction*, 29(5), 1067–75; Miller, N., Herzberger, E. H., Pasternak, Y., Klement, A. H., Shavit, T., Yaniv, R. T., Ghetler, Y., Neumark, E., Eisenberg, M. M., Berkovitz, A., & Shulman, A. (2019). Does stress affect IVF outcomes? A prospective study of physiological and psychological stress in

women undergoing IVF. *Reproductive Biomedicine Online*, 39(1), 93–101.

5. Breit, S., Kupferberg, A., Rogler, G., & Hasler, G. (2018). Vagus nerve as modulator of the brain–gut axis in psychiatric and inflammatory disorders. *Frontiers in Psychiatry*, 9, 44; Pascoe, M. C., & Bauer, I. E. (2015). A systematic review of randomised control trials on the effects of yoga on stress measures and mood. *Journal of Psychiatric Research*, 68, 270–82.

6. González-Moret, R., Cebolla, A., Cortés, X., Baños, R. M., Navarrete, J., de la Rubia, J. E., Lisón, J. F., & Soria, J. M. (2020). The effect of a mindfulness-based therapy on different biomarkers among patients with inflammatory bowel disease: A randomised controlled trial. *Scientific Reports*, 10(1), 1–7; Black, D. S., & Slavich, G. M. (2016). Mindfulness meditation and the immune system: A systematic review of randomized controlled trials. *Annals of the New York Academy of Sciences*, 1373(1), 13; Morgan, N., Irwin, M. R., Chung, M., & Wang, C. (2014). The effects of mind-body therapies on the immune system: Meta-analysis. *PloS One*, 9(7), e100903.

7. Bouya, S., Keikhaie, L. R., Hosseini, S., & Keikhaie, K. R. (2021). The effect of yoga on uterine artery Doppler indices, maternal and fetal complications in pregnant women: A quasi-experimental study. *Journal of Ayurveda and Integrative Medicine*, 12(1), 70–4; Dumbala, S., Bhargav, H., Satyanarayana, V., Arasappa, R., Varambally, S., Desai, G., & Bangalore, G. N. (2020). Effect of yoga on psychological distress among women receiving treatment for infertility. *International Journal of Yoga*, 13(2), 115.

8. Darbandi, S., Darbandi, M., Khorshid, H. R. K., & Sadeghi, M. R. (2018). Yoga can improve assisted reproduction technology outcomes in couples with infertility. *Reproductive Health*, 1, 2.

9. Verweij, L., Jørstad, H. T., Minneboo, M., Ter Riet, G., Peters, R. J., op Reimer, W. J. S., Snaterse, M., & RESPONSE-2 Study Group (2021). The influence of partners on successful lifestyle modification in patients with coronary artery disease. *International Journal of Cardiology*, 332, 195–201.

Chapter 10: Male Fertility

1. Fitzpatrick, J. L., Willis, C., Devigili, A., Young, A., Carroll, M., Hunter, H. R., & Brison, D. R. (2020). Chemical signals from eggs facilitate cryptic female choice in humans. *Proceedings of the Royal Society B, 287*(1928), 20200805.
2. Kumar, N., & Singh, A. K. (2015). Trends of male factor infertility, an important cause of infertility: A review of literature. *Journal of Human Reproductive Sciences, 8*(4), 191.
3. Fleming, T. P., Watkins, A. J., Velazquez, M. A., Mathers, J. C., Prentice, A. M., Stephenson, J., Barker, M., Saffery, R., Yajnik, C. S., Eckert, J. J., & Hanson, M. A. (2018). Origins of lifetime health around the time of conception: Causes and consequences. *Obstetrical & Gynecological Survey, 73*(10), 555–7; Colaco, S., & Sakkas, D. (2018). Paternal factors contributing to embryo quality. *Journal of Assisted Reproduction and Genetics, 35*(11), 1953–68.
4. Nargund, V. H. (2015). Effects of psychological stress on male fertility. *Nature Reviews Urology, 12*(7), 373–82.
5. Maleki, B. H., Tartibian, B., & Chehrazi, M. (2017). The effects of three different exercise modalities on markers of male reproduction in healthy subjects: a randomized controlled trial. *Reproduction, 153*(2), 157–74.
6. Salas-Huetos, A., Moraleda, R., Giardina, S., Anton, E., Blanco, J., Salas-Salvadó, J., & Bulló, M. (2018). Effect of nut consumption on semen quality and functionality in healthy men consuming a Western-style diet: A randomized controlled trial. *The American Journal of Clinical Nutrition, 108*(5), 953–62.
7. Jayasena, C. N., Radia, U. K., Figueiredo, M., Revill, L. F., Dimakopoulou, A., Osagie, M., Vessey, W., Regan, L., Rai, R., & Dhillo, W. S. (2019). Reduced testicular steroidogenesis and increased semen oxidative stress in male partners as novel markers of recurrent miscarriage. *Clinical Chemistry, 65*(1), 161–9.
8. Garolla, A., Petre, G. C., Francini-Pesenti, F., De Toni, L., Vitagliano, A., Di Nisio, A., & Foresta, C. (2020). Dietary supplements for male infertility: A critical evaluation of their composition. *Nutrients, 12*(5), 1472.

9. Williams, E. A., Parker, M., Robinson, A., Pitt, S., & Pacey, A. A. (2020). A randomized placebo-controlled trial to investigate the effect of lactolycopene on semen quality in healthy males. *European Journal of Nutrition*, *59*(2), 825–33; Ahmadi, S., Bashiri, R., Ghadiri-Anari, A., & Nadjarzadeh, A. (2016). Antioxidant supplements and semen parameters: An evidence based review. *International Journal of Reproductive BioMedicine*, *14*(12), 729; Majzoub, A., & Agarwal, A. (2018). Systematic review of antioxidant types and doses in male infertility: Benefits on semen parameters, advanced sperm function, assisted reproduction and live-birth rate. *Arab Journal of Urology*, *16*(1), 113–24.

10. Majzoub, A., & Agarwal, A. (2018). Systematic review of antioxidant types and doses in male infertility: Benefits on semen parameters, advanced sperm function, assisted reproduction and live-birth rate. *Arab Journal of Urology*, *16*(1), 113–24.

11. Durairajanayagam, D. (2018). Lifestyle causes of male infertility. *Arab Journal of Urology*, *16*(1), 10–20; Ricci, E., Viganò, P., Cipriani, S., Somigliana, E., Chiaffarino, F., Bulfoni, A., & Parazzini, F. (2017). Coffee and caffeine intake and male infertility: A systematic review. *Nutrition Journal*, *16*(1), 1–14.

12. Ricci, E., Viganò, P., Cipriani, S., Somigliana, E., Chiaffarino, F., Bulfoni, A., & Parazzini, F. (2017). Coffee and caffeine intake and male infertility: A systematic review. *Nutrition Journal*, *16*(1), 1–14; Wesselink, A. K., Wise, L. A., Rothman, K. J., Hahn, K. A., Mikkelsen, E. M., Mahalingaiah, S., & Hatch, E. E. (2016). Caffeine and caffeinated beverage consumption and fecundability in a preconception cohort. *Reproductive Toxicology*, *62*, 39–45.

13. Schmid, T. E., Eskenazi, B., Baumgartner, A., Marchetti, F., Young, S., Weldon, R., Anderson, D., & Wyrobek, A. J. (2007). The effects of male age on sperm DNA damage in healthy non-smokers. *Human Reproduction*, *22*(1), 180–7.

14. Katib, A. (2015). Mechanisms linking obesity to male infertility. *Central European Journal of Urology*, *68*(1), 79.

15. Baud, D., Pattaroni, C., Vulliemoz, N., Castella, V., Marsland, B. J., & Stojanov, M. (2019). Sperm microbiota and its impact on semen parameters. *Frontiers in Microbiology*, *10*, 234; Altmäe, S., Franasiak, J. M., & Mändar, R. (2019). The seminal

microbiome in health and disease. *Nature Reviews Urology*, *16*(12), 703–21.

16. Liu, M. M., Liu, L., Chen, L., Yin, X. J., Liu, H., Zhang, Y. H., Li, P. L., Wang, S., Li, X. X., & Yu, C. H. (2017). Sleep deprivation and late bedtime impair sperm health through increasing antisperm antibody production: A prospective study of 981 healthy men. *Medical Science Monitor: International Medical Journal of Experimental and Clinical Research*, *23*, 1842.

17. Jensen, T. K., Andersson, A. M., Skakkebæk, N. E., Joensen, U. N., Jensen, M. B., Lassen, T. H., Nordkap, L., Olesen, I. A., Hansen, Å. M., Rod, N. H., & Jørgensen, N. (2013). Association of sleep disturbances with reduced semen quality: A cross-sectional study among 953 healthy young Danish men. *American Journal of Epidemiology*, *177*(10), 1027–37.

18. Jensen, T. K., Gottschau, M., Madsen, J. O. B., Andersson, A. M., Lassen, T. H., Skakkebæk, N. E., Swan, S. H., Priskorn, L., Juul, A., & Jørgensen, N. (2014). Habitual alcohol consumption associated with reduced semen quality and changes in reproductive hormones; A cross-sectional study among 1221 young Danish men. *BMJ Open*, *4*(9).

19. Rossi, B. V., Berry, K. F., Hornstein, M. D., Cramer, D. W., Ehrlich, S., & Missmer, S. A. (2011). Effect of alcohol consumption on in vitro fertilization. *Obstetrics and Gynecology*, *117*(1), 136.

20. Presented to the European Society of Human Reproduction and Embryology, 2020.

21. Ji, B. T., Shu, X. O., Zheng, W., Ying, D. M., Linet, M. S., Wacholder, S., Gao, Y. T., & Jin, F. (1997). Paternal cigarette smoking and the risk of childhood cancer among offspring of nonsmoking mothers. *Journal of the National Cancer Institute*, *89*(3), 238–43; Liu, R., Zhang, L., McHale, C. M., & Hammond, S. K. (2011). Paternal smoking and risk of childhood acute lymphoblastic leukemia: Systematic review and meta-analysis. *Journal of Oncology*, *2011*; Gesualdo, F., Carloni, E., D'Ambrosio, A., Russo, L., Campagna, I., Pandolfi, E., & Tozzi, A. E. (2016). Investigating paternal preconception risk factors for adverse pregnancy outcomes in a population of internet users. *Reproductive Health*, *13*(1), 1–7.

22. Szumilas, K., Szumilas, P., Grzywacz, A., & Wilk, A. (2020). The effects of e-cigarette vapor components on the morphology and function of the male and female reproductive systems: A systematic review. *International Journal of Environmental Research and Public Health*, *17*(17), 6152.

23. Gundersen, T. D., Jørgensen, N., Andersson, A. M., Bang, A. K., Nordkap, L., Skakkebæk, N. E., Priskorn, L., Juul, A., & Jensen, T. K. (2015). Association between use of marijuana and male reproductive hormones and semen quality: A study among 1,215 healthy young men. *American Journal of Epidemiology*, *182*(6), 473–81.

24. Sharma, A., Mollier, J., Brocklesby, R. W., Caves, C., Jayasena, C. N., & Minhas, S. (2020). Endocrine-disrupting chemicals and male reproductive health. *Reproductive Medicine and Biology*, *19*(3), 243–53.

25. Cariati, F., D'Uonno, N., Borrillo, F., Iervolino, S., Galdiero, G., & Tomaiuolo, R. (2019). Bisphenol a: An emerging threat to male fertility. *Reproductive Biology and Endocrinology*, *17*(1), 1–8.

26. Research presented to European Society for Human Reproduction and Embryology, 2016; Marcho, C., Oluwayiose, O. A., & Pilsner, J. R. (2020). The preconception environment and sperm epigenetics. *Andrology*, *8*(4), 924–42.

27. Jurewicz, J., Dziewirska, E., Radwan, M., & Hanke, W. (2018). Air pollution from natural and anthropic sources and male fertility. *Reproductive Biology and Endocrinology*, *16*(1), 1–18.

Chapter 11: How and When to Seek Help

1. Habbema, J. D. F., Eijkemans, M. J., Leridon, H., & te Velde, E. R. (2015). Realizing a desired family size: When should couples start?. *Human Reproduction*, *30*(9), 2215–21.

Chapter 12: Investigating Female Fertility

1. Nia, S. S., Safi, F., Shoukrpour, M., & Kamali, A. (2019). An investigation into the effect of evening primrose in dilatation of

cervix and pain during and after hysterosalpingography. *Journal of Medicine and Life*, *12*(3), 284–9.

2. Isaksson, R., & Tiitinen, A. (1998). Obstetric outcome in patients with unexplained infertility: Comparison of treatment-related and spontaneous pregnancies. *Acta Obstetricia et Gynecologica Scandinavica*, *77*(8), 849–53.

3. Hull, M. G., Glazener, C. M., Kelly, N. J., Conway, D. I., Foster, P. A., Hinton, R. A., Coulson, C., Lambert, P. A., Watt, E. M., & Desai, K. M. (1985). Population study of causes, treatment, and outcome of infertility. *British Medical Journal*, *291*(6510), 1693–97.

Chapter 13: Investigating Male Fertility

1. Kohn, T. P., Ohlander, S. J., Jacob, J. S., Griffin, T. M., Lipshultz, L. I., & Pastuszak, A. W. (2018). The effect of subclinical varicocele on pregnancy rates and semen parameters: A systematic review and meta-analysis. *Current Urology Reports*, *19*(7), 53.

2. Hanson, B. M., Aston, K. I., Jenkins, T. G., Carrell, D. T., & Hotaling, J. M. (2018). The impact of ejaculatory abstinence on semen analysis parameters: A systematic review. *Journal of Assisted Reproduction and Genetics*, *35*(2), 213–20.

3. Hotaling, J. M., Smith, J. F., Rosen, M., Muller, C. H., & Walsh, T. J. (2011). The relationship between isolated teratozoospermia and clinical pregnancy after in vitro fertilization with or without intracytoplasmic sperm injection: A systematic review and meta-analysis. *Fertility and Sterility*, *95*(3), 1141–5.

4. Irani, M., Amirian, M., Sadeghi, R., Le Lez, J., & Roudsari, R. L. (2017). The effect of folate and folate plus zinc supplementation on endocrine parameters and sperm characteristics in sub-fertile men: A systematic review and meta-analysis. *Urology Journal*, *14*(5), 4069–78; Salas-Huetos, A., Bulló, M., & Salas-Salvadó, J. (2017). Dietary patterns, foods and nutrients in male fertility parameters and fecundability: A systematic review of observational studies. *Human Reproduction Update*, *23*(4), 371–89.

5. Salas-Huetos, A., Moraleda, R., Giardina, S., Anton, E., Blanco, J., Salas-Salvadó, J., & Bulló, M. (2018). Effect of nut consumption on semen quality and functionality in healthy men consuming

a Western-style diet: A randomized controlled trial. *The American Journal of Clinical Nutrition, 108*(5), 953–62.

6. Moolenaar, L. M., Cissen, M., De Bruin, J. P., Hompes, P. G., Repping, S., Van Der Veen, F., & Mol, B. W. J. (2015). Cost-effectiveness of assisted conception for male subfertility. *Reproductive Biomedicine Online, 30*(6), 659–66.

Chapter 15: Polycystic Ovary Syndrome (PCOS)

1. Shojaeian, Z., Sadeghi, R., & Roudsari, R. L. (2019). Calcium and vitamin D supplementation effects on metabolic factors, menstrual cycles and follicular responses in women with polycystic ocvary syndrome: A systematic review and meta-analysis. *Caspian Journal of Internal Medicine, 10*(4), 359–69.

2. Hager, M., Nouri, K., Imhof, M., Egarter, C., & Ott, J. (2019). The impact of a standardized micronutrient supplementation on PCOS-typical parameters: A randomized controlled trial. *Archives of Gynecology and Obstetrics, 300*(2), 455–60; Chen, J., Guo, Q., Pei, Y. H., Ren, Q. L., Chi, L., Hu, R. K., & Tan, Y. (2020). Effect of a short-term vitamin E supplementation on oxidative stress in infertile PCOS women under ovulation induction: A retrospective cohort study. *BMC Women's Health, 20*(1), 69; Jamilian, M., Shojaei, A., Samimi, M., Ebrahimi, F. A., Aghadavod, E., Karamali, M., Taghizadeh, M., Jamilian, H., Alaeinasab, S., Jafarnejad, S., & Asemi, Z. (2018). The effects of omega-3 and vitamin E co-supplementation on parameters of mental health and gene expression related to insulin and inflammation in subjects with polycystic ovary syndrome. *Journal of Affective Disorders, 229*, 41–7.

3. Azzouni, F., Godoy, A., Li, Y., & Mohler, J. (2011). The 5 alpha-reductase isozyme family: A review of basic biology and their role in human diseases. *Advances in Urology, 2012*; Aliyev, U., Pehlivantürk-Kızılkan, M., Düzçeker, Y., Kanbur, N., Aycan, Z., Akgül, S., & Derman, O. (2020). Is there any association between hirsutism and serum zinc levels in adolescents? *Biological Trace Element Research, 198*(2), 403–9.

4. Glintborg, D., Hermann, A. P., Hagen, C., Jensen, L. T., Frystyk, J., Bennett, P., Flyvbjerg, A., & Andersen, M. (2009). A randomized

placebo-controlled study on the effects of pioglitazone on cortisol metabolism in polycystic ovary syndrome. *Fertility and Sterility*, *91*(3), 842–50.

5. Unfer, V., Facchinetti, F., Orrù, B., Giordani, B., & Nestler, J. (2017). Myo-inositol effects in women with PCOS: A meta-analysis of randomized controlled trials. *Endocrine Connections*, *6*(8), 647–58.

6. Kamenov, Z., & Gateva, A. (2020). Inositols in PCOS. *Molecules*, *25*(23), 5566.

7. Wojciechowska, A., Osowski, A., Jóźwik, M., Górecki, R., Rynkiewicz, A., & Wojtkiewicz, J. (2019). Inositols' importance in the improvement of the endocrine–metabolic profile in PCOS. *International Journal of Molecular Sciences*, *20*(22), 5787.

8. Agrawal, A., Mahey, R., Kachhawa, G., Khadgawat, R., Vanamail, P., & Kriplani, A. (2019). Comparison of metformin plus myoinositol vs metformin alone in PCOS women undergoing ovulation induction cycles: Randomized controlled trial. *Gynecological Endocrinology*, *35*(6), 511–14.

9. Mendoza, N., Diaz-Ropero, M. P., Aragon, M., Maldonado, V., Llaneza, P., Lorente, J., Mendoza-Tesarik, R., Maldonado-Lobon, J., Olivares, M., & Fonolla, J. (2019). Comparison of the effect of two combinations of myo-inositol and D-chiro-inositol in women with polycystic ovary syndrome undergoing ICSI: A randomized controlled trial. *Gynecological Endocrinology*, *35*(8), 695–700.

10. Roseff, S., & Montenegro, M. (2020). Inositol treatment for PCOS should be science-based and not arbitrary. *International Journal of Endocrinology*, *2020*.

11. Tahir, F., & Majid, Z. (2019). Inositol supplementation in the prevention of gestational diabetes mellitus. *Cureus*, *11*(9), e5671.

12. Sharpe, A., Morley, L. C., Tang, T., Norman, R. J., & Balen, A. H. (2019). Metformin for ovulation induction (excluding gonadotrophins) in women with polycystic ovary syndrome. *Cochrane Database of Systematic Reviews*, (12).

Chapter 16: Pelvic Problems: Fallopian Tubes, Fibroids, Polyps and More

1. *See* Balen, A. H. (2021). *Infertility in Practice*. Informa Health-care, 5th edition.

Chapter 17: Endometriosis

1. Nirgianakis, K., Egger, K., Kalaitzopoulos, D. R., Lanz, S., Bally, L., & Mueller, M. D. (2021). Effectiveness of dietary interventions in the treatment of endometriosis: A systematic review. *Reproductive Sciences*, 1–17.
2. de Ziegler, D., Pirtea, P., Carbonnel, M., Poulain, M., Cicinelli, E., Bulletti, C., Kostaras, K., Kontopoulos, G., Keefe, D., & Ayoubi, J. M. (2019). Assisted reproduction in endometriosis. *Best Practice & Research Clinical Endocrinology & Metabolism*, 33(1), 47–59.

Chapter 18: IVF and Associated Treatments

1. Coomarasamy, A., Afnan, M., Cheema, D., van der Veen, F., Bossuyt, P. M., & van Wely, M. (2008). Urinary hMG versus recombinant FSH for controlled ovarian hyperstimulation following an agonist long down-regulation protocol in IVF or ICSI treatment: A systematic review and meta-analysis. *Human Reproduction*, 23(2), 310–5.
2. Thomsen, L. H., Kesmodel, U. S., Erb, K., Bungum, L., Pedersen, D., Hauge, B., Elbæk, H. O., Povlsen, B. B., Andersen, C. Y., & Humaidan, P. (2018). The impact of luteal serum progesterone levels on live birth rates – a prospective study of 602 IVF/ICSI cycles. *Human Reproduction*, 33(8), 1506–16.
3. Mascarenhas, M., Fox, S. J., Thompson, K., & Balen, A. H. (2019). Cumulative live birth rates and perinatal outcomes with the use of time-lapse imaging incubators for embryo culture: A retrospective cohort study of 1882 ART cycles. *BJOG: An International Journal of Obstetrics & Gynaecology*, 126(2), 280–6.
4. Harbottle, S., Hughes, C., Cutting, R., Roberts, S., Brison, D., & Association of Clinical Embryologists & The (ACE) British

Fertility Society (BFS). (2015). Elective single embryo transfer: An update to UK best practice guidelines. *Human Fertility*, *18*(3), 165–83.

5. Hart, R. J. (2019). Use of growth hormone in the IVF treatment of women with poor ovarian reserve. *Frontiers in Endocrinology*, *10*, 500.

6. Cissen, M., Wely, M. V., Scholten, I., Mansell, S., Bruin, J. P. D., Mol, B. W., Braat, D., Repping, S., & Hamer, G. (2016). Measuring sperm DNA fragmentation and clinical outcomes of medically assisted reproduction: A systematic review and meta-analysis. *PloS One*, *11*(11), e0165125.

Chapter 19: Miscarriage, Ectopic and Other Pregnancies

1. American College of Obstetricians and Gynecologists (2014). Cerclage for the management of cervical insufficiency. ACOG Practice Bulletin no. 142. *Obstetrics & Gynecology*, *123*(2 Pt 1), 372–9.

Chapter 20: Recurrent Miscarriage

1. Morley, L. C., Simpson, N., & Tang, T. (2013). Human chorionic gonadotrophin (hCG) for preventing miscarriage. *Cochrane Database of Systematic Reviews*, (1).

2. Coomarasamy, A., Devall, A. J., Brosens, J. J., Quenby, S., Stephenson, M. D., Sierra, S., Christiansen, O. B., Small, R., Brewin, J., Roberts, T. E., Dhillon-Smith, R., Harb, H., Noordali, H., Papadopoulou, A., Eapen, A., Prior, M., Di Renzo, G. C., Hinshaw, K., Mol, B. W., Lumsden, M. A., Khalaf, Y., Shennan, A., Goddijn, M., van Wely, M., Al-Memar, M., Bennett, P., Bourne, T., Rai, R., Regan, L., & Gallos, I. D. (2020). Micronized vaginal progesterone to prevent miscarriage: A critical evaluation of randomized evidence. *American Journal of Obstetrics and Gynecology*, *223*(2), 167–76.

Chapter 23: Fertility Preservation

1. Zhang, J., Chen, Q., Du, D., Wu, T., Wen, J., Wu, M., Zhang, Y., Yan, W., Zhou, S., Li, Y., Jin, Y., Luo, A., & Wang, S. (2019). Can ovarian aging be delayed by pharmacological strategies? *Aging (Albany NY)*, *11*(2), 817–32.

Chapter 24: Premature Ovarian Insufficiency

1. Eshre Guideline Group on POI, Webber, L., Davies, M., Anderson, R., Bartlett, J., Braat, D., Cartwright, B., Cifkova, R., de Muinck Keizer-Schrama, S., Hogervorst, E., & Janse, F. (2016). ESHRE Guideline: Management of women with premature ovarian insufficiency. *Human Reproduction*, *31*(5), 926–37.

Chapter 25: Alternative Therapies

1. Yun, L., Liqun, W., Shuqi, Y., Chunxiao, W., Liming, L., & Wei, Y. (2019). Acupuncture for infertile women without undergoing assisted reproductive techniques (ART): A systematic review and meta-analysis. *Medicine*, *98*(29), e16463.
2. Hullender Rubin, L. E., Anderson, B. J., & Craig, L. B. (2018). Acupuncture and *in vitro* fertilisation research: Current and future directions. *Acupuncture in Medicine*, *36*(2), 117–22.
3. Schwarze, J. E., Ceroni, J. P., Ortega-Hrepich, C., Villa, S., Crosby, J., & Pommer, R. (2018). Does acupuncture the day of embryo transfer affect the clinical pregnancy rate? Systematic review and meta-analysis. *JBRA Assisted Reproduction*, *22*(4), 363–8.

Chapter 26: The Ethics of Fertility Treatments

1. Jadva, V., Badger, S., Morrissette, M., & Golombok, S. (2009). 'Mom by choice, single by life's circumstance . . .' Findings from a large scale survey of the experiences of single mothers by choice. *Human Fertility*, *12*(4), 175–84; Murray, C., MacCallum, F., & Golombok, S. (2006). Egg donation parents and their children: Follow-up at age 12 years. *Fertility and Sterility*, *85*(3), 610–8;

Van Rijn-van Gelderen, L., Bos, H. W. M., Jorgensen, T. D., Ellis-Davies, K., Winstanley, A., Golombok, S., Rubio, B., Gross, M., Vecho, O., & Lamb, M. E. (2018). Wellbeing of gay fathers with children born through surrogacy: A comparison with lesbian-mother families and heterosexual IVF parent families. *Human Reproduction*, *33*(1), 101–8; Golombok, S., Blake, L., Slutsky, J., Raffanello, E., Roman, G. D., & Ehrhardt, A. (2018). Parenting and the adjustment of children born to gay fathers through surrogacy. *Child Development*, *89*(4), 1223–33.

Appendix 1: Female Vitamin and Mineral Intake

1. Hanson, M. A., Bardsley, A., De-Regil, L. M., Moore, S. E., Oken, E., Poston, L., Ma, R. C., McAuliffe, F. M., Maleta, K., Purandare, C. N., & Yajnik, C. S. (2015). The International Federation of Gynecology and Obstetrics (FIGO) recommendations on adolescent, preconception, and maternal nutrition: 'Think Nutrition First'. *International Journal of Gynecology & Obstetrics*, *131*, S213–53.

Appendix 3: Potential Antioxidants for Male Fertility

1. Majzoub, A., & Agarwal, A. (2018). Systematic review of antioxidant types and doses in male infertility: Benefits on semen parameters, advanced sperm function, assisted reproduction and live-birth rate. *Arab Journal of Urology*, *16*(1), 113–24.

Index

Page references in *italics* indicate images.